From UNNATURAL SELECTION

This is a tale about evolution. Not only about the evolution of our genes, although that subject was the springboard for all the current advances in genetics and is now one subtext of that progress. The more important story in these pages tells about another kind of evolution, the gradual transformation of our attitudes as a society, now that the study of our DNA has begun to present us with something far more personally meaningful than a mere theory or a rationale for museum dioramas.... Can our society's ability to understand and resolve the consequences of new genetic research keep up—can it even *catch up*—with the headlong progress of the research itself?

 . . . The problem with gene research is the same as its beauty. Its intellectual simplicity, its satisfying resolution of baffling medical puzzles with logical molecular explanations, creates the illusion that it will provide us with easy answers to larger human problems.... [We] need to understand the rock-bottom truth that most geneticists take for granted—not the molecular esoterica of how genes operate, but the reality that *genetic* only rarely implies "inevitable" or "incurable" or "fully understood." . . . We are who we are not just because of what our genes contain, but because of what has happened to us since our birth and how we use that unique genetic endowment, day after day.

"*Unnatural Selection* succeeds in presenting the fascinating issues of genetic science and ethics in a thoroughly engaging manner. By providing insights into the people behind the issues, Wingerson makes the world of genetics come alive for a wide range of readers."

—*Mark A. Rothstein*
CULLEN DISTINGUISHED PROFESSOR OF LAW
DIRECTOR, HEALTH, LAW AND POLICY INSTITUTE
UNIVERSITY OF HOUSTON LAW CENTER

By Lois Wingerson

MAPPING OUR GENES
The Genome Project and the Future of Medicine

UNNATURAL SELECTION
The Promise and the Power of Human Gene Research

UNNATURAL SELECTION

The Promise and the Power of Human Gene Research

LOIS WINGERSON

BANTAM BOOKS
New York   Toronto   London   Sydney   Auckland

This edition contains the complete text
of the original hardcover edition.
NOT ONE WORD HAS BEEN OMITTED.

UNNATURAL SELECTION
A Bantam Book

PUBLISHING HISTORY
Bantam hardcover edition published 1998
Bantam trade paperback edition / December 1999

ISBN 0-553-37515-6

Published simultaneously in the United States and Canada

Bantam Books are published by Bantam Books, a division of Random
House, Inc. Its trademark, consisting of the words "Bantam Books" and the
portrayal of a rooster, is Registered in U.S. Patent and Trademark Office
and in other countries. Marca Registraada. Bantam Books, 1540
Broadway, New York, New York 10036.

PRINTED IN THE UNITED STATES OF AMERICA

BVG   10   9   8   7   6   5   4   3   2   1

CONTENTS

INTRODUCTION

THIS IS A TALE ABOUT EVOLUTION. NOT ONLY ABOUT the evolution of our genes, although that subject was the springboard for all the current advances in genetics and is now one subtext of that progress. The more important story in these pages tells about another kind of evolution, the gradual transformation of our attitudes as a society, now that the study of our DNA has begun to present us with something far more personally meaningful than mere theory or a rationale for museum dioramas.

The matter that obsessed me as I researched and wrote these pages comes down to one simple question: Can our society's ability to understand and resolve the consequences of new genetic research keep up—can it even *catch up*—with the headlong progress of the research itself?

There's no wonder that the research has such momentum. It's scintillating stuff, DNA. Take a drop of blood, a bit of hair, maybe. Grind it up, spin it down, drop in a little of this and a little of that, and you can wind it out on a glass rod: a sparkling strand of human essence, the chemical basis of yourself or someone else.

What's in there? For someone who knows how to find the answer, the question is irresistible.

Every week some research team somewhere reports yet another discovery about the genes involved in some human quality or malady. At the end of every such report, we read that such revelations hold the prospect of providing important new clues to solving grave problems, or at least to answering deep and fascinating questions. This is true indeed.

Heart disease, diabetes, cancer—is there any major health problem that does not have a vastly different aspect now than a decade ago, because of what has been learned from genes? Huntington's disease, Parkinson's disease, Alzheimer's disease—brain disorders known only by the names of the men who described their symptoms—are gradually surrendering to new insights based on genes and molecules. Members of some families plagued with cancer now have a chance to know whether they are at risk and should be vigilant, or are likely to escape unharmed and can relax.

The benefits of coming to a deeper understanding of that long sticky strand are undeniable. We must never minimize the deep and genuinely momentous portent of these new discoveries. This line of research holds immense promise, and it justly attracts public funding.

These days the gene hackers are spinning out information about genes at a dizzying pace. The Human Genome Project—an international effort to identify and understand the contents of our entire genome,* in effect to "read" our DNA—has exceeded the expectations of everyone involved and also of its critics. The largest component of that project, coordinated from the National Human Genome Research Institute in Bethesda, Maryland, is well ahead of its own schedule for mapping the genome by the year 2005.

Of some 80,000 human genes, well more than half have now been identified, extracted, and cataloged in databases. At this writing, more than 1,200 gene segments have been implicated in more than 1,500 human disorders, and precise genes and relevant mutations have been identified for about half that number. The rest of the human genes are incubating in test tubes in laboratories around the world, and in databases, where they have been transformed.

From molecular information once intelligible only to the human body, genes have become digital and even alphabetical information, accessible on the Internet to anyone who has a computer. Geneticists can look at long sequences of those symbols, compare them with each other, and deduce from the patterns alone a tremendous amount about what they represent. As to a complete understanding of how they actually work, it is only a matter of time—and a tremendous, exciting challenge to those prepared to undertake it.

"The prospect is that in the next few years humanity will understand—and be able to control, at least in part—the fabulously intricate mechanism through which each species of living organism transmits its essential properties to the next generation," intoned an editorial in *The New York Times*. "The danger exists that the scientists will make some of these God-like powers available to us in the next few years well be-

---

*The term *genome* means the entire genetic constitution, the complete DNA code, of a single individual or of a species.

fore society—on the present evidence—is likely to be even remotely prepared for the ethical and other dilemmas with which we shall be faced."

The most striking fact about that opinion is when it was printed: November 12, 1963, ten days before President Kennedy was assassinated. Perhaps it was a bit optimistic: We are beginning to understand, and control in part, those fabulously intricate mechanisms. But those "few" years have now been more than thirty.

In the intervening years, there has been almost a fivefold increase in the number of identified genetic disorders, as well as considerable progress on the task of elucidating the public issues that surround these discoveries. Resolving them will take still longer. The problem is that much of what is written about these subjects—especially much of what is aimed at the general public—still uses that same kind of rhetoric, imputing "God-like" powers and hinting at ominous perils because of all this tinkering.

Now the Pandora's box is open. What's inside? It's time to clear aside the verbal debris and look squarely at our situation. What *precisely* intimidates us about this research? Which powers are so "God-like," and how do they differ from what we could always do in simpler ways, using natural methods of reproduction and breeding?

What are the real risks we face as a result of learning to read our genes? Many people shrink from these questions—partly out of fear that they cannot understand the scientific details (most of which are irrelevant to the ethical discussion anyway).

The head of the Human Genome Project, Francis Collins, M.D., says that even after thousands of genes have been found, he is still exhilarated by the report of a new gene discovery. But he also loses sleep sometimes over the implications, the problems these discoveries might represent for the rest of us.

"I have found this to be the most compelling, at times vexing, and overall time-consuming part of the genome project," he told me in an interview in late 1997. "I spend half my time on [these] issues. I do that by choice, because I think we have to get that right."

Collins knows there's nothing he can do at present to prevent "blatant misuses" of genetic information. He has watched with intense interest and occasional insomnia as Congress has slowly begun to turn its attention to the fundamental conflict between the rights of people with genetic risks (a number that seems to grow with every passing week and every new advance) and the economic interests of employers, the insurance industry, and even sometimes, in our current health care system, doctors themselves.

As so often happens, much of the debate on this topic that reaches the public involves propping up straw men and then shooting them down. This is especially true when Congress is listening, and especially at budget time. Often the conversation pits the heartwarming prospect of using genetic knowledge to cure fatally ill children or to prevent debilitating disease against the remote, terrifying prospect of cloning Hitlers or mass-producing men best fit to be soldiers. More subtly, members of the public are sometimes portrayed as innocent victims and corporate executives (as if they were not also people) as heartless and calculating. There are exaggeration and misinformation at both ends of that spectrum — and a wealth of important detail in between, steadfastly overlooked by both sides.

"The discoveries are just coming at an unbelievable level," DNA research pioneer James Watson told a congressional committee in 1995, during appropriations hearings. (He was no longer head of the genome project, but still — of course — a steadfast supporter.) "One week leads to one thing and now someone at Rockefeller University has found a gene that they think makes some of us fat. And a lot of people care about that.

"I can give you an instance. It's a rumor but it is reputed they want to sell the gene for close to $50 million. This just indicates there is money in these things, because we are coming really close to finding out very important things which can make our lives more pleasant by making us thin. Being able to eat and still be thin — I mean, a wonderful objective."

In a few ingenuous sentences, he touched on both the trivial and the momentous. There are "wonderful" objectives such as slender gluttons, indeed, and also massive profits to be made in due course. In that same year the molecular details about the genetic basis of immense human problems such as cancer, Alzheimer's disease, and diabetes were falling on us like manna. Or like bombs, depending on your perspective.

New knowledge of the genetic factors behind diseases means not only that they can be determined through testing, but that these findings could fall into the hands of those with the power (and the motivation) to misuse them: insurance companies linked to managed care plans, employers, adoption agencies, courts. To those who have thought about it, the prospect has been unsettling. Health insurance companies are merging with organized managed care plans, and it is perplexing to try to figure out who is paying for medical information and who actually has access to it—or takes advantage of that access.

Among the first to create guidelines for the use of specific genetic tests are not only the professional bodies but the managed care plans themselves. Of their basic motives, their intentions for the use of the testing or the use of their own guidelines, we can know little at the moment.

A now-famous survey of people who had reason to contact a genetics clinic or hereditary disease organization revealed forty-one incidents of "genetic discrimination" by insurers or employers against healthy people who were at risk of a hereditary disease. Some respondents said they had refused to participate in genetic testing because of concern about what might be done with the information.

Francis Collins alerted me to the ironic fact that the same concern now has an impact on the very research that would help to clarify the implications of genetic testing. "Already there is concrete evidence that people are afraid to participate in genetic research protocols because they're afraid the information will escape the confidentiality of the interaction," he said. In a current research project on the new-found breast cancer genes, a third of women approached to take part in the follow-up study—women already identified as having the mutation implicated in breast cancer—refused to join the project for fear that the information would fall into the wrong hands and be used against them.

In the first cohort of twenty individuals for a study of hereditary colon cancer at the National Institutes of Health, Collins added, only one person declined to participate. He was an insurance agent. Collins chuckled wryly at the memory. "And the insurance companies say, 'Oh, we wouldn't do anything bad [with genetic information],'" he said. "I don't know why this guy is worried!"

Why *are* we so worried, in the absence of any compelling and concrete evidence that the new genetics poses a real threat to us? There is an undercurrent to all of this—the memory that once, a half century ago, societies broke unwritten taboos in the name of genetics. People in Nazi Germany were tortured and killed for reasons that had to do with heredity. And well before then, also for genetic reasons, in other countries including ours, people were forcibly sterilized because they were thought to carry "bad genes." Today, as we find the genes themselves, we are learning that an immense complexity underlies their "goodness" or "badness."

If the science of genetics today is complex, the ethics surrounding it might seem to be inscrutable. But the *issues* can be explained, faced, and dealt with.

Some people have been forced to the confrontation and have grappled with the questions. Among them is Sandra Kretz, who was a vice-president at Quantum Health Resources, a company that manages health care for people with rare inherited diseases, when I met her.

At the time, Kretz's own mother resided in a nursing home, in the late stages of Alzheimer's disease. Well versed about genetics, Kretz knew that a test could determine whether her mother bore the genetic type most commonly associated with Alzheimer's disease — knowledge that might also allow Kretz to learn her own risks for the future.

It's a prospect many people shrink from, but Kretz wanted to know. "I mean, we talk about taking charge of our own lives," she said. "If there's any time for me to take charge, this is it." Kretz's mother had worked for years as a legal assistant and knew how to draft a living will. She had done so, leaving explicit and detailed instructions about her care.

Sandra Kretz was learning from experience the ways in which a living will can provide insufficient guidance. If all else were equal, she would like to write a better one for herself, armed with the knowledge of her mother's genetic type and therefore, perhaps, her own individual risk of developing Alzheimer's disease.

However, all else is hardly equal. Kretz spoke to her mother's doctor about getting the test, and the doctor advised strongly against it. "Do you know what might happen to your insurance?" he said. "Yours, and the rest of your family's?" Losing insurance coverage is evidently a risk even more frightening than facing Alzheimer's unprepared — or perhaps an ethical consideration more important than her own uncertainty.

Kretz's mother has since died. Kretz will not pursue the testing, for the time being. She can write the document anyway, if and when she chooses — and whether or not her genes predispose her to Alzheimer's disease. She has thought about her genes, and then moved beyond them. Perhaps it is a skill we as a whole community need to learn.

The scientists are busy spinning out the DNA itself. Meanwhile, a healthy new subindustry — and recently, many politicians — have begun spinning out the implications for us. Fundamentally, however, this is *our* agenda. What will the understanding of our DNA mean to us? What do we intend it to mean? What elements should enter into the process that may not occur to the doctors and scientists? If we nonprofessionals do not participate in that dialogue, or at least understand it, we cannot take a full part in crafting the shape of our own future, or that of our children.

The book that follows is divided conceptually into three parts. It begins with an account of one of the oldest and most successful genetic testing programs in the United States. The next chapter examines prenatal testing, which has taken a strong foothold in this country and many others and, although seldom purely genetic, shares all of the major issues that surround genetic testing. Because embryos and fetuses are the traditional focus of attention among medical geneticists, much of the first third of the book focuses on the unborn.

The central section looks at the motivations and activities of scientists who have studied human genes, beginning with one of the most eminent German geneticists of the Nazi era, and moving forward in time through the origins of the Human Genome Project now under way in the United States and elsewhere.

The last segment of the book examines some of the most controversial aspects of current genetic research, looking in particular at crime and human ethnic diversity. A final chapter takes a longer view, pondering the implications of current genetic research and medical progress upon human evolution.

Many other authors have written on this topic in scholarly volumes, and I am in their debt because I have drawn heavily on their ideas, as well as on interviews and on presentations at conferences. The issues are far too numerous for the pages that follow to be completely comprehensive, and events move far too quickly for such a book to remain current with genetic research. I have tried to provide the tools to examine future developments in light of past and current events.

I am neither a scientist, an ethicist, nor a historian. Members of all three professions may be uncomfortable that I have simplified details about their areas of expertise or left them out entirely. This was necessary to make the topic accessible to a wide audience. Above all I have tried to adhere to two basic tenets of my own profession of journalism: to be both accurate and fair.

UNNATURAL SELECTION

CHAPTER 1

Generation of the Upright

Unto the upright there ariseth light in the darkness.

—Psalm 112:4

WE BEGIN ONCE UPON A PLACE, IN ANOTHER WORLD. This world belongs to the children: Taylor Street, Brooklyn.

It's the Sunday before Passover. Seven-year-olds race around on junior bikes, helmets rammed down over their yarmulkes. Small boys barrel up and down the sidewalk on low-slung plastic trikes, their earlocks flying. Little girls in pigtails and parkas push their dolly strollers.

Something about what they are doing invites nostalgia. Whatever they're up to is intense, concentrated. It's serious business and not about to stop. These kids have never seen TV, and it shows.

Behind a fence three boys are fighting. It's a good solid tussle; they clutch close, arms flailing, grunting but smiling too. No karate kicks. Mom calls out at them from the balcony across the street, wearing a bathrobe and turban. They break it up.

These particular rowhouses are built of brick—but even this brand-new block is still (and yet again) the *shtetl*. Wedged between some housing projects and the Brooklyn Navy Yard, the towers of the World Trade Center looming behind them, these streets are the kind of place one reads about but never quite expects to see. The quarter of Williamsburg where the Orthodox Jews live is one part of the melting pot that did not, would not melt. The old world inhabits the new.

Were not the Jews in Egypt once saved from slavery because they held faithful to tradition in dress, names, and language? So, these people believe, must they. So they do not read *The New York Times*, they will not send their sons to any school but a yeshiva, and they speak Yiddish at home and Hebrew at worship. On the sabbath they absolutely will not push an elevator button without a special variance from the rabbi. This might seem odd to outsiders, but how could outsiders understand? Such matters go very deep.

A few blocks away, where people are busy shopping for Passover, the streets are crammed. The older children are not busy, though. They stroll about in pairs or threes, visual echoes of their parents. The girls wear long dark wool coats and calf-length dresses. Adolescent boys lean on an iron fence, talking to one another, dressed in black fedoras, white shirts buttoned to the throat, black silk vests.

All they lack that their fathers display is an exuberant beard. They're still too young for that, and too young to observe certain biblical commands, such as the one to be fruitful and multiply. That's coming, but several rites of passage lie ahead before then.

In this old, old world, one ritual of puberty is very new: the bloodletting. For the last decade, for these Hasidic Jewish schoolchildren in particular, it has become an accepted part of coming of age to give up a blood sample to someone who comes to school for the express purpose of extracting it.

Most teenagers who take part in the ritual probably understand what is happening to some degree. But they may never think about it again unless, someday in the distant future, a parent elects to tell them that the matchmaker has advised against a proposed marriage to protect the health of the prospective offspring. If the couple behave as expected, they will forget the proposed marriage (if, in fact, they ever knew about it in the first place) and look for someone else to love.

In this Orthodox Jewish community, premarital screening for certain inherited diseases is now all but universal, and also highly effective. The high-tech advances that underlie genetic screening come from the "outside" world, but oddly enough they enjoy their most unqualified success in this community of ultraorthodox Judaism, among people who otherwise shun most aspects of modern life.

"I totally, *totally* disagree with the philosophy, it's easy in that community, you can do it with arranged marriages," says Rabbi Josef Ekstein, the one person most responsible for the new ritual in Jewish Williamsburg. "Our success was not because the community was easy. We have terrible problems."

Ekstein sounds angry, and despite all of his successes, he is. His is a mission born of personal anguish, a massive and remarkably successful coming to terms with grief, a campaign against almost insurmountable odds to re-create the world so that no other parent will have to endure what he endured. That anyone could call any part of it "easy" is obviously almost too much for him to bear.

Four of Ekstein's eleven children died of Tay-Sachs disease. An evil God would be proud of creating Tay-Sachs as exquisite torture for babies and their parents, wrote one scientist who happens to be Jewish. It is a degenerative nerve disorder that slowly transforms an endearing infant of four months into a staring, drooling, immobile child with blind eyes and an overlarge head. Then, usually before the age of six, it kills him.

TAY-SACHS DISEASE

Because of a slight genetic variation, just one of thousands of brain chemicals is missing in children born with Tay-Sachs disease. The outcome is catastrophe.

The reason is that they have not inherited a copy of the gene that encodes the structure of the molecule hexosaminidase A, which would normally break down a particular fatty substance in the brain. Instead, the substance accumulates inside the nerve cells, which balloon abnormally and cannot transmit signals. Without a functioning brain, a child eventually dies.

Two physicians, Warren Tay of Great Britain and Bernard Sachs of the United States, each recognized the syndrome in the 1880s. Sachs realized it was most common among Jewish children. Before 1969, when prenatal testing became available, about sixty children with Tay-Sachs were diagnosed in the United States each year.

Beginning in 1970, because of concerted efforts by Jewish community groups and interested geneticists, screening programs for Tay-Sachs proliferated nationwide in the Jewish population in general. They have become a model for successful genetic screening.

Since 1983 fewer than five new cases have come to light each year in the United States and Canada.

Geneticists believe that the scourge of Tay-Sachs disease in the Jewish population had its origins in the historic isolation of the Jews, both geographically and culturally. The Jews spread peacefully from the Mediterranean throughout Europe and Asia Minor, but they were also often violently dispersed and isolated. Beginning in the fourteenth century, the Crusades drove them gradually east toward Poland and Russia. In many regions they were segregated into ghettos. For their own religious and cultural reasons, as well as because of discrimination, Jewish people did not often mingle or intermarry with the cultures that surrounded them.

Today some 80 percent of the 13 to 14 million Jews in the world are Ashkenazim, descendants of the Jewish families who lived in eastern Europe in the fifteenth century. Genetic isolation helped Tay-Sachs disease proliferate among the Ashkenazim, because two people at risk of passing on a hereditary disease were more likely to meet and marry in a small, isolated population than if the conditions had favored intermarriage with outsiders. For peculiar reasons having to do with the biochemistry of fat molecules, carriers of a single Tay-Sachs mutation (two are required to inherit the disease) may have had better survival odds in tuberculosis epidemics, which were relatively common in the cramped conditions of the ghettos, favoring the persistence of the deleterious gene.

Whatever the reason for its prevalence, physicians recognized a century ago that the disease was most common among Jews. This is no longer the case, however.

Ekstein and a few others have prevailed against this tragic disease, and prevailed mightily. Today in the United States Tay-Sachs disease is more common among non-Jews than among Jews.

Almost single-handedly, Rabbi Ekstein has eradicated Tay-Sachs from the Orthodox Jewish community in which it was most prevalent. The genetic screening program he founded now tests some 8,000 Orthodox Jews in the United States, Israel, and Europe each year — most of them through the schools maintained by the ultrareligious community — to see whether they are capable of passing on the disease if they conceive a child with someone who also carries the gene that confers the hereditary disorder.

About 6 million Ashkenazim now live in the United States. Ultra-orthodox sects like the one Rabbi Ekstein belongs to account for only a small fraction of this number. In Rabbi Ekstein's neighborhood, the prevalence of Tay-Sachs disease today is zero. Nil.

Rabbi Ekstein is one of many thousands of Ashkenazim who came to America from eastern Europe after escaping the cauldron of World War

II. He was born in Hungary during the war. His parents fled from Europe to Israel when he was three, and soon after to Argentina.

By the time he came to Brooklyn in 1973, Ekstein was a husband and father. One member of the family was an infant son, the fourth and last of his children born with Tay-Sachs disease. The graves of the other three are in Argentina.

Rabbi Ekstein would far rather talk about the genetic screening program he founded than about himself, and he talks only obliquely about the four children he lost to Tay-Sachs disease. "Tay-Sachs is terrible today too," he will grant, "but I can tell you, at that time it was even worse. To have a six-month-old child, you still don't know if it's healthy [and here he veers off to another subject]. . . . The biggest, biggest problem, when a sick child comes, it is a threat which is going to destroy the family [and here he veers off again]. . . . When you have a sick child, you can't believe there is nothing that will help. You will do anything."

One of the things the rabbi did, naturally, was read everything he could find about Tay-Sachs disease. It is one of those purely hereditary diseases that develop only when a child inherits the same scarce genetic variant from each parent. Recessive diseases, as these are called, are quite rare. Until a few decades ago the only way people could learn they were carriers of a recessive disease gene was to bear and then bury a child who had succumbed to it.

In the late 1960s Ekstein read about a new blood test that could detect an unusual protein variant in the blood whose presence in an adult implied the carrier state for Tay-Sachs or, in children or fetuses, could confirm the presence of the disease itself. The latter was irrelevant to Ekstein and his community, because they had a very strong taboo against abortion.

Before long it dawned on the rabbi that the test was nonetheless powerfully important. Used in adults, it could represent an almost fail-safe way to prevent the disease from occurring in the first place if it dissuaded carriers from conceiving offspring altogether. By that time, a geneticist named Michael Kaback had established a fairly successful prenatal screening program for the disease in the Baltimore area.

The community in Baltimore had actually solicited Kaback's help. But Ekstein would have no such luxury. He well knew that his own community would not be interested in testing. Far from it. They were in a deep, deep state of denial.

A geneticist at Mount Sinai Hospital in New York, Dr. Robert

WHAT IT MEANS TO BE A CARRIER

In the simplest case, like Tay-Sachs, there's only one gene to talk about. You get two chances at this gene: one from Mom's egg, one from Dad's sperm. The gene contains a molecular description of an essential protein, and if you get even one good set of instructions, from one parent or the other, you're okay.

A *carrier* is an individual who has one gene involved in an inherited disease such as Tay-Sachs. Because the disease itself has not developed, by definition he or she also has one gene with a complete set of instructions for the normal protein, so does not have the disease. The disease-related gene is invisible and recedes from view; it's *recessive*. The person, however, is a carrier of the Tay-Sachs gene.

Each carrier, logically, has fifty-fifty odds of passing on the gene. Two carriers who conceive a child have one chance in four that that child will inherit both Tay-Sachs genes and thus the disease. The Tay-Sachs gene is uncommon, and in the general population the odds that two carriers will mate are very small. The disease is rare.

Other genes are called *dominant* because they dominate the other gene of the pair passed down in egg and sperm. One dominant gene can cause a disorder all by itself. Inheriting even one copy is serious trouble. The classic example is Huntington's disease, the neurological disorder that killed the folksinger Woody Guthrie.

The plot will thicken. In other diseases the situation can be far more complex. Numerous genes may interact, and external components can get involved, such as diet, water, air, even stress. Determining all the factors that lead to such a "multifactorial" disease itself can be intricate, perhaps impossible.

Desnick, agreed to cooperate with Rabbi Ekstein in trying to set up a screening program in Williamsburg. The two men had no idea how difficult it was going to be.

"I got no cooperation at all from any source," Ekstein says. "There was *total* opposition. The entire mentality was that you couldn't even talk about screening."

On the contrary, anyone who knew about Tay-Sachs disease was obsessed with *not* telling. In a community where it is the norm to have six or seven children, if anyone knew that one child in a family had Tay-Sachs, the fact would taint the family like a curse.

In the age-old tradition of arranged marriages, love was more often than not a secondary consideration if it existed at all. What was paramount was the acceptability of the match to the rabbi, to the family, and to the community.

The matchmakers' priorities were well defined: after illegitimacy and lack of a devout character, a blemish in the family's background was the third reason to reject a match. Without question Tay-Sachs was such a blemish. Not only would it destroy children, it could easily destroy families as well. In a family known to have had one child with Tay-Sachs, it could prove nearly impossible to find matches for the others.

Ekstein's other problem was that he had to capture people for testing before the babies actually existed in any sense. In the Orthodox community, abortion is forbidden unless there is serious peril to the mother's life. Some rabbis judged that giving birth to repeated babies with Tay-Sachs was indeed such a peril, but many did not. So prenatal testing for Tay-Sachs disease was pointless. The only alternative was to test before conception and then — what? Families who were already burdened with the problem knew it all too well, while many families who were not so burdened were hardly aware the disease existed.

"At this time I was very, very sad," recalls the rabbi. "I thought they should help me." Families would come for help, he added, and then run away. Some families would actually hide their children with Tay-Sachs in Catholic hospitals before they died, Ekstein says (his voice rising), so that none of the Jews would learn about it. "It's terrible fear," he goes on. "Terrible, terrible fear."

As Ekstein speaks, he is sitting in a narrow room across the corridor from the small offices where young women are alternately speaking on the phone or poring through the files, engaged in the daily business of the screening program. He has just finished his daily hours-long call to the program's other central office, in Jerusalem.

Ekstein is interrupted midsentence by a young man in earlocks and prayer shawl; they speak hurriedly in Yiddish. It's about blood samples from Amsterdam due into Brooklyn later that day. The program he long despaired to see has now gone international and is legendary.

Besides coordinating the blood testing, Ekstein's assistants are the only link, the highly secret interface, between the test results and the people who parted with the blood samples. Everyone who is tested keeps a confidential six-digit ID number concealed somewhere at home. If a marriage is planned at some point after testing, a parent or a matchmaker, or perhaps the sample donor himself, calls the program and provides the two ID numbers, for the proposed bride and groom. As a double check, they also provide both birthdays (day and month only; no one has to tell his age), to ensure that the correct test results are being matched.

If both test results are positive for a Tay-Sachs gene, the caller is advised that the match is unacceptable. In such a case, to preserve confidentiality, the program advises the matchmaker or the parents to provide a pretext as to why the match would not be suitable, without mentioning Tay-Sachs. Genetic counseling is available afterward, also by telephone. If either sample is unaffected by the gene, the caller is advised that the marriage can proceed as planned.

Intricate and sensitive as it is, Ekstein's program has survived intense struggles within the community about whether it was morally sound. These struggles speak through its defiant name. They call the program Dor Yeshorim, from a phrase in the Talmud. It means "generation of the upright."

It took many years for Rabbi Ekstein to come up with this elaborate scheme for preventing the occurrence of Tay-Sachs disease. At first, he simply told people the test was available and faced the fact that no one cared to know.

Someone else, however, was puzzling out the same problem. At some point during those disheartening early years, Rabbi Ekstein encountered the genetic counselor and social worker who served Brooklyn's families burdened with Tay-Sachs. A compact, bright-eyed woman, Mrs. Frances Berkwits had been sharing their troubles ever since 1957, when she came to work in a Tay-Sachs ward at Kingsbrook Jewish Medical Center at the request of the families. They had not asked for testing; they had asked for support.

At that time it was the only Tay-Sachs ward in the world. "Not only were those sixteen beds filled," says Berkwits, "often there were also kids at home or in the pediatric unit." She knew all the families with Tay-Sachs whose children languished in that sixteen-bed ward, where the staff did whatever they could to make the children comfortable.

The children were not Berkwits's principal concern, of course. Her clients were the families—the parents, the grandparents, the aunts and uncles. She set up a support group and found that families involved with the unit became especially close-knit. She loved the job. She still does. Where else does a social worker get to follow the same family, year after year, generation after generation?

Little could be done for the blind and paralyzed children in the unit except to feed them, turn them to prevent bedsores, and try to control their seizures. "Basically it was a hospice," recalls a neurologist who worked there.

Not only did Kingsbrook house the world's only Tay-Sachs ward, it was also the first and preeminent source for blood tests. In the 1970s the Tay-Sachs biochemistry lab at Kingsbrook quickly became renowned for tests to detect the presence or absence of the protein implicated in Tay-Sachs disease. Berkwits's job began to "assume a different cast," as she put it.

Beyond informing individual families that they could avoid bearing children who would have the disease, she began to realize that it might be possible to begin to eradicate it in the entire community. She decided to broaden her view beyond the unit and let the wider Jewish public learn that Tay-Sachs could be prevented.

In 1974 Berkwits began to visit city schools, offering to provide Tay-Sachs testing for anyone interested. Why schools in particular? Like Rabbi Ekstein, "I felt it would be better to do this before pregnancy," she recalls. "I would go wherever I was asked."

By the mid-1970s Kingsbrook had begun conducting mass screening programs among college students at risk and for members of various Jewish organizations in the New York metropolitan area. Despite severe financial constraints, pathologist Bruno Volk, cofounder and director of the Tay-Sachs unit at Kingsbrook, was continuing his neurochemical research on the disease, testing nerve cells from fetuses aborted because of Tay-Sachs to see if they could be coaxed to ingest the missing enzyme. They couldn't.

Today Volk's old research labs at Kingsbrook are empty, locked, and layered with dust. No one there is pursuing a way to correct the disease. But the biochemistry labs there bustle, busier than ever, carrying out world-class and worldwide testing for the Tay-Sachs protein on samples from all over the globe—including those sent by Dor Yeshorim. The walls are littered with posters about Tay-Sachs. Prominent among them is one that reads: "Is there anything else on your schedule this week that is truly a matter of life and death? Prevent the tragedy of Tay-Sachs disease."

When it came to helping the families who were Orthodox, that mandate used to haunt Frances Berkwits. She knew their proscriptions about abortion, which made her own work very disheartening. "There was very little I could do to offer alternatives," she says. It took an insider, both to the community and to the disease, to figure it out.

That was Josef Ekstein's mandate too: Prevent Tay-Sachs. How did he start? He gives a morose chuckle at the memory. "It went very hard in the beginning," he says. He advertised. He cajoled. In the first year— 1983—all of forty-five people agreed to be tested. "In the first year, forty-five." He chuckles again. "In the second, 175."

"Beginners did it," he says. "Beginners—" He turns to his colleague Howard Katzenstein, searching, and says a word in Yiddish.

"They pitied him," offers Katzenstein. "They wanted to humor him, so they did it."

Mostly, the community was frightened by Ekstein's plan to provide Tay-Sachs testing, which made him very sad. "They came to me for help," he recalled, "and then they ran away." When his own brother was about to get married, Ekstein's father refused even to mention the test. Ekstein learned of a pair of brothers whose grandchildren wanted to marry. There was Tay-Sachs in both lines of descent, yet neither would mention it. "One fooled the other, and finally they both got fooled," he says. "Usually brothers in our community are more . . . *brothers* than in other communities. But with all of this they were not willing—they were not able to tell. They did not realize the importance of telling."

The kernel of the problem was obvious to Rabbi Ekstein: how to create a way around telling—some means of telling without telling. "We sat up days and nights thinking about this," he remembers. "Days and nights."

"We" was a tiny group—Ekstein (himself a merchant in religious objects by trade as well as a rabbi), a close friend who was a public relations man, and two others, an insurance broker and a dealer in venetian blinds.

"I was the heart of the program, but I needed some brains," he says. "I could not do everything alone. I needed help. The idea was, How do we take out the good parts of it without the side effects? How do we prevent children with Tay-Sachs without causing the stigma?"

Clearly, it was not working to merely announce the existence of the test and make it available. They were missing something crucial.

"We came to the conclusion that when people are already involved, it's already very, very emotional," Ekstein says. "But once we started to introduce it into the schools we thought: This is the way."

If the community revolved around respect for religious authority, Ekstein knew, the only way to proceed was to win the support of a substantial number of influential rabbis. "They threw me out the door," he says. "I came back in the window."

People outside the community might have expressed the rabbis' main concern in different words, using terms like "playing God." As expressed by members of the Orthodox Jewish community, the words were slightly different: Does genetic testing indicate a lack of faith in Divine Providence?

Ekstein spent many months seeking assurances from other rabbis that it did not and soliciting their support. Ultimately he was able to gather testimonials from a large number of religious leaders who were in favor of premarital testing.

"In light of the fact that a simple test was developed for this," wrote one of them, "one who does not make use of this test is like one who shuts his eyes to what can clearly be seen. . . . [I]t is prudent for all who are considering marriage to undergo this test."

As Ekstein knew it would, the resounding support of the religious leaders gave his program the momentum it needed. By the autumn of 1987, four years after its timid inauguration, Dor Yeshorim had tested some 4,000 individuals for the Tay-Sachs gene. Two years later the program began mass testing of twelfth graders in Orthodox Jewish schools throughout New York State.

Today Dor Yeshorim's offices in New York and Jerusalem work closely with laboratories and volunteers in England, Belgium, Switzerland, Canada, and across the United States and Israel. About 8,000 people are tested each year by and for Dor Yeshorim. Over 50,000 in total have been tested to date.

The community served by Dor Yeshorim has many remarkable qualities. Among them is its extreme deference to religious authority. This comes forth vividly in the tone of the Tay-Sachs program's promotional literature.

"This pamphlet describes a real and practical program in which you and every other Jewish parent must participate," reads one flier for Dor Yeshorim. "It is endorsed by rabbinic authorities as well as by leading medical experts. . . . Each and every parent and child has the obligation to read, understand and act on the information outlined below."

DNA AND CHROMOSOMES, GENES, AND PROTEINS

To understand gene testing, it helps to review a few basics about DNA. Physically, DNA is a twisted zipper. Functionally, it is a language.

Think first of a zipper. The molecular "teeth" in the DNA zipper — usually called bases — are not all identical: There are four different kinds. Because of their chemical structures, the bases will mesh together in only two combinations (adenosine binds only to tyrosine, and cytosine only to guanine). The zipper will close only if the teeth match. That makes a pattern.

The bases constitute a simple chemical alphabet, which creates a complicated code along the zipper. Every three consecutive bases — every set of three teeth, as it were — translates to one of the twenty amino acids that are the subunits of protein. (Some other combinations of bases signify instructions such as "start here" or "stop here.")

The DNA zipper is twisted many times, like a corkscrew. In cell division the twisted zipper — the double helix — uncoils and opens. Then the pattern on the teeth is copied, either to form a new double helix or, piecemeal, to translate a portion of the molecular code into a form it can use for its metabolic processes.

Functionally, DNA is a molecular language in which the "letters" are the chemical subunits known as bases. The "words" are genes. Most of the words are specifications for the production of proteins.

Clearly the audience will accept this directive; it already has, almost unequivocally.

The flier quotes one rabbi as saying that "every Jewish community should consider it a sacred duty to participate in the great humanitarian effort of Dor Yeshorim." The pamphlet informs readers that the risk of Tay-Sachs disease (and another hereditary illness, cystic fibrosis) is about one in 625 among members of the Ashkenazi community.

"It is quite possible you are unaware of how frequently these diseases occur in our community since, understandably, the parents often seek

A vastly diverse set of biochemicals, proteins have two primary functions in nature: to create structure (stems and leaves, bones and flesh) and to act and react (digest, process, pump, transport, move, and, by some inscrutable process, think). The proteins involved in Tay-Sachs disease, for instance, normally work to break down fats. Some proteins also regulate the function of DNA itself.

The translation process from genes to proteins is a complex series of steps. The sequence of letters (bases) in a gene is first copied and then used to create a corresponding chain of protein subunits, which are called amino acids. The chemical properties of the amino acid sequence cause the emerging protein to fold and twist in a unique way; its function is implicit in its shape. Thus the signal transmitters in the back of the eye are rods and cones, nerve fibers are cylinders, and immune cells relate to the bacteria or viruses they defeat much as keys fit into locks.

The double helix itself is also folded, coiled and recoiled, cushioned by other kinds of molecules, and packaged into the dense structures known as chromosomes. Normally people have twenty-three pairs of them, including one unmatched pair called X and Y that determine gender (XX is woman, XY is man).

Remarkably, people can survive and grow up with duplications or deletions of rather large parts of chromosomes or even, as in Down syndrome, extra copies of entire chromosomes. (People with Down syndrome have an extra copy of chromosome 21.) Still, the error rate in the system is astoundingly low. "Why the molecular strands that constitute each chromosome do not become hopelessly entangled" during any ordinary cell division, remarks geneticist James Neel, "is unknown."

to conceal what is happening to them. If, on the other hand, you know of a family struck by this tragedy, you may appreciate the enormity of its effect on the unfortunate parents and family."

How far would Dor Yeshorim take its mandate? Its development consultant, Shmuel Lefkowitz, once told *The New York Times* that the program hoped to expand testing from Tay-Sachs to "anything available."

"Hopefully, one day all recessive genetic diseases will be amenable to testing," he wrote in an article describing the program in *Genesis*, the newsletter of the Genetics Network of the New York State Department of Health. "Dor Yeshorim's dream is that blood samples could be taken from every Jewish teenager in order to test for all the relevant genetic diseases and that the technology would be available to automate this process in order to lower the cost of the multiple testing."

Exactly which are the "relevant tests," and how multiple should the testing be? This question began to concern Dor Yeshorim's leaders, as community members broadened their view of the program's purpose. Gradually they began to ask the program about the genetic basis of other misfortunes such as, say, deafness. Besides Tay-Sachs, genetic tests for a number of other serious hereditary disorders were being developed. The program had to decide on its stance.

"Whatever tragedy we can prevent without doing any harm" — that became Rabbi Ekstein's guiding principle. "Naturally every disease has to be weighed. It's not just automatically when a disease comes up, you're gonna do it. You have to weigh the cost of the test, its reliability, the frequency of the disease in the community."

In February 1995 Rabbi Ekstein traveled south on the New Jersey Turnpike with his partner in Dor Yeshorim, Howard Katzenstein. A former science teacher, Katzenstein now oversees many of the administrative duties involved in this large enterprise.

They were headed toward the Washington suburb of Bethesda, Maryland, where Ekstein was due to speak at a consensus conference at the National Institutes of Health. Several times before, Ekstein had accepted invitations to speak about genetic testing in the Jewish community, but this time he faced a special challenge. The topic of the conference was not Tay-Sachs; it was Gaucher disease. Its story was not as straightforward.

By that time Dor Yeshorim had also tested some 13,000 people for the presence of the genetic variation that underlies Gaucher disease. Some twenty-five couples who were both carriers had been identified and counseled. In twenty cases one member of a pair had later chosen to check another prospective match for genetic compatibility. Evidently they had not gone ahead with the original betrothal; even the less inevitable and less grim risk of Gaucher disease (see the box on page 15) was too great for them to hazard.

Katzenstein vividly recalls the long hours he and Rabbi Ekstein spent on the asphalt that day, not for the driving but for the intensity of their conversation. They had to resolve a delicate matter before they

GAUCHER DISEASE

Like Tay-Sachs, Gaucher disease is the result of an inherited deficiency in a chemical that would normally break down a fatty substance in the brain. Also like Tay-Sachs, the trait is recessive. A child will inherit the disease only if both his parents are carriers and both have passed on the affected gene.

Unlike Tay-Sachs, Gaucher disease is not always catastrophic. In its most severe form, which affects fewer than one in 100,000 infants (with no particular ethnic inheritance pattern), Gaucher disease causes severe neurological disease and is as rapidly fatal as Tay-Sachs. However, it also has two milder forms: one "juvenile" form (equally rare and also not particularly common among Jewish people) and an adult-onset form that *is* more common among Ashkenazim, affecting roughly one in a thousand people — an incidence about forty times higher than in the general population.

Both of the milder forms of Gaucher disease affect a variety of body systems and can cause an array of problems, from growth retardation to kidney and bone damage. Children with the juvenile form may survive into their thirties or forties. People with the adult form may live and die unaware that they have it. Neither of the milder forms causes neurological damage. Because people can live long lives with Gaucher disease, the fatty substance has a chance to accumulate outside the brain, in the spleen, liver, and bone marrow. Thus people with the disease often suffer damage to their spleen or bones and need to have their spleen removed or to have hip replacements. They also have anemia and fatigue. The most common symptom is enlargement of the spleen, which may remain undetected until autopsy or indeed forever.

In 1978 a research team at the National Institutes of Health developed a way to replace the missing enzyme in Gaucher patients through intravenous injections. Enzyme replacement therapy for Gaucher disease went on the market in 1991. The treatment does not always work and is very expensive, costing at least $100,000 per year. Gene therapy experiments now under way are trying to replace the underlying gene, not just its protein product.

reached the beltway around Washington. The prickly matter of screening would undoubtedly come up at the conference. Was it justified to test the entire U.S. population for Gaucher disease on a widespread basis, now that such testing was possible? They needed to decide on their stance.

"We asked ourselves," Katzenstein says, "do we want to ally ourselves with the people who advocate screening? These will be all the prenatal people, and that's a problem."

People who offer genetic screening for a disease like Gaucher must at least pay lip service to the option of terminating an affected pregnancy, even if they do not actually advocate it. In the United States, since *Roe v. Wade*, a couple's right to terminate has been taken for granted. But Ekstein and Katzenstein inhabit another world, in which testing is pre*marital*, not prenatal, and about as confidential as it can get.

Should they join in a consensus to encourage widespread genetic testing for a condition that in its most common form — and the only form specifically associated with the Ashkenazi Jewish ethnic heritage — is often so mild that it goes undiagnosed? Admittedly, it's *simpler* to screen for Gaucher genes in the Jewish population, because there is less variation than in the population at large. But is that in itself a good reason to do so?

By the time they left the turnpike, Katzenstein and Ekstein had made up their minds. They had decided not to cast their vote in favor of widespread screening for Gaucher disease. Those who would advocate it, Katzenstein says, were "doing something entirely different" than the leaders of Dor Yeshorim.

Their decision was rooted in the first principle of Dor Yeshorim: To test for a genetic disorder after a fetus exists is to postpone the matter too long. "Pregnancy is such an emotional imbalance," Katzenstein says. "It's not really fair. It's not the time to make such a decision."

At the conference, however, Ekstein defended the program's decision to provide testing for those families who seek it. "While we recognize that Gaucher and other diseases present more complexities with regard to variability in the way the disease is manifested, we and our advisers believe that people are able to understand and have the right to know such complex risk information," Ekstein told the conference.

The purpose of an NIH consensus conference is to collect a diverse

NONMALEFICENCE

Rabbi Ekstein's guiding principle for Dor Yeshorim is the most ancient canon of biomedical ethics, which dates back to the Hippocratic oath: *Primum non nocere.* First, do no harm.

The sanction against abortion in the Hasidic community makes it relatively straightforward for Dor Yeshorim to apply this value. No conceivable harm could come to a child through Ekstein's strategy — unless never being conceived in the first place is considered harm. Most bioethicists (and clearly Ekstein and the other rabbis) do not consider this a harm worthy of serious consideration.

The more serious potential harm was the stigma that might attach to testing, and Ekstein's ingenious system avoids it. As to the harm of preventing a marriage, Ekstein weighs it rather lightly: "Considering that we are not dealing with Adam and Eve," he says, "it's no great tragedy to tell John and Jane that they are better off not marrying each other."

The principle of nonmaleficence, doing no harm, is the flip side of beneficence, doing good. Rabbi Ekstein is deeply gratified to be able to satisfy both. In other contexts, it becomes more troublesome.

Prenatal testing for genetic disorders is a prime example, because it forces us to decide what is good and what is harm, whose good outweighs whose harms, and even whose interests to consider. Aborting a fetus with a genetic disease confers benefit upon the family by sparing it cost, effort, and intense anguish, but some would argue it harms the fetus by denying it life. In the case of Tay-Sachs, the arguments against giving too much weight to this harm are compelling. The disease is a death sentence of itself, executed after a few painful years.

Dr. Michael Kaback, a pioneer in prenatal testing for Tay-Sachs disease, would place another element on the benefit side of the balance. Before prenatal testing, most families just stopped having children if they lost one to Tay-Sachs disease. Now they can safely try again. Against the fetuses lost to Tay-Sachs testing, Kaback places the many thousands born healthy.

group of interested parties, let them listen to presentations by experts, and then ask them to deliberate and eventually formulate recommendations about the detection and treatment of certain medical problems. As it turns out, the bulk of the participants agreed with Ekstein on the issue of screening. "Widespread application of genetic screening to detect either presymptomatic patients with Gaucher disease or ... carriers is not appropriate at this time," reads the final report of the conference. The "medical value" of such screening, the participants concluded, "has not been established."

In the case of Gaucher disease, at least, the enclave of Dor Yeshorim and the much larger, less ordered society outside it conform to the same principle: Genetic testing should be fully voluntary, and the initiative should rest with individuals.

Thinking about the conference afterward, Katzenstein remembered the turnpike debate about screening, but Rabbi Ekstein focused on another memory entirely. What burns in his memory was the deeply foreboding tone of the entire conference, even though its subject was a matter about which he is personally, defiantly optimistic. As he speaks of it, his voice rises.

"I was very aggravated by this meeting, because everybody was painting dark," he says, gesturing broadly with his hands. "Why didn't I hear one word about the good side of this? Where is the bright side of the story?"

Ekstein had been invited to speak about Dor Yeshorim, but as he sees it, his most important contribution was a larger one. Baffled by the turn in the deliberations, he rose from his seat and spoke a word of thanks to the researchers who had found the genes behind Gaucher disease and created a test for them. As Ekstein sees it, saying this was a courageous act that no one else had been willing to dare.

"Everything can be used in a good way or a wrong way," he says, in the same insistent tone one would use to tell a child why he should not chase a ball into the street. "You can get in a car and drive where you want to go. Sure, you can drive up on the sidewalk and kill somebody. Does that mean a car's a bad thing?"

The question poses itself: Who is blinded to what? Is Ekstein so devoted to his cause that he underestimates the perils that genetic testing could present in a different context, outside the invisible walls of Williamsburg? Or are those who focus on the perils of the new genetics chasing after phantoms that exist only in their own imaginations?

Frances Berkwits, who has worked as genetic counselor for Dor Yeshorim since the program's inception, has a broader perspective on the issues, and her outlook is somewhat darker than the rabbi's. "I do think our society has to begin to deal with the issue of how we should deal with genetics," she said recently. "I've been told people come in and say, 'I want to be tested for everything you can test for.' We can test for things we don't have treatments for. What are the benefits? . . . In testing for Gaucher disease, we find not only carriers but some affected people. What is our obligation to them? How do we inform them? If we're dealing with this, it's time for the program to find out: What are the results we are getting? What are the problems that confront us?"

Within only a few years, her question would take on a much sharper focus as Ashkenazi women would be shown to be at uniquely high risk of breast and ovarian cancer — and some would begin to worry not just about cancer, but about their marriageability.

To Rabbi Josef Ekstein, it is a conundrum that so many people choose to focus on the dilemmas that surround genetic testing. "Negative, always negative," he says. "We're missing a balance." Even in "liberal" America, where matters are more "complicated," he insists, "there are still people who value what their future generation will look like. For those people, I think you can educate them, to be protected so they can't have this problem."

The medical geneticist who helped to found Dor Yeshorim, Dr. Robert Desnick, is no longer involved with the program. But he continues actively to test methods of genetic screening in other communities within New York's Ashkenazi population, and he shares Ekstein's enthusiasm.

"Although this population is unique, it will serve as a gold standard" for developing methods for the delivery of genetic screening, he wrote in a grant application. "Clearly, the lessons learned . . . in this receptive and health-oriented population should prove instructive to future prospective genetic screening programs."

Perhaps. Certainly Dor Yeshorim, and similar programs in other Jewish communities, offer brilliant lessons in how to carry out genetic screening, beginning with a full and deeply sensitive understanding of the nature and needs of the community involved. Would an equal sensitivity to the nature and needs of other communities lead to similarly successful outcomes?

An approach like Ekstein's might somehow work for the rest of us too — if we could drag our sensibilities back a century or so, overlook our tremendous diversities, and unite in giving great deference to authority.

Perhaps. But more likely, we and our children will have to deal with the new realities that the genetic revolution brings to us in our own way, as the individuals we are, in the kind of world that surrounds us. It will not prove simple for us either.

CHAPTER 2

The Stress Test

I don't have time to worry about things that may or may not be.
There's enough that *is* to worry about.

— Folksinger Arlo Guthrie, perhaps at risk of Huntington's disease

HOW CURIOUS IT SEEMS: THAT ADOLESCENT BLOOD-letting, the clandestine telephone calls, the matchmakers—as exotic, all of it, as prayer shawls and earlocks. Intrigued, the rest of us stand outside the invisible fence around Dor Yeshorim and peer inside. Other cultures are indeed fascinating.

As is ours to Anna W. What we undertake without thinking is remarkable to her. Anna worked as a baby-sitter and housekeeper for a wealthy family in Brooklyn—not very far from Williamsburg, in fact. As she saw it, she had become party to a peculiar state of affairs.

Where Anna comes from back in Poland, there are no such things as baby-sitters and housekeepers. Parents do not stay at work until dark and leave their children in the care of others. They come home in midafternoon and play with their children. If they can't, the grandparents are always there. Late afternoons are for bicycle trips to the countryside, not for conference calls.

But Anna did not find this eccentricity about New York at all intimidating, any more than the crime or the cockroaches. She would not have come to New York in the first place unless she were the sort of person who is excited by the unfamiliar. While her friends in Poland were getting married and having children, Anna was traveling alone to China and Turkey, to Malaysia and Singapore. New York was just another great adventure.

She and her husband came to New York to make enough money to build a house back in Poland. Although she has a master's degree in economics, Anna took a job caring for children because it was quick, easy, and lucrative. Her husband, a mining engineer by training, got a job in construction.

Their pregnancy was planned. What they were not prepared for was the experience.

The routine prenatal testing that we take for granted now was alien and bizarre to Anna. Her doctors seemed to be searching doggedly to find something wrong with her baby, which came to her as a surprise and something of a violation. But what happened to her during the course of that experience is a metaphor for the shape that genetic testing has begun to assume in general: the ability to search for things amiss.

"We're not so stupid," Anna said at one point during her pregnancy. Spending any time with her, that's obvious—although her slight but unmistakable accent and her imperfect English may have left a different impression with certain people, including her doctors.

Even newer to the New World than the people of Dor Yeshorim, Anna also gave blood to be tested for Tay-Sachs disease—but only after she was pregnant, not before. As a result, she found herself caught up in what Rabbi Ekstein's business manager would call an emotional situation.

There were certain things she kept trying very hard not to think about.

"I'm kind of a pessimist," she said, furrows in her forehead, her face long and drawn. "I tend to see the glass as half empty." As she spoke, she was six months pregnant. As she put it, she had started off on the left foot, and after that everything went wrong.

"I know that's not rational," she went on. "It's just the way I'm thinking now." Her own mother had said prenatal testing was a mistake, that if you worried too much, the worry would affect the baby. Anna didn't really agree with her—but that was something else to worry about.

Anna had two options, according to her doctor's advice. She could have an amniocentesis; fluid would be withdrawn from her womb through a long needle and sampled directly for damage to the chromosomes inside cells from the fetus, which are routinely shed into amniotic fluid. There is a small but definite risk, about one in 200, that a woman undergoing amniocentesis will have a miscarriage as a result. (Anna's risk of having a baby with either Down syndrome or spina bifida, a neural tube defect, was itself about one in 200.) Alternatively, Anna could have a more or less harmless ultrasound scan to look for visible signs of malformation.

Anna was puzzled by her predicament and almost as puzzled by the strange culture that had put her into it. But as an economist by training, she well understood risk. She saw that for amniocentesis, the odds were even. Rather than endanger the baby (who might or might not be normal) with the procedure, she chose to endure the uncertainty.

Three months earlier and three months pregnant, Anna had fallen ill and had been advised to take some medication. Not at all stupid, she inquired whether the medicine could endanger her baby. Her doctor didn't know and referred her to a genetic counselor who would know how to answer her question.

Anna loved the counselor. She took time and listened carefully, didn't look at her watch once, and took an extensive family history. During the interview Anna revealed something that was a deep secret a half century ago: Although the family was Roman Catholic, one of her grandmothers was Jewish. Anna had grown up in Oswiecim, the very town where the Auschwitz concentration camp had been located a quarter century before she was born. Her grandmother's true ethnic history, once a lethal piece of information, seemed a benign detail here and now, in America in the 1990s.

The counselor checked her references and told Anna quickly that she had no need to worry that the medication might endanger the baby. But in her report to the obstetrician, she added that there might be cause to worry about the ethnic history.

"Ms. W. is of Polish descent and her grandmother is of Jewish descent," wrote the counselor. "I discussed the autosomal recessive inheritance pattern of Tay-Sachs disease. Ms. W. appeared to understand that in order for a baby to have a 25 percent chance of having Tay-Sachs disease, both parents must be carrying the Tay-Sachs gene. We would recommend screening for Tay-Sachs."

The counselor may have mentioned Tay-Sachs to Anna, but she didn't focus on it. Obviously her eastern European origins and her grandmother's ethnicity didn't have the same significance to her as they did to the counselor. All she recalls is astonishment when, at her next visit, the obstetrician suggested she should have a test for Tay-Sachs.

Anna's immediate reaction was negative. Her husband, who is of a calmer temperament, offered to be tested instead. If he was not a carrier, after all, there would be no reason to inquire further. He went to the lab and had blood drawn.

Four days later, on a Friday, the doctor called to say they needed to return and both take the test. Mr. W.'s result was inconclusive. The doctor suggested that they might also want to have Anna's blood drawn for a test that could give information about the risk of other defects, such as Down syndrome.

"She didn't say, 'You *have* to have the test,'" Anna recalled. "She said, 'Almost everyone does it. I can't tell you, you should or you shouldn't. You decide.'"

The following weekend was horrible for Anna, who sees glasses as half empty. On Monday, rigid with concern, she returned to the doctor's office with her husband to have blood drawn for the follow-up tests. The wait in the outer office was interminable.

At one point her husband rose to ask the receptionist why his first test had been inconclusive. "I don't know," she responded. "Probably someone got drunk and spilled the sample." Anna's husband asked for a copy of the test result, and she made a photocopy for him. He put it in his pocket.

Later, at home, they got out the dictionary and studied every word in the report. Peculiar: no matter how they read the document and the numbers, it seemed obvious that Mr. W.'s result fell into the normal range. For some reason the word *inconclusive* was underlined, but the result clearly fell outside the range of numbers corresponding to that category.

Perplexed, they called an American friend who is a psychiatrist, then went to his house with the puzzling report. The friend read it the same way: Judging from the numbers, the lab result was normal. Perhaps the doctor had looked at the report too hastily, seen that inexplicable line under the word *inconclusive*, and jumped to the wrong conclusion. Actually, it didn't look like an underscore at all. It was more like a scratch or a crease.

On Tuesday they called the doctor and asked for an appointment. Impossible, the receptionist said. The doctor was booked up. They took another day off from work and went to the doctor's office, prepared to sit there until she would see them. They sat all day.

Finally, the doctor ushered them into her office. Anna's husband showed her the photocopy, and the doctor acknowledged that his interpretation was correct. "Okay, you're not a carrier," she said abruptly. "Now what's your next question?" From that moment on, Anna says, the doctor's demeanor was frozen and very formal.

At her next scheduled visit, the news was truly bad: The result of the second test, the level of a fetal protein known as AFP, was out of the normal range. Naturally, she asked to see the report, but no mistake had been made this time.

The AFP test measures levels of alpha-fetoprotein, a substance made by the fetus that makes its way into the mother's blood; most commonly obstetricians test at the same time for AFP and two other substances in blood. Levels of these substances that are higher or lower than the normal range are read out as degrees of risk for having a baby with Down syndrome or spina bifida. The normal risk figure for a twenty-nine-year-old woman is one in 780. Anna's results indicated a risk of one in 200.

Having banished from her imagination the possibility that the unseen creature inside her was doomed by Tay-Sachs disease, Anna now began to envision a child with almond eyes and limited intellect, or else some sort of opening around the spinal cord. That last image haunted her during the final few months of her pregnancy: an infant with a grotesque protrusion somewhere in its back.

Something else played at the edges of her mind: "One thing I was really concerned about was, why bother with the test? Because even if you're okay, it doesn't tell you everything is fine. What's the point of doing this?"

Even if the fetus is found to be free of Down syndrome and spina bifida, hundreds of other things might still be wrong: heart defects, shrunken limbs, a cleft palate, a huge birthmark on the face — the list goes on and on. Many things can go wrong that aren't even genetic. Why expose oneself to the possibility of these two bits of bad news, spina bifida and Down syndrome, in particular? Just because those tests happen to exist? Because they are the most common of serious birth defects? What about testing for the others? Where should one stop?

Virginia Corson, a genetic counselor at Johns Hopkins University Medical Center in Baltimore, says many of her clients go through a similar kind of inner turmoil during the course of prenatal testing. "In medicine you don't usually make your own decisions," she says. "You usually get the advice of your doctor. I don't know what to advise people. . . . Some people have great, *great* difficulty making these decisions. What if I *don't* have the test and then there's an abnormality? What if I *do* have the test, and then there's a miscarriage? How will I deal with that? What if I *do* have the test and there's an abnormality? What will I do then? Somehow, people do muddle through and make a decision. But it's not easy."

Despite her misgivings, Anna went through the testing. When asked why, she shrugged. "I did it because I was hoping everything was normal." What she had now wasn't really good news or bad news. It was merely the *possibility* of bad news, with a number pinned to it.

Anna put the situation in economic terms. If she entered a lottery that gave her one chance in 200 of winning, she would hardly take out her credit card and buy something in anticipation of the prize money. If she were thirty-five and not twenty-nine, she knew, a risk of one in 200 in an AFP test would be considered normal. Would she worry about the same risk if she were six years older? Probably not. Why was it so fearsome now? If she *were* stupid, perhaps she would have spent less time wandering about in the hypothetical.

Would Anna and her husband terminate an affected pregnancy? The question is easy to ask but was powerfully difficult for them to answer in the abstract. Affected with what? How *definitely* affected? With levels of risk that balanced each other, and a planned and welcome pregnancy, neither termination nor continuing the pregnancy was easy to contemplate.

One thing they could do was seek a second opinion. By this point Anna and her husband did not trust the original doctor at all. Perhaps she had misjudged the stage of Anna's pregnancy, which would alter the risk levels indicated by the result of the blood test. On that slim possibility they asked their psychiatrist friend to refer them to a different obstetrician.

"The second doctor said what we already knew: It's only a screening test," Anna recalled. "It doesn't mean anything is wrong. But because he's a doctor he has to take it under consideration."

Evidently Anna's second doctor was careful to leave the choices up to her; but sometimes doctors may subtly pressure patients to have amniocentesis, says Suzanne Carter, who works as a genetic counselor at Albert Einstein Medical Center in New York.

"For example," she says, "the provider may tell the patient not to schedule her next prenatal visit until the amniocentesis results are available. Although patients will still have their usual pregnancy worries, relief is greatly apparent after genetic counseling, even if they decline the amniocentesis." Unfortunately Anna, like many women, did not have the benefit of another session with the genetic counselor as she was feeling her way toward a decision.

But she did have recourse to Aunt Sophia back in Poland, who is a

GENES AND RISK

Anna alluded to the lottery. Most clients in genetic counseling anchor their thoughts in the same way. They're like gamblers who focus on extreme ends of the scale—winning big or losing everything—and to judge their risk based on what has happened lately.

Parents-to-be tend to have extreme visions of Down syndrome. "My child will be severely retarded and live in an institution," says one pair. "My child will grow up to be kind and good-humored and work in a grocery store," thinks another. As with many genetic conditions, the range of outcomes between these extremes is wide.

Clients appear to find genetic risks much less threatening than environmental risks, such as carcinogens, because they are in control of the outcome and it involves only them, not everyone in town. Surveys show that they tend to view the same risk figure as less serious than a doctor or counselor would. (To a doctor, a 20 percent risk is high. Clients see it as moderate.)

Clients tend not to change their minds about what to do based on the counseling session, perhaps because they and their counselors talk past each other. When the risk is worth talking about at all, clients want to cut to the chase. If the risk is above 10 percent (that is, not negligible), they want to talk about the possible consequences: the nature of the problem, the cost of care, options for education, and effects on the family. Traditionally counselors have focused on making sure clients understand their level of risk.

This information comes from a study of hour-long counseling sessions. If doctors do the counseling and want to limit the length of the session, as is often the case, patients who want to spend time talking about their options, rather than their exact risk figure, had better say so out loud.

Very often risk figures based on genetic tests are estimates of uncertain accuracy and value. Even people who understand the dimensions of their risk will be left up in the air.

doctor. Aunt Sophia was growing accustomed to these calls by now — Anna had consulted her at every turn of events, and with every call the story they told sounded stranger.

"Every time I had a question, the answer was always amnio," Anna said. "Amnio amnio amnio! In Poland, they don't do amnio unless you're over forty. They don't even do an AFP blood test unless someone in the family already had a problem."

With nothing to lose, she and her husband opted for ultrasound, which both doctors had suggested. The result was reassuringly normal. The fetus even turned over at a critical moment, so they could see a profile. But Anna did not carry a snapshot of the scan afterward, as some other prospective parents do, so she could show off the baby even before it made an appearance.

Anna had difficulty thinking of the baby who would soon emerge as hers, or as real, or as an individual of any kind. "I don't want to be the greatest," she said near the end of her pregnancy, unaware that she was speaking about results of tests relating to her infant as if they reflected on herself. "I don't want to be perfect," she went on. "I just want to be normal."

An American-born lawyer once expressed directly the conflict that Anna herself didn't recognize. "I was hoping I'd never have to make this choice, to become responsible for choosing the kind of baby I'd get, the kind of baby we'd accept," she told anthropologist Rayna Rapp. "But everyone — my doctor, my parents, my friends — everyone urged me to come for genetic counseling and have amniocentesis. . . . And they all told me I'd feel more in control. But in some ways I feel less in control. Oh, it's still my baby, but only if it's good enough to be our baby, if you see what I mean."

As her original doctor must have seen the situation, Anna is a high-strung woman who was having unusual difficulty with the emotional aspects of her first pregnancy. As Anna herself sees it, a sensible question about the possible risks of medication led to a dreamworld of perils and possibilities that clouded the rest of her pregnancy and left her with no real options except worry.

Originally, amniocentesis was developed as a way to resolve uncertainty for parents who were at known risk of having a child with genetic disease, because it could allow direct study of fetal chromosomes. Its use later spread to all pregnant women over the age of thirty-five, because older women are more likely to have babies with chromosomal defects that amniocentesis can detect. For younger pregnant women, like Anna, it is often also recommended as a follow-up test, when other

WHAT IS VOLUNTARY?

Liberty and freedom are fundamental values in American culture, and the medical profession pays constant lip service to the idea that we should undertake all tests and treatments of our own free will. In prenatal testing and screening, however, as a number of critics have commented, the nature of the word *voluntary* is open to question. Women who would prefer not to consider terminating their pregnancies may agree to testing for financial and societal reasons, or to defer to their husbands or other relatives—or just to conform.

After surveying women who, like Anna, decided not to have amniocentesis, sociologist Troy Duster wrote that "the mere existence of the new technology, and the social distribution of knowledge about its availability, act together as twin pressures on a potential client." One interviewee said her friends implied "that any sane woman over thirty-five with an ounce of brains would have amniocentesis."

If a test is seen as routine and its emotional consequences are not laid out, women will likely take the course of least resistance and go through with it. In California, where AFP testing is routine unless a woman signs a *refusal* form, anthropologist Nancy Press found that some receptionists described it as "just a simple blood test" to "show how your baby is developing." This description is deceptive. Its implication: To resist would be weird.

"Society does not truly accept children with disabilities or provide assistance for their nurturance," observes Canadian epidemiologist Abby Lippman, probably the most outspoken voice on the question. "Thus, a woman may see no realistic alternative to diagnosing and aborting a fetus likely to be affected."

"We need to reassess what 'choice' is for women," writes psychologist Robyn Rowland. "In gaining the choice to control the quality of our children, we may lose the choice *not* to control the quality; the choice of simply accepting them as they are."

tests raise a suspicion that the fetus may have a hereditary defect that could be detected by microscopic study of the chromosomes.

It is easier to justify the widespread dissemination of AFP testing, as well as the so-called triple marker test, which analyzes the pregnancy-related hormones estradiol and human chorionic gonadotropin in addition to AFP. Both can be done without risk to the infant, because all they entail is taking a drop of blood from the mother's finger. Thus they offer a relatively safe way to screen the fetuses of younger women for Down syndrome and spina bifida.

In August 1994 the American College of Obstetricians and Gynecologists issued a statement advising obstetricians to offer AFP screening to *all* their patients. The American College of Medical Genetics followed suit in the same year.

Triple marker screening has become an integral part of ordinary obstetrics practice in America, perhaps less to "reassure" pregnant women — as the people who provide the testing often say — than for another reason, unstated in either of the societies' guidelines: to protect doctors against the risk of "wrongful birth" lawsuits, should a child with either condition be born to a woman who has not been offered the test.

Prenatal testing deserves our attention here not so much in its own right but as an archetype, because it is in this setting that genetics has already permeated society, almost unremarked. One who is not pregnant, not a mother, not a feminist, even someone who loathes children, would do well to consider the case of prenatal testing, because it has all the hallmarks of the ingenuous acceptance of genetic technology that our own society wishes upon us.

Any woman facing prenatal testing has to come to grips with (or suppress) the idea of terminating a wanted pregnancy. Anyone facing a test for a predisposition to any trait with a hereditary component will have to grapple with all the implications of the fact that an entire medical and diagnostic testing industry has decided that such a trait is worthy of detection. On what basis was this decision made? Who wants to know the test results, and why?

One recent survey of obstetricians in suburbs north of New York City found that more than half felt it was not necessary even to tell a woman, let alone gain her consent, before her blood is tested for signs of fetal abnormalities. In many cases, therefore, it appears that women are being told they have a risk of a fetal abnormality without being asked whether they want to know. Although 99 percent of these obstetricians say they would tell patients that the blood test is only a screening test and does not make a firm diagnosis, only 51 percent would inform them that results of a follow-up test such as amniocentesis might require them to decide whether to have an abortion.

In another recent survey of American health care providers who offer AFP testing, more than a third of obstetricians did not mention to their patients that such testing was voluntary, and 32 percent made recommendations to patients as part of reporting the result. When discussing amniocentesis, four of ten doctors mentioned abortion. Only 27 percent discussed the possibility of continuing the pregnancy.

"Many women are not given an informed choice," declares geneticist Golder Wilson, M.D., of the Dallas Children's Medical Center. "They're not [even] told the test was done until they get the results. Mandatory screening without counseling is not my idea of good genetics."

In Anna's case, the blood test had raised a theoretical specter, but a later test reassured her somewhat by contradicting the first result. She was dubious about the whole process.

Anna may be more willing than most women to comment about this situation, coming as she does from another culture. But many ordinary American mothers would recognize it, particularly those who had their first baby before 1994 and then another afterward. From the first pregnancy, they got a child. With the second pregnancy, they got choices. They had *freedom* of choice, of course, but may not have found it especially liberating.

"Among ourselves," says genetic counselor Carter, "we have nicknamed the AFP test the stress test, because of the undue tension surrounding a positive result." In subsequent pregnancies, she adds, some women who have had AFP testing before will refuse it entirely. "They want to avoid the uncertainty of a positive screen," Carter explains, "or, more simply put, 'I don't want to go through that AFP test again that you can't tell me if my baby has Down syndrome.'"

It should be pointed out that the AFP and the triple marker screen are not true genetic tests because they detect proteins in the blood, not the genes that direct production of the proteins. They are *like* many genetic tests, however, in that they tell only the risk of a future event, rather than make a positive diagnosis of an existing condition. (Cytogenetic tests done after amniocentesis — microscopic studies of chromosomes within fetal cells, which *are* true genetic tests — can determine whether large sections of DNA have been deleted, duplicated, or rearranged, information that is truly diagnostic of a fetal condition. This certainty, however, comes at a risk to the fetus.)

It should also be pointed out that, shortly before Christmas 1995, Anna gave birth to a normal, healthy baby girl.

CHAPTER 3

Choices

For his birthday, Daddy gave him a time bomb.
Britain's #1 killer can be hereditary.
Help us fight it.

— British Heart Foundation billboard

FOR SOME COUPLES THE NEWS IS REAL, IT'S BAD, AND IT won't be gone by morning. Consider now Jonathan and Kris Vander Plaat. They are here because they have faced a genetic verdict — a final, unequivocal verdict — and carried on, and because they are willing to share the experience.

For one week in April 1993, while he drove back and forth every day between his home in Bergen County, New Jersey, and Columbia-Presbyterian Medical Center in New York City to visit his baby, Jonathan Vander Plaat told himself there was still hope that it was all a terrible mistake. Everyone knows the feeling: *I can cope with this. Yes, I can. Here is what comes now — one foot, and then the other.*

Because of the temporary commute and his own state of mind, Jonathan completely missed the sad news back home. A different set of parents were burying an eighteen-year-old son, who had died the day before he was due to give the valedictory speech at his high school graduation.

The teenage boy died in the same hospital where Jonathan's infant daughter, Meghan, was now staying, of the same illness that kept her there: cystic fibrosis. Jonathan's own brothers were the undertakers who buried the young man that week. (The Vander Plaat family operates three funeral homes in Bergen County.) They certainly didn't involve Jonathan in *that* particular funeral.

He learned about it only several weeks later. The owner of a luncheonette near the Vander Plaat funeral home asked Jonathan how he had ever handled burying that high school kid, knowing he had cystic fibrosis just like little Meghan.

Afterward, Jonathan blew up at his father. "You had no right!" he said. "I'm going to have to deal with things like that!" Jonathan's daily labor involves embalming the dead and counseling their families. He knows well enough to keep an eye out for those families who seem to go on after a funeral as if nothing is wrong. He knows he has to try to find a way to help them get started on the hard work of grief. Secrecy and pretending are out of the question. Living in the dark is no strategy.

In addition to their regular duties, the Vander Plaats inter, free of charge, miscarried fetuses—small bodies who are mourned for who they might have been rather than for who they are. Asked how his profession has affected his attitude toward his little girl's illness, Jonathan responds without a pause.

"I guess I value each day more than I would if I were not a funeral director," he says, "and I value infants even more."

That doesn't mean he will ever coddle Meghan. Quite the contrary: just a month after her illness was diagnosed, when Jonathan and his wife Kris were certain at last that their three-month-old daughter had cystic fibrosis, they took her on a camping trip. They did come home earlier than planned, because the baby coughed too much and no one was having fun. But what obviously matters to Jonathan Vander Plaat is that they went in the first place.

"A lot of people are consumed with the disease," he says. "They don't let their child who has it have a life. There are those who build their life around the disease. We want to build the disease around our life."

At two, Meghan Vander Plaat is enchanting and wispy-haired, quite a talker. Her father, a pragmatic man, makes the path that led up to the present sound almost easy. Not so Kris Vander Plaat, who sits beside him at the dining table and apologizes for feeling guilty about her daughter's condition.

"I knew I couldn't help but feel guilty," she says. "I knew there was no way I could change it. I'm a carrier. I have no symptoms, but she's the one who's going to suffer."

Except for her brief hospital stay in 1993, Meghan does not actually seem to have suffered much. She evidently enjoys the gentle pounding she gets, on her upper chest and back and underarms, several times daily, as well as her regular sessions breathing in from the nebulizer, all of it necessary to break up the mucus that builds in her lungs. As far as she knows, the enzymes she must take to help her faulty digestion are

WHAT IT MEANS TO BE
A CARRIER, PART II

Carrier status is invisible, but it's hardly insignificant. To many carriers of the cystic fibrosis (CF) gene, like Kris Vander Plaat, the ambiguities are painful.

Studies of CF testing programs show that when people are found to be carriers, they have an immediate depression and may have anxiety for long periods afterward. Carrier status implies possessing a flaw and the ability to pass it on, without oneself suffering the consequences of the flaw. Thus carriers may, like Kris, experience survivor syndrome—guilt for having gone untouched by something that has harmed or even killed a loved one.

Carrier status can easily affect relationships—especially future relationships, if the carrier is not currently involved. Outside Dor Yeshorim, the world leaves carriers with the full burden of deciding whether, when, and how to raise the issue. Carrier status may also threaten someone's insurance coverage.

Studies by psychologist Joanna Fanos show that even people who are tested and shown *not* to be carriers can experience survivor guilt and may even wish they were carriers after all. "I felt like, God, why do I get off scot-free?" said one subject who had a sibling with cystic fibrosis. "Give me some burden to carry. I still feel bad about it."

just pretty sprinkles on her yogurt. If anything, other children might have reason to envy Meghan all that loving attention.

Meghan does not live inside a glass ball—far from it. She goes into the nursery at church. She has regular contact with other children. Her mother has long since put away the bib that reads "Look but don't touch."

Meghan has been so robust that Kris once actually contemplated asking the doctors whether she could have outgrown cystic fibrosis. But at heart, she knew better. It's in the genes.

Judging from the recent past, Meghan's prospects look quite rosy. In the less than two decades that separate her from the young man who died before he could graduate from high school, improved medical care has transformed the prognosis for children born with cystic fibrosis.

"My view and that of most CF specialists is extremely different than even ten years ago," says Meghan's doctor at Columbia-Presbyterian, Lynne Quittell. "Now it's not necessary to have to present parents with a death sentence for their children, the way it was ten years ago."

As she speaks, Dr. Quittell is in charge of the care of a sixty-year-old man with cystic fibrosis—an exception, someone at the far edge of the statistical curve, but also a testament to the variability of the disease. She says that one of the leading research scientists in the field, a man old enough to have earned a Ph.D., himself has cystic fibrosis. A 1995 survey showed that one in three young adults with cystic fibrosis worked full time and 90 percent finished high school. Ten years ago, the average life expectancy for cystic fibrosis was about seventeen. Today Meghan can expect to live beyond thirty.

"That may sound like a horrible number to you," says Dr. Quittell, who herself passed that birthday the previous year. "To me it's amazing." Because a field once so desperate is now so full of hope, she adds, "it's a fair statement that most cystic fibrosis caretakers find a death now much more frustrating than it ever was. We're always on the cusp of being able to save them. It's harder to accept the natural history of the disease."

Medication for cystic fibrosis was improving dramatically even before the gene responsible for the condition was discovered in 1989. Isolation of the gene led directly to the root problem: a molecular defect in a channel that carries salts across cell membranes. It may be that the change in salt concentration inactivates a natural antibiotic that protects body fluids.

That knowledge should lead to even better medicines in the near term. Then there's always the possibility, somewhere just over the horizon, that a child like Meghan can benefit from gene therapy—if researchers can find a way to deliver to her cells a functional gene for this channel.

In the same month that Meghan entered Columbia-Presbyterian, Dr. Ronald Crystal began testing gene therapy on a few children with cystic fibrosis, down and across town at the New York Hospital-Cornell Medical Center. Earlier, he had tried out his strategy on rats, and found that the gene transfer worked safely. After gaining approval from the hospital ethics board, he proceeded to try the transfer strategy on humans. He infected nine children with a cousin of the cold virus, which he had engineered so that it became a sort of drug delivery system: genetically altered so that it could not cause disease but was able to infect a cell with the gene that creates a normal salt channel across membranes.

"Have we cured the disease? Absolutely not," Dr. Crystal says. "It will take years to prove it." That will require trials in hundreds of patients. "Don't take this as anything but anecdotes," he goes on. There are still many technical problems to resolve and questions to answer. Gene therapy to date has not improved salt transport, and of course the immune system responds to the virus that carries the beneficial gene. What exists now, he adds, is the *potential*.

"In the same way we knew in the 1980s that finding the gene was going to be a reality, only we didn't know when," says Dr. Quittell, "one day, we're going to wake up and find that gene therapy is a reality." Awaiting that day, she keeps after her families to be faithful in doing the therapy that exists for them today, to use antibiotics and pummel the child's back to help keep the lungs clear. "They have to be well!"

Dr. Quittell's brightness and optimism helped the Vander Plaats begin to regain the equilibrium they had lost on the evening of income tax day, when two-month-old Meghan suddenly stopped coughing. It was cold and snowy. Jonathan was standing at the living room door, ready to go out to play tennis. Meghan was in her grandfather's arms.

"Already at two months," Jonathan says, "she was very verbal. I mean she babbled all the time. Suddenly, everything just stopped. You could say she was just—stuck. . . . She was coughing and coughing." All of a sudden she stopped.

Jonathan flipped Meghan over and pounded her back. He was afraid she had stopped breathing. She gasped and seemed to gulp for air. They bundled her against the snow and drove straight to the pediatrician, who examined her and told the couple to take her home. Everything appeared to be fine, he said.

Jonathan was not reassured. "Can you guarantee us she will live through the night?" he asked the doctor. He would not say. Rather than returning home, they drove to the local hospital. The doctor who examined Meghan there ran down a list of possible explanations for her breathing problem. The last item on the list was cystic fibrosis. He passed over it quickly.

"Don't even think it could be CF," he said. "It's a horrible, horrible, horrible disease." Kris remembers clearly: he repeated "horrible" three times.

CYSTIC FIBROSIS

It was the kiss of death: if kissing a child on the forehead left a salty taste, said an ancient European proverb, the child was bewitched and would soon die.

The modern version of that test for cystic fibrosis is the sweat test, which measures the amount of chloride (a component of salt) in the perspiration. CF is a defect in the transport of chloride into and out of cells. It disrupts the secretion of digestive enzymes, endangering the pancreas and liver; of mucus in the lungs, making breathing labored and encouraging infections; and of fluid in the reproductive tract, rendering many CF patients infertile.

CF children no longer die early, and the course of the disease is highly variable. Many now survive well into their twenties or longer, because they can take antibiotics for infections and digestive enzymes in pill form. They also need to have their chests pounded on a regular basis, to loosen mucus in the lungs.

About 30,000 Americans live with cystic fibrosis. Another 5 percent of the population are carriers of a cystic fibrosis mutation— capable of conceiving a child who will have cystic fibrosis, if the other parent is also a carrier with the same mutation. Some 650 different mutations have now been identified that can cause CF, but geneticists know the list is not yet complete. Therefore testing will not leave someone in the clear about carrier status unless doctors know the precise mutation passed down in his own family.

Three nights later Meghan was still in the hospital, and all the other possibilities had been ruled out. No alternative remained except the time-honored diagnostic for cystic fibrosis: the sweat test, a check for excess salt in the perspiration on the surface of her skin. Kris and Jonathan were in the waiting room when the phone call came from the doctor in charge of her case.

Looking back now, Kris can remember noticing the classic symptoms of CF from the first few weeks of her baby's life: the salt taste on her lips when she kissed Meghan's forehead, and her distended abdomen. But until that moment, she says now, she had been certain the problem would be "something they could cure."

Jonathan came back to the waiting room after taking the doctor's call. "I knew the result by his face," says Kris. "He was glassy-eyed." In that instant she sketched out for herself a bleak image of the future. Her first child would die by the age of three or four. There would be no tearful first day at kindergarten. *I'm never going to be able to handle this*, she thought.

The next morning the Vander Plaats grimly checked Meghan out of the local hospital and drove her a half hour into Manhattan, to the specialty clinic at Columbia-Presbyterian Medical Center. There they met Dr. Quittell, who had to start them all over and guide them, step by step, to a new understanding of their situation. She gave them brochures about the disease, and a coloring book that would explain it to Meghan's cousins. She told them what could be done.

"Suddenly everything was so much more relaxed," recalls Kris. "She talked to us about patients she has that are over forty years old. She told us that some patients do really well. She kept repeating over and over the fact that Meghan was only two months old, that we could take control and slow the progression of the lung damage."

To the Vander Plaats, Dr. Quittell talked about the nature of the disease. To herself, she muses about the nature of the Vander Plaats. What determined Meghan's general good health in her early years? Perhaps something about her genes. Perhaps the large extended family that enveloped her, the hopeful resolve with which her parents managed the extra chores involved in caring for a child with cystic fibrosis. Lucky child. Wonderful family. Variable condition.

Responses to the situation are also variable. Although the rest of the Vander Plaat family is dealing admirably with the reality of Meghan's illness, one member of the extended family cannot bear even to see a photograph of Meghan. For some reason that puzzles Kris and Jonathan, he can't handle the thought of it.

Genetic risks "tend to make ourselves 'the enemy,' and we are not conditioned to enjoy that message," observes one visionary geneticist, Charles Scriver. "We have been taught to wage war upon disease; and why not? Past crusades and campaigns against scourges have been very successful. . . . We use the language of World War I to describe our victorious attack on disease."

But now, he went on, "how do we understand the enemy when it is partly ourselves? Our cherished medical paradigms fail us when we try to understand." How can one vanquish a genetic disease without somehow threatening the one who bears it in the process? Who is the enemy, the disease or the diseased?

Once when Meghan was still in the hospital, Kris Vander Plaat asked Dr. Quittell about their risk of bearing another child with the same disease. "Don't worry about that yet," she replied. "Let's get through this, and then we'll go through the options."

They were ready to think seriously about it when Meghan was two. The fact of her illness dramatically altered the elements of the reproductive question for them. The fuzzy hypotheticals that haunt ordinary expectant couples now coalesced into some firm realities. She and Jonathan had only a few possible rolls of the genetic dice: a healthy child (three chances in four, either a carrier or a totally unaffected child) or another child with CF (one chance in four).

When they returned to Dr. Quittell to talk about it, she presented them with four options. They could conceive the usual way, have prenatal testing, and if they chose, terminate the pregnancy if the fetus was affected with CF. They could play it completely safe and adopt their second child. Or Kris could be artificially inseminated with sperm from a man who was not a carrier of the cystic fibrosis gene.

Finally, the truly high-tech alternative was: preimplantation diagnosis. They could opt for in vitro fertilization, supplemented by a DNA test on the fertilized eggs in that laboratory dish. Based on the results of the test, they could choose which embryos to reimplant. Kris and Jonathan took note of their options and went home to think.

Adoption was out of the question. The reasons had nothing whatever to do with a preference for their own genes. Rather, Kris's sister and her husband were trying to adopt. What if the Vander Plaats somehow managed to adopt a second child before the sister received her first? "Maybe it was a naive train of thought," says Jonathan, "but we knew that wasn't the way to go."

The artificial insemination option was an equally delicate issue for them. "Neither of us were really comfortable about that," Kris admits.

As to the possibility of terminating an affected fetus, this was another non-option, because of their religious faith. "We would go to a long length [to avoid aborting a fetus]," says Jonathan. "Let's talk about quality of life. I think the quality of life of my daughter is just fantastic."

What if Meghan had been sicker? What if, like other children they know, she was in and out of the hospital every few weeks? What if the option that faced them was a child who would live for a few years and then, for certain, die? "That is one of those [questions that] I don't know if I can answer," says Kris. "It would have been a lot harder."

"If my child had been very, very ill," Jonathan says, "that doesn't mean the second child would be that ill. I could still probably have played it out."

The way Kris sees it, once sperm and egg have joined, they form a human life. At least it has that potential, Jonathan says. Jonathan talked about the matter of abortion with several ministers, who told him that nothing in the New Testament forbids it. Still, it was not an alternative he and Kris could choose.

In vitro fertilization was "a real big moral issue," Jonathan says. "What do you do with the ones that come out positive [for CF]? . . . Who are we to say, 'Sorry, you're not what we wanted'?"

"Then we look at Meghan," Kris breaks in. "She's such a joy. That would be like saying her life wasn't worth it." At some stage they asked Dr. Quittell if in vitro testing could assure, with hundred-percent odds, that their fetus would be normal. Not a hundred percent, she replied. "That's when we stopped troubling about it," Jonathan says.

They don't even mention whether they ever discussed with Dr. Quittell a different option entirely, the one they finally chose. As Kris puts it, they looked to their faith. They decided just to go for it, to put the matter in God's hands. They would conceive a child, and they would bear it. Come what may, they would bear it.

"Human nature tells us we want to have a healthy child," Jonathan says. "By the same token, who are we to decide?"

"God knows what we can handle," Kris adds quietly. "And He won't give us what we can't handle." What God gave them, almost as soon as they had resolved the matter in their own minds, was a pregnancy.

God did not give them peace of mind, however. It was, in Jonathan's words, a rough decision. They knew they could deal with whatever happened, but they were desperate to know what they would be dealing with.

As soon as possible after Kris conceived, they traveled to Philadelphia for CVS, chorionic villus sampling. This is a test similar to amniocentesis, but it can be done earlier. A couple can get results within eight weeks of conception. It poses some additional risk to the fetus, but Jonathan and Kris were told that the center where they would have the CVS test had one of the best records for not harming a pregnancy. Knowing the outcome would be important even for the fetus itself, because in the delivery of a child with cystic fibrosis, special matters need to be attended to.

The Vander Plaats placed the matter in God's hands, and as they see

ABORTION

Americans have not changed their minds about abortion since it became legal in 1973. In poll after poll, the split in our opinions about abortion remains all but unchanged.

Nine in ten of us feel abortion should be legal to save the mother's life. But on abortions for reasons of convenience or cost, we are split right down the middle. At least three-fourths of Americans favor legal abortion of a fetus with a "serious defect." Still, 46 percent of Americans in one recent poll said abortion is the same as murder.

We are torn asunder on this question. It touches almost all of the deeply rooted values in American society: life, liberty, the pursuit of happiness, privacy, and fairness. For some Americans, the issue is rooted and intertwined with their religious beliefs. No wonder it remains unresolved: The two sides argue from opposite premises about who owns a person (God, society, or herself). That issue is also fundamental to genetics.

Like many deeply felt issues, attitudes about abortion are emotional as well as rational. Where we stand depends in part on where we came from. Thus our attitudes may not be subject to rational discussion.

Prenatal diagnosis is enmeshed in these attitudes, but almost no one likes to talk about that officially. In California's screening program for neural tube defects such as spina bifida, the education brochure pre-

it, God spared them the same challenge again. Their genes recombined such that their second child is not affected with cystic fibrosis. Ryan Kristopher was born in May 1994, as healthy as predicted, but also (as predicted) a carrier, inheriting Jonathan's gene for CF.

As carefully and seriously as anyone on earth could have done, one couple from New Jersey faced up to their options. And now Jonathan Vander Plaat is exercising another option.

"I'm done having kids," he says bluntly. "That's it."

So far, we have dwelt on nothing especially exotic — nothing, that is, beyond the ironclad resolve of a rabbi, the uneasy forbearance of an impared by the state says that "different options" should be "discussed" and that staff should "support whatever decision the woman makes." That's the only official hint that the AFP test may lead to an abortion decision. Women undergoing the testing seldom raise the issue on their own, and many may try to avoid grappling with it.

Harvard law professor Laurence Tribe points out that the abortion debate arose only after scientists learned the facts of fertilization in the late nineteenth century. At that point, the Church then moved the emergence of the "soul" from quickening back to fertilization. Late-nineteenth-century doctors tended to favor restrictions on abortion, to discourage it among women of "high repute" who, they felt, were endangering the fitness of the population by reducing the size of their families while the poor and immigrants continued to breed.

In the early twentieth century debate about abortion was remarkably scarce in the United States, and physicians quietly performed it for many women; poverty and maternal psychiatric problems were seen as good reasons to terminate a pregnancy. Although abortions were illegal—and women did die from them—prosecutions and convictions for abortion were not common. In Michigan, for instance, there were only forty convictions for unlawful abortion between 1893 and 1932.

After about 1950 doctors began to focus on the health threats of pregnancy and the relative safety of the abortion procedure thanks to medical advances. But only after a German measles epidemic in the mid-1960s threatened to create a surge in birth defects did the medical profession begin to favor legalizing abortion.

migrant woman, and the ordeal of a funeral director and his wife. The blue-ribbon technical heroics belong to people like Michelle and Paul O'Brien of Burnley, England, and to the doctors who helped them.

Like the Vander Plaats, the O'Briens are both carriers of the cystic fibrosis gene and have had one child with the disease. Their second child, their daughter Chloe, is completely free of cystic fibrosis. For Chloe's conception, they chose the high-tech option.

In March 1992 Chloe was conceived by IVF; her mother's egg and her father's sperm were joined in a petri dish. There is nothing very unusual about that today. IVF began and is still used most often as a means of achieving pregnancy for couples who are unable to do so through simple intercourse, but today the method is also an essential component of the earliest interventions to avoid bearing a child with a hereditary illness.

When Chloe was no more than an eight-cell embryo (what many scientists refer to as a "pre-embryo"), a researcher flew to London from the Baylor College of Medicine in Texas for the express purpose of removing one of those eight cells and analyzing its DNA for the genes implicated in cystic fibrosis. Mark Hughes carried out the same DNA tests on cells from each of the other embryos the O'Briens had conceived, in a thin glass dish, at the same time.

The conception itself had been engineered by Alan Handyside at the Hammersmith Hospital in London, a pioneer in the fledgling field of preimplantation genetic diagnosis. Until then, Handyside had been able to use IVF only to circumvent genetic disease for one of the sex-linked disorders, such as muscular dystrophy, where a condition is inherited only by boys. He could determine the gender of the embryo and limit the implantation to the females.

The O'Briens were the first couple for whom Handyside and Hughes had the opportunity to test embryos at the very level of the gene, because new techniques allowed finer discrimination of the DNA. This broadened the scope of preimplantation diagnosis greatly, because now it could be used for diseases such as cystic fibrosis, which had no link whatever to gender.

DNA from the lone cell taken away from Chloe-to-be did not contain any genes that would confer a risk of CF. Hughes could tell that the fetus that would develop from that embryo would not even be a CF carrier. He determined that some of the other pre-embryos would have become children with cystic fibrosis, and some would not. Only the unaffected embryos made the move from glass to womb. They were transferred to Michelle's uterus, and Michelle went home.

Naturally, as the O'Briens were their first such case, Handyside and Hughes were eager to confirm that the fetus they had created was in fact free of cystic fibrosis. They asked Michelle to return to London, as her pregnancy progressed, for the earliest possible prenatal test, CVS. To their chagrin, when they called Michelle to remind her, she said she didn't want to have the test.

After that, Hughes recalls, Michelle seemed to want nothing further to do with the doctors in London. They hoped they had actually guaranteed her a healthy baby.

"We left her alone until it was time for the amniocentesis," recalls

Hughes. "She said she didn't want to have that either. She said later that she just didn't want to know."

The scientists, the two men who had created Chloe O'Brien in a glass dish and probed her outer membrane and extracted a cell of her, were desperately eager to know whether their gene tests had been accurate, or they had made a terrible mistake. But Michelle, in whom Chloe was visibly growing, did not want to doubt.

Hughes recalls that Michelle placed more faith in the bands on the DNA tests than even the doctors did. Beyond a certain point, she suspended disbelief.

For the Vander Plaats in New Jersey and the O'Briens in England, the outcome was identical. Each couple, once thunderstruck by the hard reality of genetic disease, now has a second child who is not affected by it. But there is a difference — some might say an ethical seismic fault of a difference — between them.

Ryan Vander Plaat, Meghan's little brother, came to be and was found to be healthy after conception. Chloe O'Brien, her life begun as part of a high-technology medical intervention, was selected. Some of her potential siblings were not.

We have new choices. The choices begin with embryos but expand in all directions.

They also resonate painfully — like it or not — with a horrible episode in recent history when genetic choices involved preventing illness by either sterilizing people or killing them outright. We will consider this history later in detail. For now, however, it is well to bear in mind that the options offered by modern genetics also involve certain kinds of termination and exclusion, which may be less brutal but are perhaps no different in their fundamental nature.

Who should be allowed to use genes to decide between individuals? Which genes, when, and how? That's the crux of the issue behind the new genetics — for us as individuals and as a society as well.

CHAPTER 4

The Faulkner Conference

I'm also very concerned about what society says to a parent who says,
"You know what, my kid's going to be a dwarf, and that's okay with me."
And other parents or other people in society looking and saying,
"My goodness, why did you decide to do this? Why—why did you
bring this—this child into the world?"

—Equal Employment Opportunity Commissioner Paul Steven Miller
(himself a dwarf)

THE MATTER OF THESE CHOICES GOES RIGHT TO THE
core for Ruth Ricker, an articulate and forthright woman who happens
to be about as tall as a third-grader. Ricker has achondroplasia, an inherited form of dwarfism, and is president of a special interest group
known as Little People of America. One March Saturday in 1995, she
had occasion to speculate in public about what the future could hold
for people with her particular body dimensions.

"What are the chances that a couple of generations from now there's
going to be a lot fewer healthy dwarfs?" she mused. "In our culture that's
the outcome people have been trying to deal with," she said. Now parents with achondroplasia too could face the dilemma of prenatal testing, because the gene involved in her condition had been discovered
the previous year. One form is recessive, and fatal.

That afternoon, at a public symposium in Boston, Ricker's chief
concern was rather different. "It concerns me what the rest of society
considers as normal and healthy," she said. "A few years from now,
when average people are going to be able to screen for this, you know
there's going to be a shopping list. We're going to see a whole lot less
of [dwarfs]—and I'm not necessarily comfortable with that."

Ricker well understands the reasons why someone might not want to
bring a dwarf child into the world. Sometimes, she granted, life has
been pretty crummy for dwarf children. "But it will be crummy for my
children too," she added, "if they're the last generation."

It was a unique occasion, that symposium. The venue was Faulkner

Hospital, a small institution on the outskirts of Boston that includes a fertility center. Doctors there had their toes in the water of pre-embryo testing, the same novel technology that Mark Hughes had pioneered with the embryo that would become Chloe O'Brien. Before plunging in altogether, the Faulkner Hospital had convened a daylong workshop, open to anyone who chose to come, to probe what people thought about the merits and possible perils of removing cells from embryos in vitro, testing them, and using the results as the basis for making decisions about whether to nurture the embryo.

The Faulkner conference attracted some 125 people, genetic counselors and doctors, professional ethicists, members of support groups for the disabled, and high school teachers, a diverse group of individuals who were interested enough to give up a Saturday to deliberate about the issues surrounding pre-embryo genetic testing. The moderator was a television reporter.

The exemplar of the subject under discussion, Mark Hughes, was also present. Often scientists who are invited to speak at sessions that focus on ethics will show up, present their work, and then leave immediately, missing all the deliberations about what they are up to. Hughes didn't do that. He described his techniques, the advantages they offer, and some of the dilemmas they present. Then he stayed until the end, often taking a lively part in the dialogue.

"Technology drives science," Hughes declared at the outset. "Science pushes medicine. And medicine pushes us all into making decisions we never thought of."

These are unusual times, and almost every day some new development gives people the opportunity to think about a situation that has never occurred before. A whiff of this was in the air that morning, a feeling of standing over a chasm and wondering whether it would be safe to leap. In fact, the reproductive specialists at Faulkner Hospital had already leaped: They had performed one pre-embryo genetic diagnosis, and two more couples were waiting to have it happen to them.

However, the symposium had been in planning for some time. The man behind it, medical director Machelle Seibel, had been working with an ethics panel at the center for five years, and had just coauthored a book on the ethics of reproduction. Both this history, and his opening comments, suggested he was looking before he leaped.

"This is not a time when we should look back later and say what should not have been done," Seibel said.

Just because something *can* be done, Mark Hughes added at the start of his presentation, doesn't mean it *should* be done. Hughes is opposed to prenatal testing for the purpose of gender selection; he calls it "abuse." He also grants that preimplantation diagnosis is "just a stopgap method," and that an effective treatment for the disease in question would be far preferable. He also, however, seemed puzzled by the discomfort people felt about the procedure.

"Just because it can be abused doesn't mean it's bad," he argued at one point. A trim and energetic man who seldom minces words, Hughes used vivid images in describing his craft. He characterized one molecular method he uses as "Jurassic Park technology" and chose to display an eight-celled embryo, the object of his studies, in a photograph taken by an electron microscope. It balanced precariously along one slope of a massive promontory: the tip of a sewing needle.

This is all we're debating about, he meant. The pre-embryo on the slide looked nothing at all like a miniature baby. It did not even resem-

HUMAN EMBRYOGENESIS

1. **Contact**: Sperm penetrates egg. Fertilization begins, a process that will take roughly an entire day. Male and female chromosomes mingle. The product is a single cell called a *zygote*.

2. **Cleavage**: The zygote travels down the fallopian tube and divides into two identical cells, called *blastomeres*. The mother's genes still control the process.

3. **Redivisions**: The blastomeres divide again at about eighteen-hour intervals, becoming four cells, then eight. This is a *preimplantation embryo* or *pre-embryo*. At the four- and eight-cell stage, individual cells can be removed without apparent harm to the embryo. During this period, the embryo's own mingled genes gradually begin to take control of its development.

4. **Specialization**: The embryo divides again, to a sixteen-cell stage, barely visible to the naked eye. The resulting *morula*, for reasons of sheer geometry, now has some specialization: Some cells are on the inside,

ble the snail-like object most people recognize as a developing fetus. It was most reminiscent of a raspberry, eight identical globules adhering to each other. Its newly crafted name, "pre-embryo," is perhaps meant to convey the comforting thought that the entity in question was created outside the human body and has yet to find a place inside it, all of which tends to free any discussion about what is done with it—sustaining it, ending its existence, or simply *using* it for something—from the emotional ramifications that might arise.

Hughes proceeded to explain how, after such a pre-embryo is created by in vitro fertilization, he can use the finest of needles to extract only one of these eight cells, break it apart, remove the DNA, and test the DNA for the presence of a particular gene of interest. That's his specialty: finding genes within single cells. After one cell is lifted away, the remaining seven cells in the "raspberry" can grow quite normally into a fetus and a full-fledged child, if they are implanted in the uterus of a

---

some are on the outside. (At this point, cells could no longer be removed from embryos created in a laboratory dish by IVF without affecting their ongoing development.)

5. Differentiation: Beginning about four days after fertilization, cells on the outside of the embryo flatten; they will become the placenta. Inner cells will become the embryo proper. The embryo now looks like a fluid-filled balloon. It is called a *blastocyst*.

6. Implantation: At around day six the blastocyst, some 120 cells large, arrives in the uterus. About a day later, it begins to implant itself in the uterine wall, where it can connect with maternal blood circulation. By day fourteen, the embryo is completely buried in the wall of the uterus. Inner cells begin to organize into two distinct layers, called *ectoderm* and *endoderm*.

7. Gastrulation: A few rapidly dividing cells edge between the two layers to form a middle layer, or *mesoderm*. The center of this mass of moving cells, the *primitive streak*, gives the embryo a head and tail, a left side and a right side. Its appearance signals the start of development of individual organs. The embryo can no longer divide to become twins.

woman treated with the right combination of hormones to make it receptive to and capable of sustaining the pregnancy.

Generally, women undergoing pre-embryonic testing have taken hormones that stimulate their ovaries to release more than one egg. Because several eggs are fertilized in vitro, as with Chloe O'Brien, there is an opportunity to select for implantation only those pre-embryos that are not affected by the genetic defect of concern. Demonstrably, some couples find it easier to contemplate choosing from among eight-cell pre-embryos created in a laboratory dish than aborting a later-stage fetus or rearing a child with that condition.

In fact, many of the couples who had come to Hughes for preimplantation diagnosis were not opposed to abortion. They had already endured several terminations, and they were sick of it. Hughes doesn't like the term *preimplantation diagnosis*. He prefers to call it *blastomere analysis before injection*: BABI.

By the time of the Faulkner Hospital symposium, thirty-three babies had been born worldwide as a result of preimplantation diagnosis. At that moment it was possible to test a single cell from a pre-embryo for twenty-eight genetic conditions, from Tay-Sachs disease and cystic fibrosis to the bleeders' disease, hemophilia, and Huntington's disease.

An additional condition now amenable to preimplantation diagnosis is Lesch-Nyhan syndrome, a neurological disorder with bizarre manifestations. Children with Lesch-Nyhan syndrome mutilate themselves compulsively and are often retarded. Hughes showed a slide of a woman with a boy on her lap who had a vacant expression on his face. She loves her son very deeply, Hughes told the audience. She would never, never wish he had not been born. Still, she could not face the thought of bearing another child with Lesch-Nyhan syndrome. BABI had helped her to conceive again, without fear.

Hughes hastened to say that it would be "ridiculous" to test an embryo for all twenty-eight diseases at once, or indeed for any disease for which a family was not known to be at risk. He had named the list only to show the potential power of the technique.

But with the power comes dilemmas. "You can go from diseases to traits, and that's the gray area," he acknowledged. "Few people would say avoiding Tay-Sachs is a bad idea, but what about cystic fibrosis? What about Down syndrome?" What about (we're fantasizing now) a short temper or even short stature?

The moral dilemma does not even stop at deciding which embryos to reject. Hughes concluded by discussing a predicament that had been troubling him for more than a year. Meanwhile, the couple who posed it were waiting for him to decide whether he could grant their wish.

They already had a daughter with a hereditary immune-system disorder called ADA deficiency. Setting aside all the emotional consequences of this problem, her medical bills had come to $1.6 million. The couple came to Hughes for preimplantation diagnosis, hoping to avoid having another child with their daughter's condition. The request was simple enough, in a manner of speaking, but they also presented Hughes with an extraordinary proposal.

"If you can give us an embryo that doesn't have the disease," Hughes said they told him, "that's great. But while you're at it, maybe you can stack the deck." They asked him to look in particular for embryos that had the same tissue type as their daughter.

ADA DEFICIENCY

Because of a small alteration in their genes, children with ADA deficiency cannot produce the enzyme adenosine deaminase (ADA), and a substance accumulates in their blood that is toxic to cells of the immune system. Because they suffer repeated infections, in the past all such children — even the famous "bubble boy" who lived isolated inside a plastic tent in a Texas hospital — would eventually succumb.

That death may no longer be inevitable. In the late 1970s injections of the enzyme became available. And in the mid-1980s a few children with ADA deficiency took part in the first human gene therapy experiment. Researchers at the National Institutes of Health injected them with their own blood cells, which had been removed and gene-engineered so they could produce the missing enzyme.

At this writing, twelve patients worldwide had received gene therapy for ADA deficiency. For three, due to technical problems, the experiments were not a success. But nine of the children (including all those who live in the United States) are still healthy, living at home and going to school. Their immune functions are not as strong as usual for children of their age, and some of them still need to take medications, but researchers now judge the gene therapy a success.

What they proposed would not harm the second child in any way whatever — it would not have any of its blood withdrawn or be subjected to surgery for the sake of the older sibling. All they wanted was to have doctors extract some fetal stem cells from the blood in the umbilical cord during childbirth, blood cells that would normally go into the trash bin along with the severed umbilical cord. Stem cells from blood are like seeds, undifferentiated but able to flower into mature, competent immune cells. These could be maintained for transfusion into their older child.

The request sent Hughes to medical ethicists — and kept him stalling the couple for eighteen months.

The odds were nine to one, Hughes said, that fetal stem cells from a younger sibling who had the same tissue type would allow the older sister's body to generate a vigorous new immune system. Would this process harm the newborn? No way.

The difficult question Hughes confronted, with the guidance of the ethicists, was the motives of the couple with regard to the younger child. They were asking Hughes, if he could, to select their fetus not only for the absence of disease but for a value-free trait, a mere tissue type, ordinarily something no more meaningful than eye color or handedness. Here it had gained a meaning.

They desired the fetus for a particular purpose, something beyond its own existence. Even before its birth, they had begun planning to use a baby as a source of cells. They would value it, at least in part, for its blood type.

Hughes had thought about the problem long and hard. Children are often wanted for something other than themselves — to fulfill unrealized ambitions, to inherit wealth or position, to hold a relationship together. But few couples explicitly involve the medical profession when they select a child for the qualities necessary to fulfill the ulterior motive — even where the intent might be considered high-minded. It sounded like a slippery slope. Unnatural selection, pure and simple.

"You can imagine all sorts of people who want to have a healthy second child but also want a bone marrow donor in case the older child develops leukemia," he says. "Now we've crossed a barrier. We're not selecting against a lethal mutation. We're selecting *for* a trait. Is that right or not?"

The participants at the conference quickly responded to his challenge. They seemed immediately to grasp the undercurrent that roils current discussions about prenatal diagnosis. If we set aside heartwarming cases like Chloe O'Brien, what are the odds that people will begin to use testing for less compelling choices, options far beyond Tay-Sachs and cystic fibrosis? To identify a fetus who would be taller? Shorter? Deaf? Obese? Left-handed? Prone to acne? Given the options, are there limits to what people will find acceptable? How long is the step from a case like Chloe O'Brien to a vending machine for embryos?

Judging from what Hughes said at the podium, one might think these speculations were far-fetched. After all, in order to sidestep the ordinary process of prenatal diagnosis and termination, the comparatively few women who have used preimplantation diagnosis have had to undergo cycles of hormone treatment and minor surgery to extract eggs from their ovaries, and to endure tests of the pre-embryo to ascertain its "health" as well as the uncertainty of waiting to see whether the fertilized embryo "took." How many couples would undergo all this for more "trivial" causes?

But the question is not outrageous, as Hughes himself implied. In part because of the invasiveness of this procedure, researchers are working to develop ways to flush fertilized embryos out of the uterus for testing. A couple could conceive at home — "the fun way," as Hughes put it — and then have their embryo retrieved, genetically tested, and finally reimplanted. Noninvasive and benign for everyone involved (except possibly the embryo), this technique could ultimately make preimplantation diagnosis a test for the masses.

Meanwhile, the technique Hughes liked to call BABI would be limited to patients facing presumably serious conditions. But what is "serious"? Sociologist Dorothy Wertz rose from the middle of the audience to pose the question, and to provide an answer that itself is a conundrum.

For fifteen years Wertz had been surveying specialists and the public on issues surrounding genetics. In one recent questionnaire she had asked geneticists in a number of countries around the world to name hereditary conditions and to rate them as lethal, serious, or not serious.

"Over six hundred conditions were listed," she said, "and many appeared in all three categories." Cystic fibrosis was one of them. In the vicinity of 30 percent of geneticists, she added, would abort a fetus if it had a gene for obesity. For the achondroplasia that affects Ruth Ricker, the proportion would be "even higher."

"Most people say it should be up to the parents," she went on, "which means that once pre-embryo genetic diagnosis is no longer research, it is up to the parents to define what is serious."

BLAINE'S BIOLOGY PROJECT

In the spring of 1995, as a school project, fifteen-year-old Blaine Deatherage-Newsom conducted a survey on the Internet. He sent it to twenty-five newsgroups focused on a wide variety of topics, from "biology:chromosome" to ethics, from spina bifida and cerebral palsy to Tourette's syndrome, from white power to Buddhism and Islam.

Blaine posed five questions: "If we had the technology to eliminate disabilities from the population, would that be good public policy to do so? What are the Pros? What are the Cons? What is your answer? Why do you feel the way you do?"

Blaine added that he has spina bifida and hydrocephalus (the accumulation of fluid on the brain), "so I have my own feelings and answers to these questions." Afterward, he wondered whether that statement had biased the outcome of the survey.

Several factors prompted Blaine to choose the Internet survey for his project. He had heard that 95 percent of couples who learn their unborn child would have spina bifida choose to have an abortion. Also, he went to an exhibit at a science museum that asked visitors to vote on whether a child born with spina bifida should live or die. When he saw the exhibit, Blaine said, "the child was losing by quite a few votes."

The results of Blaine's survey were mixed. When the time came to write his report, he had received about ninety responses from many countries and many newsgroups. Nineteen of the respondents said they themselves were disabled, and thirteen had a child with disabilities.

All together 40 percent of respondents felt that we should not use technologies to eliminate disabilities; 23 percent said we should do so, and 29 percent were undecided or equivocal. The parents of disabled children were much more united on the question: 62 percent would not take public-policy steps to wipe out disabilities. However, people who did not say they had any close connection with a disabled person were almost evenly divided on the issue between yes (33 percent), no (28 percent), and "it depends" or "I don't know" (39 percent).

That uncertainty generated interesting comments. Some people wanted to know just what Blaine meant by "eliminate" (he had been thinking of genetic engineering) and by "disabled."

"I have certainly learned that no two people may agree on what counts as a disability," he wrote later. One person asked if frizzy hair is a disability, or being ugly. The survey also provoked responses on both sides of the issue about whether deafness is a disability or a separate language and culture.

"Few people are born to the image that they would prefer," remarked the father of a twenty-two-year-old woman with Down syndrome. "All struggle against some handicap and wish that they could somehow change their genetic makeup and be stronger, more beautiful, smarter, etc. We all have to learn to live with what we are. That is harder for some than others."

Several respondents questioned whether the world would be better off without people with disabilities. They invoked great historical figures who endured physical or mental handicaps, such as Beethoven, Blake, van Gogh, Franklin Roosevelt. "People with disabilities are different," wrote one parent of a disabled child. "They have unique experiences. Sometimes their brains are different, which gives them different ways of experiencing and learning. We can all benefit from being around these people and learning from them."

Some asked whether helping disabled people was worth the cost. "Should we spend millions on one disabled patient if it means ignoring hundreds of other patients with equally fatal but more easily cured problems?" wrote another. "I do not think I could wholeheartedly support the fitting of a prosthesis if it meant that 100 children would go untreated for leukemia, for example." Several asked whether the same options would be available to rich and poor, and the mother of an autistic child worried online what would happen to her child if she died.

What could Blaine make of all this? Certainly his conclusions must have been colored by the perspective he stated at the outset of his report.

"I wonder if people are saying that they think the world would be a better place without me," he wrote. "I wonder if people just think the lives of people with disabilities are so full of misery and suffering that they think we would be better off dead. . . . Most of the time I am very happy and I like my life very much." (Blaine spends his days in a wheelchair, cannot make most people understand what he says aloud, and had undergone surgery eleven times by the time he conducted the survey.)

"My mom says she can't imagine the world without me," he went on, "and she is convinced that everyone who has a chance to know me thinks that the world is a far better place because I'm in it. Maybe she thinks this because she's my mother, but she may be right. People do seem to like me, and I think I'm a pretty good person. I don't think I'd want to change."

Although the statistical outcomes of his survey were very indecisive, Blaine pointed out, the verbal responses included more arguments against eliminating disability than in favor of it. But he was troubled by the obvious differences between people who were closely involved with disability and those who didn't appear to be. "I feel a bit concerned that a decision like this might be up to the general population," he wrote. "It seems like those who best understand what the decision involves would be best equipped to make the decision about it."

Blaine says he wishes he could repeat his survey without revealing his own situation, and he's aware that his respondents were not a random, scientifically valid sample of the population. Nonetheless, he says, a more rigorous survey might come up with quite similar results. "I think we should be very, very careful to make sure people making decisions like these actually know what they're talking about, and what they're voting on," he concluded.

Blaine's teacher gave him an A+ on the project.

Someone else in the audience spoke up: "If medicine pursues this, it sends a message that this is legitimate — to screen embryos for which are right and which are not. This whole realm is going to take on a new social acceptance if people view this as the right thing to do."

Families like the Vander Plaats would not consider rejecting an affected fetus, because to do so might be the same as saying they wished Meghan didn't exist. If this is so, what will it say to the community of the disabled when tests proliferate that will make it simple for couples to rule out essentially any characteristic that science can identify? Preventing births is only one end of a continuum.

"If insurance companies and employers, for instance, use recently developed diagnostic genetic techniques to weed out those they do not wish to insure or employ, namely people with genetic disorders," wrote the president of the National Neurofibromatosis Foundation in a letter to *The New York Times*, "... then the very best the human mind is able to produce will be used not to reduce human suffering but to exploit it."

There is no best solution to such a question. Deep matters of justice are involved. Can we make a future for prenatal testing that is kind and good, for parents like the Vander Plaats and the O'Briens, but that is also just and fair, so that we do not come to see the likes of Ruth Ricker as somehow undesirable?

The Faulkner conference was a start, at least, at groping toward a consensus. Or rather a wish list and a warning, which the chairman of the summary discussion scrawled onto a blackboard at the front of the room. Let us not "lessen what we tolerate and enjoy in our society" by trying to end variation, those present decided. Let us remain aware that disability is not the same as illness, and that there is a wide variation in the way people experience it.

A long list of "shoulds" followed: Couples about to undergo preimplantation genetic testing should be informed of the physical and emotional costs as well as the financial costs, and of the limitations of the diagnostic tests and the fact that they do not rule out other birth defects; they should be referred to support groups and given follow-up throughout pregnancy and even longer. Quality assurance in IVF clinics and laboratories should be addressed, the education and skills of people who provide the tests should be improved, and who decides to order a test — the doctor, the patient, the insurance company—should be determined; far too much, and too intricate, for one roomful of people to resolve in one day.

Theirs was hardly the last word on the subject. A year later, with funding from the National Center for Human Genome Research (the home of the U.S. branch of the international genome effort), the discussion resumed in a more formal fashion at a bioethics institute just north of New York City. The Hastings Center launched a three-year project on the ethical and social values around prenatal testing and their implications, which would involve some of the speakers at the Faulkner conference and many others besides — not only experts on genetics and ethics but members of the disability community too.

Over the course of many meetings, the group focused on well-defined questions surrounding the prospect of prenatal testing, using seven conditions as case studies: sickle cell anemia, Down syndrome, early-onset Alzheimer's disease, schizophrenia, deafness, male homosexuality, and female gender. (Some of these are strictly speaking not disabilities, but each of them can be disabling in certain contexts.)

"What are the goods in familial and social life that people believe to be—and are—thwarted by the presence of some forms of disability?"

principal investigator Philip Boyle had asked in the grant application. "How ought society to change its response to people with disabilities as it comes to understand the genetic roots of disabilities that can be tested for?"

John Hasler, whose business is embryos, has a certain perspective on all these developments. Hasler heads a company called Emtran, which operates nationwide from Pennsylvania Dutch country, providing embryo transfer services for dairy farmers wishing to optimize their herds. Today Emtran provides bovine IVF for farmers whose cows have a blocked oviduct. It also freezes bovine embryos so they can be sold.

When the company started operations eighteen years ago, Emtran could do no more than take embryos out of a valuable cow after her once-a-year ovulation and shift them to a less valuable cow, in order to protect the valuable cow's health. That was before it became possible to superovulate cows, using hormones to increase by a hundredfold the number of eggs they can produce, and therefore their potential value.

"In a relatively short time, a superior bull can be sure of thousands of calves," says Hasler. "But until embryo transfer, the reproductive potential of a superior cow was infinitesimal." It's relatively simple these days to superovulate a cow, artificially inseminate her, and flush out the embryos.

In his own industry defining "superiority" is value free and also quite straightforward. The genetic value of a cow derives from a formula, based on a sophisticated statistical analysis of her milk yield, the fat percentage and protein content of the milk, her age, and the performance of other cows in her lineage. Hasler knows of a Dutch dairy farmer who has sold $20 million worth of semen from one of his bulls, based on the genetic value of one of the daughters it sired.

"It's not all that different from trying to breed athletes," Hasler says. "If you look at the ability to run and their distance, you would very quickly be able to pull out of the population of humans the individuals who ought to be selectively bred — ignoring the other 98 percent of the population. It's really not all that different. Of course, we don't do that."

There's a bovine genome project too, and that genome is also being mapped. If researchers in livestock genetics can tease out the factors that control milk quality or yield, it will revolutionize the industry. "You could literally start removing eggs from calves, or just take a piece of embryo and test a cell or two," Hasler muses. "Of course, that's way down the road."

The field of theriogenology—the study of reproduction in beasts—is thriving. Bovine embryos can be a cheap way for farmers to improve their stock. IVF and embryo transfer are also an effective (if expensive) way to preserve endangered species.

Ten or twenty years ago human reproductive scientists watched in some awe as their colleagues in animal husbandry poked needles into the center of animal ova and talked of cloning livestock embryos to create entire herds of identical animals. More recently they cheered the birth of Dolly, the cloned sheep. Cloning had been tried in cattle for many years but it hadn't worked well. A cloned calf was finally born in early 1997 at an animal breeding farm in Wisconsin.

Throughout the history of attempts to clone livestock, "the yield was not necessarily very great, and because of all the variations you may mate a supersire and a superdam and get an average calf," says Roger Perkins of the animal products program at the U.S. Department of Agriculture. "There have been some aberrations. Frequently one calf becomes oversized in utero. Generally these have to be delivered by cesarean section, and they're not normal." A year after Dolly's birth, several more cloned farm animals were in existence, and Dolly herself was pregnant. But the yield of healthy cloned animals was still, on balance, miniscule.

The truly bizarre is also technically possible. Hasler says a few calves have actually been created from fourth-generation embryos (fertilizing ova from fetuses, creating more fetuses from those embryos and extracting their ova, and so on repeatedly, without ever growing the whole parent animal to maturity). The offspring that result from this process are rare and often defective; still, he adds, the people in the human IVF business, even in these days of their own heady progress, could probably learn a thing or two from the dairy industry.

At the same time Hasler is disquieted by the popularity of human IVF and the lack of any systematic effort to assess the results. He wonders whether children born to infertile parents because of medical technology are themselves at increased risk of infertility. He's troubled that there is as yet no reputable census of the health of former IVF babies, and while he has no problem with the idea of terminating fetuses that have inherited a grave medical condition, Hasler is disturbed by our increasing ability to pinpoint human genes that govern the development of traits—which borders on defining the kind of people we prefer to create, in the same way one bets on a racehorse. "It's coming," he says.

"We're going to know. We're going to nail down genes for hair color, and for aspects of intelligence.

"Man has the ability to develop incredibly powerful technology, and somebody always misuses it," Hasler adds. "I don't see that ending. We can't feed all the people in the world. We can't even protect them from malaria, but we can do genetic analysis on a wealthy woman's embryo. We really kind of misuse our resources."

University of Pennsylvania bioethicist Arthur Caplan made the same point in a recent lecture. "Part of what we think of as disease is what others persuade us to [regard as] unattractive, dysfunctional. But then there are another set of diseases—the inability to walk, the inability to properly metabolize food, the inability to do something with oxygen—that are clearly deleterious. . . . I think the way to answer this is to force medicine on the carpet and say, Could you define for us exactly what we see as disease, dysfunction, and impairment?

"There are other days in which I think: Half the world is still dying from diarrhea. We could do better than this kind of mission. Couldn't we say, Let's get at the basic kind of diseases, morbidity and mortality, and say that's what the job is?

"I think it's going to be on medicine's plate to answer the question [about] where the line is. If it doesn't draw any line, the individual . . . is going to do all of this."

The issues are cut-and-dried when the market is livestock, slippery and messy when the focus is not on markets but on patients or even populations. There is a medical "market" too, after all, and new genetic tests may be attractive targets for speculators interested in investing in it.

Genetic tests demand considerably less time and commitment to develop than new drugs, notes Houston consultant Michael Rusnak in a 1995 article in *Biotechnology*. In general diagnostics undergo a less stringent and quicker approval process in the Food and Drug Administration. In the particular case of genetic diagnostics, the new technologies provide both a new product and a potential for drug discovery, because they may point the way to correcting the disorder that underlies the test.

"It is little wonder that larger diagnostic companies are either buying, merging, or partnering with biotechnology start-ups," writes Rusnak. In theory, a genetic testing market without external restraints could target the end customer directly. The technology is becoming almost simple enough to leave specialists out of the picture entirely.

DETERMINISM

In exploring the contents of our genes, perhaps we are setting ourselves up to replay a centuries-old philosophical argument, this time with Nature instead of God at its center. If our fate is predetermined by our genes, what room is left for free will? Is our script written the day we are conceived?

Upon reflection, the dilemma vanishes. For one thing, no one yet knows nearly enough to determine the course of an entire life based on genes. Also, even when it does become possible to read the entire text of an individual human genome, the genetic script will tell only part of the story.

There is tremendous variability in the onset and course of most hereditary diseases. In the case of sickle cell disease, for instance, the same molecular variant is associated with a wide range of severity. The experience of disease (or of anything else, for that matter) involves subtleties of physiology beyond our knowledge, as well as social factors such as mental outlook, family support, and other external factors beyond our control.

"Knowing the complete genetic makeup of an individual would not tell you what kind of person that individual would become," wrote the National Bioethics Advisory Commission in its 1997 report on human cloning. "Even identical twins who grow up together and thus share the same genes and a similar home environment have different likes and dislikes, and can have very different talents. The increasingly sophisticated studies coming out of human genetic research are showing that the better we understand gene function, the less likely it is we will ever be able to produce at will a person with any given complex trait."

Life has a way of intervening at unexpected moments and playing havoc with our expectations. This is as true of genetic prediction as it is of anything else. Perhaps what usually happens in genetic diagnosis is that we give a name to a possibility.

For instance, a test first developed to detect chromosome abnormalities in human embryos created by in vitro fertilization (known as FISH, for fluorescent in situ hybridization) could be combined with tests that isolate fetal blood cells in maternal blood samples, to provide a simple pinprick method of prenatal diagnosis. Unlike amniocentesis, this test would be simple (from the mother's point of view) and safe for the fetus. It would also broaden the market for prenatal testing considerably.

Rusnak foresees that such tests will expand into the home, much as pregnancy testing has done in recent decades. On the face of it, there is no technical reason why women could not send samples of their own blood to a genetic testing lab and receive results by phone or mail.

FISH

A quarter-century ago, a doctor could remove some of the amniotic fluid bathing a fetus, test some fetal cells by amniocentesis, and tell the anxious woman — a month or so later (when she was twenty weeks pregnant) — whether her fetus had too many or too few chromosomes. Today the results of amniocentesis tests are available in about a week. But an even quicker option is also available: fluorescent in situ hybridization, or FISH.

Fluorescent markers light up the test probes, which are chemical mirror images of parts of chromosomes. Mixed with DNA from a fetal cell, under the microscope, the markers will bind to the fetal chromosomes and light up; there is no need to grow the fetal cells in a culture dish, or to stain and identify all the chromosomes. The cytogeneticist just counts the tiny spots of light (hoping they all show up in pairs). It's easy and fast — results are available in two to four days.

FISH tests are available to count those chromosomes involved in the most common syndromes involving large-scale errors in genetic duplication — 13, 18, and 21 — as well as to identify the sex-determining chromosomes, X and Y. Newer FISH tests can also detect the smaller deletions that lead to certain well-known hereditary syndromes.

A pinprick blood test involving FISH, were it to expand to the entire prenatal market, "would rival any biopharmaceutical product," Rusnak predicts, "with a market opportunity in excess of $500 million."

In *Brave New World* Aldous Huxley foresaw ranks and ranks of genetically engineered babies in incubators. Consider the more likely possibility: gene tests for an array of disease conditions and physical traits in the form of a relatively simple blood (or even urine) test, and an elective abortion.

Envision a woman sitting in her own bedchamber, pondering the result of a test she has just carried out on herself, without the benefit (or burden) of counseling. This is true freedom of choice. Mark Hughes

At first FISH was used for women at known risk of passing on a genetic disease. Now it is often used to test embryos created by in vitro fertilization, usually those of older women whose eggs are at higher risk of having chromosome duplications or deletions. FISH can even be used to test single cells, and the hot prospect for the future is using it to analyze fetal cells in blood extracted by pinprick from a pregnant woman's fingertip.

In 1992 a report in *The New England Journal of Medicine* told the tale of a woman whose fetus was misdiagnosed by FISH, undertaken after an ultrasound test raised suspicions. The FISH test suggested the fetus was missing one of its sex chromosomes entirely and that the child would have Turner's syndrome. Later amniocentesis proved that the FISH test had simply missed the Y chromosome. The woman gave birth to a normal boy.

A year later the American College of Medical Genetics released a statement that FISH was not ready to be a stand-alone test, and that women should be told it was experimental. Nonetheless, suggested geneticist Gorden Dewald of the Mayo Clinic in 1995, some labs are better at pursuing genetics than at following policy recommendations.

"The correct procedure, if you're using testing that is not approved by the FDA, is that you're supposed to use it in conjunction with other tests," he added. "Whether that comes through to the patient, I don't know."

refers to such a possibility as "boutique medicine" and asks himself if that is the business his professional research is aiding.

The technology to allow such a scenario does not exist now—it is some unmeasurable distance over the horizon. But all the elements are there. Home test kits for a wide variety of conditions (HIV, blood glucose, cholesterol, and anticoagulant levels, not to mention pregnancy and infertility) are on the market now. Urine-based tests for pregnancy hormone levels are the most popular and are easily available over the counter at pharmacies. Short DNA strands are being put on computer chips to speed and miniaturize the testing procedures, and some researchers have begun experimenting with urine as an alternative to blood for AFP testing.

In late 1996 the same researchers who first used genetic testing to inquire whether a fetus had sickle cell disease announced that they had accomplished the same result using a pinprick of blood from a woman who was ten weeks pregnant. The result may be "the long-awaited noninvasive method to offer safe antenatal diagnosis" for single-gene disorders, predicted an editorial in the journal *Nature* that accompanied the report.

Science News went further, quoting an expert from the University of California, Los Angeles, who alluded to the potential of microchips loaded with hundreds of mutations as well as the possibility of screening from pinpricks. It "could usher in a new era of prenatal diagnosis," predicted the article. Hundreds of genetic variants could be screened at once, from a single pinprick. The possibilities are impressive.

The biotechnology firm Integrated Genetics, based in Framingham, Massachusetts, has created DNA testing technology that in a single test can simultaneously analyze patient DNA samples for more than a hundred mutations. The technique "brings two capabilities together which have heretofore been mutually exclusive," says a press announcement from the company, "the ability to test large numbers of samples cost-effectively, and the ability to ask hundreds of complex genetic questions about each sample."

The system subjects each one of dozens of tiny samples of a patient's blood to a different specific DNA segment, to see whether they are similar to the DNA pattern for a known mutation. Only those specks of blood that match are tested further for their exact DNA sequence, to define the mutation precisely.

MULTIPLEX TESTING

Triple marker screening in prenatal diagnosis was a preview of the future. Recent advances in miniaturization and gene technology have now made it possible to create arrays of DNA samples that can be tested for hundreds or even thousands of genetic variations at once. The variations most likely to be studied, naturally, are the ones that would lead to disease.

The possibility of such "multiplex" testing raises important and troubling issues about autonomy and informed consent, as an expert panel from the National Academy of Sciences pointed out in its 1994 report *Assessing Genetic Risks*. The panel argued that multiplex testing should never be undertaken simply because it is possible, and it advised that tests should be combined only when the groups of tests raise related issues in terms of the severity of the conditions being tested for, the variability of symptoms, and the availability of effective treatment.

One analyst has estimated that once a multiplex testing system is set up (at considerable expense), it costs about fourteen cents to create one chip. Naturally the ideal outcome of such testing would rest on clear, careful explanations of the issues and possibilities, about each of those hundreds or thousands of conditions (or at least the ones that raised red flags during the test), as well as informed counseling. Is such counseling going to be available when the chips are?

Initially Integrated Genetics promoted the technology as a way to define which of many mutations for a particular disorder—breast cancer, say—appear in a particular sample. But the company also said it was "talking to potential partners" about extending the method to other diagnostic areas. There is no technical reason why it could not be applied to mutations for a number of diseases at once, or to prenatal testing.

Persuading both professional bodies and government agencies to endorse such a concept as in-home genetic testing would be a substantial hurdle. It is an outlandish idea—but so are many developments that have already come to pass: ovum banks, embryos in freezers, cold viruses used to correct cystic fibrosis. Why not women gene-testing their fetuses in total privacy?

In fact, several technical hurdles also remain in the interim: from one test to hundreds at once, and from blood to urine. (Experience shows that people are very reluctant to prick themselves at home, especially in search of news that might be bad.) The lack of "customer support" is not such a hurdle: some existing diagnostic home-test services offer confidential results via a code number and a toll-free telephone line, and provide counseling via telephone. With all of today's economic incentives to reduce visits to the doctor, home genetic testing paired with telephone counseling begins to sound less like a wild idea and more like a real prospect for the future.

What if a test result shows that the fetus is affected? Will a telephone counselor be good enough? Where would someone go for emotional support if she had misgivings about her decision? Even now, the emotional consequences of learning of an affected fetus are hardly simple. Unlike the patient who hears a diagnosis of cancer or heart disease, a couple facing the prospect of a fetus affected with a genetic disorder will have no caring doctor to put his arm around them and guide them gently toward a decision about what to do next. In the field of medical genetics, as nowhere else in health care, many professionals characteristically avoid giving direct advice. Indeed, they are discouraged from intruding into private reproductive decisions. Instead, they present risks and options. But it's a no-win situation, because it perforce leaves couples on their own with the task of choosing life or death for someone else, often someone they have longed for and someone they already care about.

For a substantial proportion of American women, deciding what to do about an affected fetus is a no-brainer. When social worker Jeannie Evans of New York City, for example, was expecting her first baby at the age of twenty-eight, she opted immediately for amniocentesis, with the implicit understanding that she would terminate the pregnancy if the result was abnormal.

"I didn't feel the trauma of losing a pregnancy was the same as the trauma of having an abnormal baby," she told *The New York Times*. "Even one in 1,500 isn't a very comforting risk if you're that one. I don't think that I'm equipped to handle a baby with severe disability." The options mean different things to different women.

To a woman who has given birth to several other children, who herself comes from a family of five or six, and who lives as part of a large extended family, the fact that increasing age slightly hikes the risk of having an infant with Down syndrome may not loom very large. In her particular culture, "special needs" children may be seen as a fact of life. On the other hand, for a maturing professional woman who expects to have one child, or at most two, who must fit into her busy professional and social life, a risk of one in 300 may seem extremely high.

These issues are decidedly personal, but they also touch on many matters that are broadly societal. On one level (as the bulk of Americans and our current law agree), the fetus is the responsibility of the woman who is carrying it. But on another level — a level that geneticists have chosen to occupy through much of their history, and to which they still elevate the discussion from time to time — fetuses and our attitudes about them embody the future of our society.

In other areas of social action, we often pay lip service to the idea that our actions determine what kind of world our children will have. With prenatal diagnosis now widespread, we are also taking actions that determine what kind of children our world will have.

For two decades, since the advent of amniocentesis, it has been a simple matter to determine the gender of a fetus. For many Americans in the late twentieth century, this possibility sets the image of prenatal testing in high contrast: Is it acceptable to eliminate a fetus simply because you'd like the other sex?

Societies take different positions on the question. Some nations have actually outlawed abortions for gender choice. Many, like ours, tacitly ignore the practice. Others very nearly endorse it. In China, where widespread abortions have led to about 1.7 million fewer girls than boys being born each year, sex screening of fetuses was banned in 1994 because of the imbalance. (In the same edict, the Chinese government banned marriage and procreation among couples diagnosed with diseases that "may totally or partially deprive the victim of the ability to live independently, that are highly possible to recur in generations to come.")

To activists in the disability rights movement, the trend toward prenatal diagnosis of disabilities is a grave political challenge, worthy of organized opposition. They argue that, if we can stand aside from our visceral prejudices, we will have to acknowledge that even major disabilities are compatible with a rich and full life and can be seen as just one of many possible circumstances an individual has to deal with in growing and maturing.

GRIEVING A WANTED CHILD

Often health care workers and women themselves speak in code — if at all — about the possibility that genetic testing will have an unwelcome outcome. If no one wants to talk about "genetic terminations" beforehand, very few people want to examine the psychological aftermath either. Studies of women who abort a wanted fetus are rare.

The few that do exist show that genetic terminations are more traumatic than are truly elective abortions. They "dash dreams and hopes," write the authors of one study, forcing a mother to take an active part in the death of a child she had in mind.

Whatever support might take place during genetic counseling is "part of the distressing diagnostic routine and not perceived as helpful for the future," reports a research team from the University of Wales. They portray the aftermath of genetic abortion as an "acute grief reaction" with no grave, no baby, and no photograph, an occasion often regarded by others as a failure and greeted with silence. One of four women in that study had not embarked on a subsequent pregnancy six months later, and one in six still had severe grief reactions.

All women who terminate pregnancies for genetic reasons should have counseling within three months, the Welsh doctors advised. Yet eight years later, in 1993, authors of another report said that "there is little societal understanding and minimal support for such women" among their families, friends, or in the health care profession. Women often have no support in confronting the dark side of genetic diagnosis, it seems, either beforehand or afterward.

Concerned about such reports, genetic counselors at Yale University began a support program, involving clergy as well as genetic counselors. Couples are given a choice to view and hold the fetus after termination, or to talk with other women who have been through the same experience. Genetic counselors follow up several days after the abortion.

The Yale team compared the effects of genetic terminations done late, after amniocentesis, with those carried out in the first few weeks. "The grieving process appears to be equally as intense and complicated as it is later in pregnancy," they reported. In either case, they added, a support group helps a lot.

Rather than "preventing" disability by eliminating fetuses, they argue, we should accept the disabled as our human equals and their disabilities as fundamentally unremarkable. Public buildings have levers rather than doorknobs, large flippers instead of light switches, larger toilet stalls, and ramps beside stairways to accommodate wheelchairs. They are a convenience to us all; we don't notice them anymore.

The irony in all this is that at the psychic level, many people with disabilities and their families are not necessarily very different from the rest of us. For instance, studies indicate that families whose children have mental retardation are as satisfied with their lives as anyone else. How well a family functions seems to correlate with the parents' orientation to life more than with the level of disability among the children. (More important factors in family satisfaction or dissatisfaction were whether the mental retardation syndrome involved behavioral problems such as aggression, and whether the parents were socially isolated or impoverished.)

At the opposite end of the spectrum of opinion are those who argue that nothing is new about eliminating unacceptable or unwanted infants. For thousands of years, human beings have killed babies they didn't want, often systematically and with the implicit approval of society. Now we forbid the murder of children, but many of us (and the law) endorse a woman's private decision to rid herself of a pregnancy for her own reasons. However, when an entire medical industry and whole administrative structures exist to help a woman find reasons why she *might* want to be rid of her fetus, perhaps there is cause to stand back and think about it.

For several years, the triple marker test has been hailed at medical meetings as an advance because it is cost-effective. But doctors now define its "effectiveness" in this context not with regard to parents' choices but with regard to the cost savings from terminating an affected pregnancy, write obstetrician Thomas Elkins and his coauthor in *Clinical Obstetrics and Gynecology*. "Triple screening is not finally about good medicine or economics," they add. "Triple screening . . . is about our social character."

In 1980 only 5 percent of American births were subject to prenatal testing. By 1993 that proportion had doubled. In this decade prenatal triple marker testing followed by amniocentesis has become routine. "We didn't understand until recently that we were doing it as a screening test," remarked James Haddow, a geneticist with the Foundation for Blood Research in Scarborough, Maine, during the annual meeting of the American Society of Human Genetics in 1995. "That's what is most likely going to be a reality."

By then the accepted standard of practice was to perform amniocentesis on all pregnant women older than thirty-five, in search of genetic defects, and to give women under thirty-five the AFP or triple marker test for the same purpose. Doctors in California are now required by law to offer triple marker screening to all pregnant women before the twentieth week of gestation. The state health department sends preaddressed self-adhesive mailing labels to doctors, so they can easily send the blood samples to the lab. When the results are in, the lab calls a diagnostic center, which calls the doctor, who informs the family. The center itself sends a letter to the family as well, stating results of the test.

In 1992 some 60 percent of pregnant Californians got a triple marker test, compared with about 15 percent in the nation as a whole. The four in ten California women who refuse the testing do so because their health plan will not pay for it, because they are suspicious of the technology, or for moral or religious reasons. Nonetheless, the testing system is long-standing and well entrenched.

Bioethicist Arthur Caplan alludes to current medical practice as "bullying" women to have prenatal testing. Will the same become true, in time, for genetic testing of adults for conditions to which they may be susceptible?

Early in this century, eugenics—the intent to create a healthy society by actively promoting the survival of "healthy genes"—was the socially correct credo, widely encouraged by a variety of prominent thinkers and political groups (as we will consider in detail later). The focus was on society; individual choice was seen as subordinate.

Today we tend toward the opposite opinion. We Americans now have a devotion to individual choice, which suffuses our attitudes about everything from reproduction and sexual orientation to the uses of intensive care. The mind-set of the day is that the rights and needs of individuals, insofar as is possible, outweigh those of society at large. This does not mean that eugenics is no longer a concern, however, especially with regard to the unborn but also potentially with regard to adults at risk of disability or illness.

"In coming to believe that 'individuals' should make decisions about genetic destiny, we can be blinded and then broadsided by the social frame of these decisions," writes sociologist Troy Duster. He has predicted that progress in genetic research will lead those nations that place great weight on individual choice to a difficult dilemma: whether to try to control explicitly the choices presented by the new technology, or to watch them being manipulated by forces with interests that don't necessarily align with those of the individuals involved. Perhaps the strongest of those interests are economic: the sick and disabled are expensive, and genetic prediction can provide a way to eliminate those costs (while couching the issue in terms of public health).

The U.S. government official who may be closest to such issues — the chief of genetic services for the U.S. Maternal and Child Health Bureau, Dr. Jane Lin-Fu — has been troubled for some time by the conflict between public health priorities and genetic testing. As a member of a national task force on genetic testing, she raised the issue several times. She said no one responded to her concerns during the meetings.

"Primary prevention [efforts to prevent diseases from occurring in the first place] has always been stressed in public health as preferable to secondary and tertiary [efforts to ameliorate their effects once they exist]," Dr. Lin-Fu said at the final meeting of the task force in 1997. "We never have considered the issues of eugenics. . . . We have no time to debate it." Again, there was no debate, not even a response.

There is no question that eugenics is still with us. We just don't call it by that name anymore. The gathering in the basement of Faulkner Hospital could not resolve this issue in a single day. It will be with us, no doubt, for decades.

CHAPTER 5

Regarding Borderlines

Not really. I MAKE friends. They're toys. I make them.
It's a hobby. I'm a genetic designer.

— J. F. Sebastian in the film *Blade Runner*, 1982

BRIGID HOGAN, THE HORTENSE B. INGRAM PROFESSOR
of cell biology at Vanderbilt University, sat at the head of a conference
table with her brows furrowed and her mouth curved down. She would
spend much of the next two days with that dour expression on her face.
She was facing another battle in a long campaign. It was not a pleasant
prospect.

The subject of the conflict was an entity no larger, as she would
point out, than the dot at the end of a sentence. Later, even that observation would generate some verbal sparring: Was it an insult to use
a mere ink dot as a symbol for an early human embryo? Some parties
in the feud—Hogan among them—regard the pre-embryo itself as a
sort of symbol (granted, a symbol of something rather important) and
an object of considerable intellectual interest. To others, especially
those vehemently opposed to abortion, it actually *embodies* something.
Or someone.

This was December 1994—more than two years before Dolly the
sheep was cloned, fanning into flames a long-smoldering public debate
about cloning. Hogan was awaiting the start of a two-day hearing at the
National Institutes of Health, during which she and the eighteen other
members of an expert panel would present to the NIH their views on
when and how scientists should be granted public funds (and therefore
official permission) to use brand-new human embryos for research.
Whether they should do so wasn't really at issue. No one who objected
to the whole idea of such research had been invited to join the panel.

Several critics had objected to this omission. Shortly after the Human Embryo Research Panel was appointed, a private foundation in Pittsburgh, claiming to represent parents of children with birth defects, had filed suit against the NIH and the panel members. The foundation argued that panel members should be prevented from judging the ethics of human embryo research if they in fact were directly involved in this type of research. They claimed that the members were biased because they would benefit from such research.

Indeed, the members had some rather noteworthy affiliations. Hogan had a stake in a company that hoped to be able to store and market lines of cells from aborted fetuses (but not embryos). Another was Mark Hughes, whose BABI procedure (which would be the subject of much interest at the Faulkner conference a few months later) was exactly the sort of research that the panel was meant to advise about. At one meeting, while discussing possible guidelines about preimplantation genetic diagnosis, a fellow panelist would speculate about trying to find "a way of protecting some of Mark's work."

What could be closer to a conflict of interest? On the other hand, argued not only panel members but also the head of the NIH, Harold Varmus, who could advise the government better about the merits of research than researchers themselves? On some level, a dialogue with those who were dead set against doing any research on embryos at all seemed pointless.

The subtext of the dispute was an issue that seldom arose as such during the two-day presentation to Varmus and his advisers: abortion. Perhaps bioethics bodies must "simply steer clear" of issues in which abortion is a factor, argued a later report from the Institute of Medicine (IOM), a congressional advisory body and an affiliate of the National Academy of Sciences. "Even if competing biases were equally balanced on a commission," it added, "opinions about abortion are usually so strongly held that it is unlikely that significant movement toward a middle ground could occur." Bioethical issues that touch on abortion might be ripe for consensus in the future, the IOM report added, but not now.

In late 1994, as the Human Embryo Research Panel was concluding its deliberations, the state of affairs in America was a positive insult to Brigid Hogan and other eminent embryologists, and it had been for a long time. For fifteen years they had been denied access to the human embryo.

For reasons peculiar to American politics, the elite among scientists — those working at universities, usually with federal grants — were implicitly denied permission to study human embryos in tissue culture. In 1974 Congress had ruled that institutions that receive federal funding could not allow embryo research without approval from an ethics board. Then in 1990, during the Reagan administration, Congress did not act to renew authorization for the ethics board that could grant such approval, and it was disbanded. Catch-22: no approval, no research.

Meanwhile, no one seemed to have much idea about (let alone any control over) what the staff at the nation's private fertility clinics were doing with the embryos they were creating in the interests of helping would-be parents. The American Fertility Society (AFS) had issued extensive guidelines to direct their behavior, but these were entirely voluntary and there was no mechanism for oversight.

In 1992 infertile women underwent some 30,000 cycles of in vitro fertilization, according to the AFS. That same year, responding to reports of abuses at some clinics (inflated or distorted IVF success rates, and one instance of a fertility specialist who repeatedly used his own sperm for artificial inseminations), Congress had set up a watchdog mechanism to monitor fertility clinics. But it later failed to provide enough funding, so the watchdog, the Centers for Disease Control, never actually went on guard.

Meanwhile fertility experts were gleefully announcing innovations in "assisted reproduction": freezing, thawing, assisted hatching, sperm microinjection, zona drilling, zygote intrafallopian tube transfer. At medical specialty meetings they would describe these new procedures and reveal how many babies had been born as a result (or would claim high success rates even though many "chemical pregnancies" defined by hormone levels never progressed past the initial stages).

Whatever the private fertility specialists were up to, Hogan argued, if they were calling it science, it was not very *good* science. The researchers didn't really understand what constituted a good experiment, how many subjects you needed for validity or what kind of comparisons were enlightening, she said later. They didn't know much about the molecular events in development. They were not really scientists interested in pure research to elucidate the phenomena of nature; they were medical specialists, intent on achieving pregnancy for specific patients. (In fact, in order to avoid oversight, IVF doctors sometimes argued that their efforts were explicitly *not* research but innovative medical practice.)

The process could not improve without good basic research on embryos. And those who knew best how to do such research were forbidden to carry it out.

Embryologists like Hogan are imbued with an insatiable wonder and curiosity about the early embryo and the mysteries it holds about matters that are almost philosophical: Where do we come from? How do we start?

To scientists like her, in vitro fertilization opens an almost endless array of possibilities for research. One could look for cellular signals on the surface of a fertilized egg and discover which nutrients it needs to mature to the stage where it is capable of implanting itself in the wall of a uterus. One could also split the egg as it divides, creating identical twin or even quadruplet embryos. In theory, one could then expose some of them to chemicals, to compare the effect on the exposed cells with the fate of the unaffected ones.

At long last, however, the long research hiatus seemed about to end. In January 1993, on the twentieth anniversary of *Roe v. Wade*, President Clinton had lifted the requirement for ethics board approval before government-supported scientists could pursue embryo research. It was one of his first official acts as president.

A few grant applications for embryo research soon dropped into the NIH mailbox. The head of the agency that would have to approve such funding, the National Institute of Child Health and Human Development, was apprehensive about making such weighty judgments all by himself. He asked that a panel be formed to guide decisions about embryo research. The Human Embryo Research Panel met for the first time in February 1994.

Ten months later, by the time the NIH director met with the panel to hear its conclusions, seventy-one grant applications had come across the transom. Harold Varmus and his advisers sat around a huge oval table in an upstairs conference room at the NIH, waiting to hear the Human Embryo Research Panel say how the NIH should judge these research proposals.

After an introduction, the panel's chairman, Steven Muller, who is president emeritus of Johns Hopkins University, rose to the podium. He began by describing the panel's working process and went on to relate how it had solicited input from the public.

For most ordinary people, he noted, discussions of research on embryos created outside the womb are "incomprehensible gobbledygook in a foreign language." To many members of the public, he added, the phrase "human embryo research" conjures up an image of "ripping living flesh from the womb." This invites exploitation by opponents of human embryo research, he went on, noting that the bulk of the "flood of

mail" opposing its work that the panel received had been prepared responses—postcards and petitions—generated by organized campaigns.

In fact, the proposed research would not rip anything from anywhere.
Brigid Hogan began her remarks by describing the work in question,
much of which involved peering through microscopes at barely visible
blobs of indistinct cells. The last stage of development that an early embryo can attain in a laboratory dish is a blastocyst, a mass of about twenty
cells. At that size, Hogan said, it's about a half-millimeter in diameter—
roughly the breadth of an eyelash.

Hogan spoke quickly and intensely, illustrating her words with slides
on a projector screen. Varmus and his advisers listened carefully. It
would be up to them to decide which particulars the NIH should accept among the panel's recommendations about research on such an
object.

In making its decisions on this point, Hogan said, the Human Embryo Research Panel had governed itself according to three "overarching considerations." First: To be approved, research on an early
embryo must promise "significant" benefits. Second: The pre-embryo
warrants "serious moral consideration," but not as much respect as a
person or a fetus. Third (and really, one could argue, another significant benefit for the public): Setting rules for government-sponsored
embryo research might encourage ethical behavior in those private fertility clinics.

Hogan proceeded to list the numerous areas of medicine that qualified under the first of those considerations, significant benefit: infertility, repeated miscarriage, contraception, inherited genetic disorders,
birth defects, and cancer. She described a number of ways in which embryo research could improve the rather dismal results of current infertility treatments. It could also improve techniques for preimplantation
diagnosis of genetic abnormalities.

Hogan went on to give several examples of questions about in vitro
fertilization that could be answered definitively only if researchers were
allowed to fertilize human eggs as part of the research process. English
embryologists had done so before they proceeded with the first successful IVF, Hogan noted, and current researchers would miss a "very
important part about this research, this basic research," she said, if they
were denied the ability to determine the best conditions for culturing
eggs to maturity by fertilizing them in vitro. But the products of the experiment might well be tainted by the process; one could not let them
develop and be born.

"Another area in which deliberate fertilization of oocytes [precursor eggs] would be necessary would be to get increased knowledge about the process of fertilization," she went on. "The exciting thing," she had observed, is that fertilization triggers a cascade of events, such as a massive influx of calcium into the egg. Why? What happens afterward? Very little is known about it, she said.

In her research Hogan had been doing exactly what a good scientist is supposed to do. She had observed a phenomenon and raised various questions aimed at understanding it better. The most straightforward way to obtain the answers she sought would be to create early embryos and study them in various ways. As things stood at that moment, as a university researcher she was forbidden to take that next logical step.

Meanwhile, exciting events had been transpiring in animal research. On the very day the panel was presenting the report of its recommendations, an article in the journal *Science* reported an experiment that one embryologist described as a "remarkable feat." (The researcher himself portrayed it as letting a genie out of a bottle.)

Ralph Brinster and his team at the University of Pennsylvania School of Veterinary Medicine were the same group who had made headlines in 1982, when they created a superlarge mouse by transferring into a mouse embryo the growth hormone gene from a rat. Now they had transferred into sterile male mice the precursor sperm cells from fertile males. The transferred cells had matured into sperm; the recipient mice became fertile and impregnated females.

On the face of it, this feat may not sound particularly astonishing. But like the cloning that later created Dolly, it could be seen as paving the way for a giant step over what had been an ethical borderline: such experiments foreshadowed making intentional, permanent changes in the genome. Altering blood cells or nonreproductive body cells for the purposes of gene therapy (as is being done to treat ADA and cystic fibrosis) would have no direct impact on future generations. But altering the genes in the precursors of human sperm, then using them for artificial insemination, could theoretically make a permanent change in the genetic composition of an entire family line.

A subtle interpretation of an ordinary experiment, perhaps, except that generations of geneticists had said that making such alterations in the *human* germ line—the genome itself—should not even be under consideration. We owed it to future generations to understand a great deal more about the risks, many people felt, before we began making irrevocable changes in our germ line.

SHALL WE CHANGE THE BASIC TEXT?

Perhaps more than any other idea in genetics, the thought of making direct changes to the DNA within reproductive cells raises a red flag. It is, as ethicist Eric Juengst observes, an "aboriginal subject in bioethics." The concept comes closer than almost anything else to hubris—to playing God, as it were.

On a visceral level, do we have the right to tinker directly with our actual genetic endowment, to change the program? On a practical level, can we do so without wreaking some unforeseeable havoc on future generations? Biologists are adventuring in the germ lines of mice and other lab animals. We could try it in humans. Should we?

The ethical arguments turn on whether genetic manipulations should be permitted to change the DNA of sperm or eggs, presumably to "improve" them. This is already being done indirectly in pre-embryo genetic testing, where embryos are being selected for the absence of certain genetic attributes. But no direct actions are being taken to alter the genes of human sperm or eggs or embryos.

That kind of germ-line alteration is no more sophisticated than the outright termination of a pregnancy because of a genetic problem. For whatever it's worth, it is not a very efficient way to bring about changes in the human genetic endowment as a whole. They are too slow and too piecemeal.

Could we ever predict the impact that changes in the germ line might have on future generations? Ethicist Marc Lappe has argued that it would take at least two generations to resolve the question, until an embryo subject to germ-line alterations could mature and have children of its own who might be tested. It would be impossible to obtain informed consent from parents anticipating such an experiment on such an em-

What transpires in laboratory mice, history shows, is often echoed soon afterward in humans. Ralph Brinster, interviewed about his achievement in *The New York Times*, said, "I don't think there is any way to hold back knowledge." It's best to know what's coming, he said, "so we can decide how to handle it." Fine words, although it was hard

bryo. Given this level of difficulty, should we even worry about the in-ability of future generations to give consent?

The question also raises the issue of instrumentalism, of using a hu-man being (or a potential one) as a vehicle for someone else's purpose, a sort of arm's-length slavery. Adding it all up, concludes Lappe, "germ-line engineering as a directed attempt to change the genotype of future gen-erations cannot ethically be justified." He echoes generations of others who have written on the point. Still, some enthusiasts have begun to ar-gue that, as medical science has the obligation to try to cure all diseases, it has a positive mandate to pursue germ-line therapy.

In theory, alterations in the germ line could already be taking place in current gene therapy experiments aimed at blood or lung cells, be-cause the introduced genes may somehow be making their way to the sperm or eggs. At the moment there is no evidence, either positive or negative, to answer the concern. We may not know for several genera-tions.

In any case, the argument may be academic for some time. What we would need for true alteration of genes in the germ line would be a way to target specific genes and then replace them. All we can do at the mo-ment is *add* genes into cells, and even so we cannot target the location where they insert themselves.

Starting well ahead of time — now, presumably — we could take steps to assure that when the technology matures, it is monitored over the long term, both by qualified scientists and by experts in policy and ethics, to detect any serious consequences and to ensure that the subjects of the therapy and their possible offspring are guaranteed both social and fi-nancial support. For the time being, however, there does not seem to be any impetus to create legislation or policies with real teeth that would address the ability we already possess to make genetic alterations in our own germ cells.

to take them seriously given the fact that revelations about embryo re-search kept appearing. But debate about them never seemed to go any-where.

Back then, the furor died quickly after a rather startling report of cloning a human pre-embryo. The outcry was brief and muted compared to what greeted Dolly's birth, but at the time it happened, embryologists called it a "hullabaloo." In late 1993 two scientists from George Washington University in Washington, D.C., announced that they had split a living human pre-embryo into eight individual cells and allowed them to continue developing in tissue culture into eight identical embryos.

Embryologists Jerry Hall and Robert Stillman used the word *cloning* to describe this embryo manipulation, although what they had done was different from the process that created Dolly. (They had sectioned an intact embryo; Dolly was the result of replacing an embryo's own nucleus with one from an adult cell. Both manipulations can go by the same name.)

Hall and Stillman could have used less emotive characterizations—*blastomere separation* is the term of art and is less likely to conjure up images of multiple Hitlers—so their choice of words seemed calculated to provoke controversy. (Indeed, Hall and Stillman later said they meant to inspire ethical debate.) The Vatican quickly responded, calling the experiment "perverse."

"This is the experiment we were never going to do," said Boston University ethicist George Annas. He noted that the development raised the possibility of allowing one embryo to mature long enough to discover what it was like, then freezing the rest and selling them based on their characteristics. A market already existed for human sperm and eggs, he pointed out; why not for embryos?

Another medical ethicist, John Fletcher of the University of Virginia, said the experiment "shows again why there needs to be a public forum. Our policy on embryo research is in total disarray."

In fact, except for the provocative detail that Hall and Stillman's experiment involved a *human* embryo, there was nothing particularly new or exciting about it at all. A researcher in England had reported doing the same with sheep embryos in 1979, and "blastomere separation" had been achieved with rats several decades before that. Other researchers had used the same technique to create twin calves and lambs.

Should work like Stillman and Hall's experiment be stopped? Three pioneering embryologists—including Robert Edwards of Cambridge, England, who was responsible for the first successful human IVF attempt—posed that question in the journal *Fertility and Sterility* in March 1994, then gave themselves an unsurprising answer: Not at all.

"Guidelines are in place," they went on. "The guidelines were followed."

As it turned out, they were mistaken on this point. Many months after the revelation about Hall and Stillman, it came out in the science press that they had never sought approval from their own institution's ethics board before doing the "cloning" experiment, as they were required to do by law. George Washington University censured them verbally afterward. The National Institutes of Health chose not to impose its ultimate penalty, the withdrawal of government funding for their ongoing research.

The next embryologist to test the rules would not fare so well.

After Brigid Hogan had finished speaking to Varmus and his advisers, other members of the embryo research panel elaborated on the ways in which studying the early human embryo could prove advantageous to medicine—enlightening cancer specialists about cell growth and regulation, for instance, or revealing episodes of early development that played a role in the development of later diseases. But plainly, and for good reason, the prospects for fertility treatments were always at the forefront.

That year alone, some 5,000 children would be born in the United States as a result of in vitro fertilization, and an estimated three hundred clinics were carrying out the technique. Some 2.3 million infertile couples in the nation had at least some reason for an interest in in vitro fertilization.

The claims of all of these people, and of infants and children who could also benefit from embryo research, easily outweigh those of the developing embryo, said Ronald Green, head of the Ethics Institute at Dartmouth College and the panel's medical ethicist, when he followed Hogan at the podium. As to the panel's second "overarching consideration," the respect due the preimplantation embryo as a form of human life, Green listed several realities that limit its claim to our respect.

Individual cells within a pre-embryo do not begin to differentiate—to shift and change form in ways that determine their future fate within the growing fetus—until about fourteen days after fertilization. Until then, evidently, every cell is identical. After fourteen days the first primitive signs of a nervous system appear, when a band of cells emerges that is known as the primitive streak. Before this stage, there is no chance that an embryo has any sense of its own existence. Nor can it feel pain.

Therefore, placing a fourteen-day age limit should make it acceptable to do research on embryos that has no possible benefit for the embryos themselves, the panel felt. (The limit "may appear somewhat arbitrary,"

Green said, but the panel believed "a clear time limit should be set.")

However, said Green, because the preimplantation embryo is a developing form of human life, the Human Embryo Research Panel favored imposing stringent restraints on experiments that involved deliberately fertilizing an egg, such as those that Hogan had just described. The panel would reserve this for only the most "compelling" examples of studies with "outstanding scientific and therapeutic value." Thus, the panel members felt, rules they had set for moral reasons should be somewhat pliable, depending on their own judgments of the merits of proposed research.

"Urgent medical research of value to citizens," Green said, should not be regarded as an "unworthy" reason for deliberately fertilizing embryos, because it had the potential "to answer crucial questions in reproductive medicine that directly affect people's lives and health." Those who oppose the development of embryos for research, he had argued forcibly in an editorial in *The Washington Post*, would have to accept the idea of using untested procedures on embryos that would later be born.

On this point—the proposal to create embryos deliberately for research purposes and destroy them later—the panel deviated farthest from existing guidelines about research on human fetuses. Those rules, laid down by an earlier ethics panel in 1974 and still in effect, had forbidden fetal research that was not clearly beneficial either to the fetus or to the mother, or was at least harmless. Tissue from aborted fetuses could be used for research, but then aborted fetuses were already dead and could not suffer further harm. And no researcher, obviously, could abort a fetus for the purpose of using its tissue. Much embryo research—and especially deliberate creation and then destruction—was potentially harmful to the embryo itself.

The Human Embryo Research Panel recognized that some people felt that intentionally fertilizing embryos for research was to stand at the top of a slippery slope, Green told Varmus and his advisers. But he noted that many infertile couples undergoing IVF routinely discard some of their embryos that reach this stage, that such research went on in private clinics in the United States all the time, and that some other countries do allow creation of embryos for the purpose of research.

"We were unanimous in our belief that some development of research embryos must be permitted," Green concluded, "if we're to obtain scientific and medical knowledge of great value to many persons."

However, the panel's cochairman for policy, Georgetown University law professor Patricia King, had been so troubled by the proposition that she had written a dissenting document as an appendix to the panel's recommendations. (King was no novice to such issues; she had served on the recombinant DNA advisory committee, which had long counseled the NIH about genetic engineering, and also on two bioethics commissions formed by the U.S. government.)

The proposition of fertilizing human ova expressly for research was "unnerving," King wrote, "because human life is being created solely for human use. I do not believe that this society has developed the conceptual frameworks necessary to guide us down this slope." The panelists' rationale that it should be allowed because not enough "spare" embryos were left over from commercial IVF "is to my mind not compelling," she added, "and carries us perilously close to fertilizing oocytes for no other reason than scarcity of spare embryos."

At the panel's final open meeting, the previous June, Richard Doerflinger, the associate director of the National Conference of Catholic Bishops Secretariat for Pro-Life Activities in Washington, D.C., had specifically targeted this issue. There can be no "legitimacy of non-therapeutic experimentation on live embryos," he said, because nothing in existing law or precedent said that the embryo outside the womb deserved less protection than the unborn fetus.

Other objections came from people who had no titles. At the outset of the meeting, panel chairman Muller had pointed out the thousands of petitions and preprinted postcards that had been sent by people who "make no distinction between the embryo and the fetus." But a look at the files shows that some of the dissenting letters from ordinary people revealed a clear understanding that the subject of discussion was a newly fertilized human egg.

"An embryo is totally human from the moment of conception," wrote members of a church in Commack, New York. ". . . The idea of creating human life for the express purpose of experimentation and then to be discarded after it is no longer useful to us should be absolutely immoral." A man from Garland, Texas, wrote that he was "troubled by the fact that human life would be created for the express purpose of being experimented on and then destroyed." A student from Pennsylvania State University argued that debating the "moral status of a laboratory-created person" was ". . . a step too far in the work of applied science."

Another letter of opposition, from a physician engaged in medical genetics at a hospital affiliated with Harvard University, argued that trying to rank early embryos as less worthy than others was standing atop a slippery slope, at the bottom of which was devaluing actual people. Much as the panel tried to argue a benefit to society, the debate would continue to return to the other consideration: the value, or non-value, of that embryo.

One of the most powerful opposing statements came from a physician and professor of medical ethics at Georgetown University, Edward Pellegrino. "To treat any part of the human species as a mere means to the ends of others is morally indefensible," he wrote to the panel. He also argued forcefully against choosing the fourteen-day appearance of the primitive streak as the moment when an embryo becomes an indi-

MAJOR RECOMMENDATIONS OF THE NIH HUMAN EMBRYO RESEARCH PANEL

All embryo research, the panel said, should be done by qualified scientists and should promise to be of "significant scientific or clinical benefit," using a valid research plan. Animals should be used instead, if possible, and donors must not be paid for eggs or sperm. Researchers must gain informed consent from donors. For now, research would be allowed on embryos only within fourteen days after fertilization.

The panel would forbid certain kinds of research but would allow:

- Research on parthenotes (eggs artificially stimulated to begin dividing without fertilization), which cannot survive

- Research to study normality of embryos derived from eggs fertilized after freezing

- Preimplantation genetic diagnosis

- Development of embryonic "stem cells" (which could be harvested as sources for transplant into people with illnesses such as Parkinson's disease)

vidual. "What is to prevent a subsequent panel from choosing a more convenient time," he asked, if there were "compelling" reasons that research on a later embryo or a fetus could also be useful?

Pellegrino, who had been vice-chair of that ill-fated bioethics advisory committee whose demise had created the de facto ban on embryo research, also rejected the argument that early embryo research should be permitted in order to raise standards in private fertility clinics. "If certain types of embryo research are wrong in the first place," he argued, "they ought to be prevented—not given limited sanction."

Of course, the panel also received many letters of support for embryo research. A member of Varmus's standing advisory committee,

- Replacing the DNA of a fertilized or unfertilized egg with DNA from a different embryo or germ cell (approved by a "narrow majority")

- Intentional fertilization for research "when a compelling case can be made" that it is necessary for research that is "potentially of outstanding therapeutic value"

After further study, the panel said, it would be willing to reconsider allowing:

- Research on embryos after fourteen days but before the neural tube closes

- Cloning by blastomere separation (but such embryos could not be transferred to develop into babies)

- Replacing the contents of the nucleus of a fertilized or unfertilized egg and then implanting the egg, to circumvent inherited defects

- Developing embryonic stem cells from eggs fertilized just for this reason (approved for further consideration by a "narrow majority")

- Research that fertilizes eggs removed from aborted fetuses, without subsequent transfer into a woman (some panel members would never rescind the ban on this idea)

Duke University president Nannerl Keohane, took special note of the "most thoughtful comments . . . from women coming in proudly with their children, saying if it were not for these techniques, little Joshua would not exist. Very powerful, very eloquent, but very simple statements of support." Poignant pleas from infertile couples also appeared in a background file provided to members of the advisory committee, along with supporting letters from numerous researchers in the field of infertility.

Setting aside the aforementioned postcards and petitions, the panel had received 217 letters in favor of permitting federal funding for research on preimplantation embryos, and 9,354 opposing it. They heard twelve oral arguments in favor of the proposal, and twenty-nine against it. Whatever the merits of their arguments, the opponents were clearly the most vocal.

The most worrisome among them were right across town, in Congress. A group of thirty-five members of Congress, headed by conservative California representative Robert K. Dornan and including Newt Gingrich, had engaged Varmus in a volley of letters. Their first one had demanded to know, among other things, what the NIH had done to assure that the panel members had no conflicts of interest, why the panel included no one avowedly opposed to research on pre-embryos, and by what authority the NIH proposed to exempt embryos in laboratory dishes from the protections Congress had earlier afforded to fetuses in utero.

The responses they received from Varmus evidently had left them unmoved. In the latest letter, Dornan had vowed to use "every legislative means available" to prevent the use of federal funds for "grotesque research of this nature."

"The American people will be justifiably outraged and appalled," said Dornan in a public statement, "if their tax dollars are used to create human life in a laboratory dish only to have it thrown out with the trash when the scientists are finished with their bizarre experiments." The threat, warned a member of Varmus's advisory committee near the end of that day's meeting, should be taken very, very seriously.

Varmus's advisory committee spent the rest of the afternoon pondering what to do about the report. "What you are into is controversy," panel chairman Muller said as they began their discussion. "We stood the heat and stayed in the kitchen. It is your choice whether you want to do that or not."

The conversation began with how Dornan, or in fact the president, might react the following morning. "Anything is possible," warned King. "There is something that stirs the blood here."

Quickly discussion turned to how to "inform the public" about the recommendations, how to calm the blood that would stir at the thought of embryo research. Don't discount the signatures and postcards, urged one member of Varmus's advisory group; show those who sent them the negative impact of *failing* to do this research. After all, someone else argued later, what would be the moral consequences of failing to do embryo research that would allow later embryos to be born healthy?

"There will be people concerned and worried about slippery slopes, people of all stripes," remarked the panel's bioethicist, Dr. Green. Only "moving forward with research that proves truly beneficial, or that shows its medical and practical benefits, and shows that we can practice research of this sort responsibly, without undermining our humanity," would cause the critics to moderate their views, he added.

Another member of Varmus's advisory committee countered with a proposal that the advisers should consider "doing things incrementally"—accepting the least controversial of the panel's recommendations first, and reconsidering the others in future years, as research proceeded. But which recommendations were least controversial? Should they start with parthenogenesis (a laboratory process by which eggs can be provoked briefly and temporarily into further development without being fertilized), or did that seem too ghoulish? Would approving the use of spare embryos only—and forbidding researchers from fertilizing ova on purpose—allow the proposal to pass muster with Congress?

"As a scientist," said biochemist Terry Krulwich of New York's Mount Sinai Medical Center, it was easy to develop "tremendous enthusiasm" both for the pure science and for the therapeutic potential of embryo research. But if the committee members themselves felt uncomfortable with some of the ideas, how on earth would they ever gain public acceptance?

The advisers' discussion sounds like just what we have been arguing for eight months, interjected one member of the embryo research panel. "The effort to anticipate what would be incremental doesn't work very well in this area," Dr. Green agreed. "People are broadly offended on a variety of grounds, including those who feel that any research on the early embryo is impermissible, those who are concerned about slippery slopes and means-ends issues. If you try to tailor some-

thing to meet each of those concerns, you end up giving up." Several
times later, he urged Varmus's advisers not to try to distill the report into
its least controversial parts.

Several people around the table suggested ways to win approval for
the recommendations from both Congress and the public. One could
seek support from members of Congress who had family members with
infertility or genetic problems. One could also seek statements of support from outside organizations such as the American Medical Association. One could rewrite the report in simpler language. One could
publicize the needs of infertile couples. Or one could hold a public
conference on the issues.

The only approach "that is going to be able to sell" on the floor of
Congress, argued a representative from the National Institute of Dental Research, would be to allow research on spare embryos in order to
find ways to reduce the need for late abortions. "That is the only approach that we have left," he added.

"Congressional staffs, the lay public, and Congress all have to be
sold it or educated very, very thoroughly in terms of the benefits to
mankind of this kind of research," agreed Duke University cancer specialist Barbara Rimer, who was present on behalf of the National Cancer Advisory Board.

Later, Rimer echoed several other speakers who felt it was important to identify key community leaders and professional groups for such
education. "I think it's important to create a sense of involvement on
the part of the public," she added. "We have been talking about how we
think people will react based on the kinds of letters that we saw, but I'm
not sure we know really what the public thinks."

"We can't keep hearing the term 'sell the report,'" broke in Dr.
David Guyton, a professor of ophthalmology at Johns Hopkins Hospital. "I think that is perhaps an unfortunate use of the term, because we
really ought to be talking about informing or educating. Selling implies
something a little bit scandalous or something under the table. I think
that is not what we want."

"There's a great risk here that this whole process that moves along
can look like another scientific railroad job, to coin a term," said Dr.
Edward Stemmler, head of the Association of American Medical Col-
leges, when the discussion continued the next morning. "I think we
want to make sure that people understand that's not what we're doing,
that that is not the context of this discussion — that the discussion has
risen to a much higher plane than that."

*   *   *

After a day and a half of deliberation, the advisory committee to the director of the National Institutes of Health voted unanimously to support the panel's recommendations for his consideration. As to how Varmus should get them past the thirty-five angry members of Congress, the committee had only a few words of advice: Hold public meetings to bring the public along, and seek the influence of members of Congress who have had a family history of birth defects or infertility.

The worst that could happen, one attendee had warned on the first day, would be "legislation or some sort of Executive Order that puts us back to square one." That, in fact, is what happened, beginning only hours after Varmus's advisers approved the panel's report.

That same afternoon the White House issued a statement: Federal funding would be barred for experiments in which embryos were created merely in order to study them. "I don't believe that federal funds should be used to support the creation of human embryos for research purposes," wrote President Clinton, "and I have directed that NIH not allocate any resources for such research."

The chairman of the embryo research panel, Steven Muller, responded afterward that he was surprised by the speed of the White House announcement and concluded that it was "primarily politically motivated." But at least one panel member, cochairman for policy Patricia King, who had dissented from the panel's support for creating embryos for research, must have been relieved. However, having experienced similar failures of compromise on the same topic as a member of an earlier bioethics panel, she must not have been surprised.

A few days after the president rejected the panel's recommendation on the creation of embryos for research purposes, the head of the NIH under President Bush, Bernardine Healy, spoke heatedly on public television, on the *McNeil-Lehrer NewsHour*. "You have to draw a line somewhere," she said. "We do not have to [intentionally fertilize ova] to achieve these goals. That's the kind of talk that's used to bring the public on board, but what I did not see after reading six different transcripts from these meetings was a definitive answer as to why this work could not be done in other systems. They did not provide a moral imperative to use human embryos cultivated in the laboratory.

"You are commanding living human life to the custody of science solely to do science," she added. "I think that is an extraordinary if not profound step that I don't believe should be taken."

Panel member Ronald Green, speaking on the same program, was more reserved. "I regret there was not more of a dialogue," he said, "so that the president could have been educated as we were educated."

A month after the Human Embryo Research Panel released its recommendations, a number of scathing responses appeared in the journal of the Hastings Center, a bioethics think tank in a suburb of New York City. (The journal, *The Hastings Center Report*, is well known in the bioethics and health policy communities.) A medical ethicist from Oregon State University, Courtney Campbell, noted that the panel saw embryos as interesting not in their own right but because of their usefulness, which "renders the serious moral consideration attributed to the embryo morally meaningless." He called the panel's report "political rhetoric that invites us to engage in science without humanity."

The center's own director, medical ethicist Daniel Callahan, wrote most pointedly of all. Though he himself had long argued that embryos, although not fully human individuals, deserved "profound respect," he admitted in print, "I have always felt a nagging uneasiness at trying to rationalize the killing of something for which I claim to have a 'profound respect.'" What on earth could that kind of "respect" mean? Wafting the term about, he decided, "at least makes me feel a little better about it all.

"I have wondered for twenty-five years whether this is profound wisdom or profound self-deception," Callahan went on. "How does one tell? Now we as a society are asked to take a further step down that road of respect."

Callahan questioned whether it was valid to designate the primitive streak, that first sign of nervous system development, as the paramount milestone in embryonic development. If the primitive streak is so important, he wondered, why is it unethical to carry out certain research before fourteen days—but acceptable to abort a fetus for personal reasons afterward? If research needs are so great, he asked, why not draw the line much later in gestation?

The congressional opponents of embryo research took somewhat longer than the president to respond. Two months later, on February 8, 1995, Representative Dornan wrote to the chairman of the House commerce and health subcommittee, calling it an "absolute outrage" to pay scientists with taxpayer dollars to manipulate and then destroy embryos, and requesting federal hearings.

Almost a year later, in January 1996, when Congress was entangled in an intractable budget debate, a ban on embryo research was attached as a rider to a budget bill. It prohibited using federal funds for "research in which a human embryo or embryos are destroyed, discarded, or knowingly subjected to risk of injury or death greater than that allowed for research on fetuses."

It was not clear how long the ban would stay in effect, said NIH director Varmus, but in the meantime eight groups that had received grants to study fertilization were restricted to using animal material or stopping short of full fertilization. On this score the NIH was back where it started: in limbo. In the meantime, Varmus added, he hoped to "do a better job of educating the public."

If the outcome of the process was a victory for the opponents of embryo research, it was a rather lame one. As the panel members had repeated over and over, whatever research was not funded and regulated by the government would surely continue, unrestrained and without oversight, in private hands.

A few months before the Human Embryo Research Panel concluded its work, Mark Hughes had relocated from Baylor University to Washington, D.C., where he became a contract investigator at Georgetown University. There he intended to continue his research into methods of pre-embryo genetic diagnosis, under NIH funding. He also set up a laboratory at an independent hospital across the street from the NIH campus.

Unfortunately, in one case his tests erroneously misdiagnosed an embryo that was affected with cystic fibrosis; the parents were told, wrongly, that their baby would be unaffected. According to a report in *Science*, postdoctoral fellows working in his lab at the private hospital became concerned that they were violating the ban on embryo research, once it went into effect, because they were being paid by the NIH. Apparently Hughes conceded the point and took to doing all research that might be questioned himself, across the street.

Nonetheless, the NIH cut off Hughes's funding in October 1996 and ended its relationship with his work, citing violations of the ban. Later, in a statement in congressional hearings about the experiments, Hughes denied that the NIH had ever directly communicated news of the ban on pre-embryo research in the wake of the passage of the congressional rider. "I believed in good faith that I was permitted to continue my . . . research," Hughes said.

Questions were also raised about some equipment that Hughes was suspected of diverting. All of this put him in a tenuous position with Georgetown University, a Catholic institution that also had policies

FEDERAL GOVERNMENT BIOETHICS PANELS

In recent decades, Congress and the president have appointed numerous expert panels to deliberate and report on topics in bioethics:

**National Commission for the Protection of Human Subjects of
Biomedical and Behavioral Research (1974–78):** Established
local-level boards to review research involving human beings. Issued nineteen reports, including the oft-cited "Belmont Report"
(1978) on protection of human subjects, and reports on research
involving fetuses (1975) and children (1977).

Ethics Advisory Board (1978–80): Created to review and advise
on proposals for research involving fetuses. Issued one report: *Support of Research Involving Human In Vitro Fertilization and Embryo
Transfer* (1979).

**President's Commission for the Study of Ethical Problems in
Medicine and Biomedical and Behavioral Research (1980–83):**
Created to advise the president and Congress on bioethical issues.
Released fifteen reports, including one on the definition of death
(1981) and another on decisions to forgo life-sustaining treatment.
Also: *Splicing Life: A Report on the Social and Ethical Issues of*

against research that would lead to discarding embryos. If Hughes had
come to Washington expecting to be allowed to continue his research,
the efforts of the embryo research panel to generate funding for that research had failed him.

The panel had also failed the public, judging by the criteria set up
for bioethics advisory committees in a report issued by the Institute of
Medicine in 1995. The panel did not create useful new policy and did
not move the debate forward. It fell short on several of the IOM's criteria. It failed to create an "appropriate and fruitful balance" between interests, disciplines, and cultures in American society. The members did
not grapple seriously with opposing views but "advanc[ed] their own

Genetic Engineering and Human Beings (1982) and *Screening and Counseling for Genetic Conditions* (1983).

NIH Recombinant DNA Advisory Panel (1975–present): Established to guide NIH and review research protocols about research involving DNA transfer. Issued one report.

Working Group on Ethical, Legal, and Social Implications of the Human Genome Project (1988–96): Very broad mandate involving genetic research (see Chapter 13). Issued reports on genes and disabilities (1991), genes and insurance (1993), and genetic testing (1997), among others.

Biomedical Ethics Advisory Committee (1988–89): Created by Congress to report on ethical issues in biomedical research and health care. Committee was paralyzed by the abortion issue. Congress took more than two years to decide on the membership and let it die before it could issue any reports.

National Bioethics Advisory Commission (1996–present): Impaneled by President Clinton in mid-1996, this fifteen-member body has several special charges: To consider the protection of human research subjects, the proper use and management of genetic information, and the implications of patenting human genes. Within weeks of its creation, the commission was also assigned to make recommendations about the potential and risks of human cloning.

preferred approach." Perhaps one reason why it failed was that the issue under its purview was simply not yet "ripe" for resolution. For several years afterward, panel members were defending their work against articles in medical and ethical journals that criticized both their methods and their conclusions.

The ink had barely had time to dry on these debates when Scottish embryologist Ian Wilmut introduced Dolly, the cloned lamb, to the world on February 23, 1997. President Clinton's response was even swifter this time. The day after Dolly made the news, he asked the head of his newly created National Bioethics Advisory Commission to give him its advice on the subject within ninety days. Barely a week later, on

THE BARE BONES OF CONTENTION

The dispute about embryo research could be resolved in one of three ways: by pronouncement from above (witness President Clinton's ruling against creating embryos for the purpose of research), by compromise (witness the recommendations of the Human Embryo Research Panel), or by impasse, which is the state of the dispute at the time of writing.

The debate is thorny because the various parties differ deeply at every level of discussion:

1. *Information.* Some of the loudest critics of embryo research obviously misunderstand the entity being discussed. They think the entity is the formed fetus, not an undifferentiated mass the size of the dot on the letter *i*. Other people may have less obvious misconceptions about the nature of the embryo or fertilization. This difference is the one most easily resolved: Inform the misinformed. If they continue to argue from ignorance, ignore them.

2. *Premises.* Some disputants disagree about the value of that mass of cells, about how to define human life, and about when it starts. This difference is far less easy, perhaps impossible, to resolve.

March 4, the president announced that he would ban using federal funds to clone adult human cells.

Embryo researchers leaped to respond as well, urging regulators not to rush to judgment and create a ban that might have a chilling effect on responsible research, simply by using the term *cloning*. After all, the cloning that created Dolly (inserting DNA from an adult cell into an embryo whose own DNA had been micro-vacuumed out) was not the same as the cloning that Hall and Stillman had tried on abnormal human embryos (sectioning into separate cells), which in turn was not at all the same cloning that molecular researchers use to create many copies of a single gene (inserting it into intact cells of almost any kind, blood cells or tumor cells or animal cells, often in order to preserve the gene in the laboratory for further study).

The risk of another Hitler re-creating himself by cloning was a titil-

3. *Values.* To some disputants, progress in science is the paramount concern. To others, the needs of infertile couples are most important. Others (like Patricia King) feel a fundamental but less defined disquiet about the direction in which our society may be moving in some of its bioethical judgments. This difference is deeply felt, but is perhaps subject to some compromise.

4. *Consequences.* Some parties decry the continued lack of regulation of the private fertility industry. Others fear that if science or society continues to push forward the stage before which embryos can be used for research, we will eventually lose any age limit beyond which the unborn or even the newly born may not be subjects for intentional, directed research—a development that would threaten our concept of human dignity. Another possible consequence is the prospect that results of IVF could improve quickly, or remain forever as poor as they are now. The disputants can argue about the relative value of these possible consequences of embryo research but cannot predict any of them with certainty.

lating diversion to think about, but in the light of other realities, it was perhaps not a very worthy one after all. "Just how dangerous are really stupid ideas?" asked Eric Parens of the Hastings Center, shaking his head, at a press conference shortly after Wilmut's announcement. "Does the proliferation of stupid ideas have an effect on society? I fear it does." Would controversy over such outlandish concerns trigger unwise legislation or muffle more questions?

Rabbi Marc Gellman of New York's Temple Beth Torah, who has a Ph.D. in medical ethics, responded with some considerations that were anything but trivial. For what illness, he asked, would human cloning be a therapy? Grief at the loss of a child, perhaps, or at the prospect of one's own impending death?

"Grief is not an illness," Gellman answered himself, "but a form of growth." He also mused that in our individualistic society, some would argue that because they own their own body, they have the right to clone their own DNA, and that ultimately "a horrific argument will be made that a clone is not a human being" because someone else had created him.

The National Bioethics Advisory Commission worked feverishly in its first three months of existence to arrive at a consensus about human cloning. Were researchers in private clinics already trying to duplicate what Wilmut had done in sheep? Not likely, the commission argued; their mission was to create pregnancies, not to re-create identical copies of adults.

Even so, they must not be allowed to venture into such terrain, the new commission warned, recommending in a report of June 7, 1997, that laws be passed making it illegal to clone adult human cells — at least for three years. Some members of the commission had felt that in a free society scientists and individuals should be at liberty to proceed as they wished. Others felt just as deeply that cloning adult humans would threaten fundamental concepts about family, individuality, and even humanity.

The commission members concurred on at least one point: that cloning might not be safe for the individuals it created. And the only way to stop it would be to pass a law. This, at last, might be something Congress could agree on as well.

In pondering the issue of cloning, the National Bioethics Advisory Commission took care to solicit and document the opinions of religious thinkers who had written and spoken on the subject. Its report cites Protestant theologian Ted Peters saying that, as creatures made in the image of God, we are responsible for using our creativity and freedom to improve our destiny, and nothing requires us to leave human nature unchanged. It quotes Sheikh Fadlallah, a Shiite Muslim jurist, and Abdulaziz Sachedina, an Islamic scholar, saying that God allowed Dolly to be created and may have intended her as a divine lesson of sorts. It also quotes testimony by one rabbi that humans are God's "partners" in improving our lot; another rabbi notes that God commanded Adam to take dominion over nature.

Both rabbis testified, however, that human clones should be regarded as full human beings and that there is a potential for discrimination against them. The report cites numerous opinions from Roman Catholic sources that cloning would involve treating human beings as commodities, because it so closely controls the nature of an unborn being.

One of the rabbis declared in his testimony that "risks to persons created through cloning are now so unknown that we should virtually rule out human cloning for the present, because those who create children in this manner could not be sure that they are 'doing no evil.'" This was one point upon which the commission members could reach a firm consensus, and it agreed with the rabbi that human cloning should be banned, for now.

By issuing its conclusions about cloning, the commission tried to buy the rest of us time to think and to learn. Unlike the Human Embryo Research Panel, it recommended saying a simple and definitive no to researchers and would-be patients who want to pursue a new kind of genetic research. No—or at least, not now.

"Banning human cloning reflects our humanity," said President Clinton when the report was released. "It is the right thing to do. Creating a child through this new method calls into question our most fundamental beliefs."

Barely a month later the news emerged quietly that scientists might have found a way to make an end run around the whole debate. A developmental biologist from Johns Hopkins Medical Institutions in Baltimore, John Gearhart, announced that he had kept precursor sperm and egg cells from aborted human fetuses alive in tissue culture for more than seven months. These cells could probably be grown into many kinds of human tissues for medical research. In theory, perhaps they could also be implanted into a woman's womb to create a baby.

It was an echo of Ralph Brinster's 1994 feat using mice—this time using human tissue. An article in *Science News* reporting the development acknowledged that there were ethical issues, but it quoted Ronald Green (the ethicist on the embryo research panel) saying that the technique might not raise as many ethical questions as cloning.

"Gearhart himself wonders who, if anyone, will regulate the use" of these precursor sperm and egg cells, the article said. "Johns Hopkins University officials have already filed for patents on the cells and the procedures used to create them. One or more companies may soon buy the rights to their research, adds Gearhart, noting that the . . . research has been conducted without any federal funding."

All of this fades in the light of the revelations of Richard Seed, the Chicago physicist who has promised to offer human cloning to tens of thousands of eager volunteers, with the help of some anonymous doctor friends. If American authorities threatened to thwart his plans, he said, he would open up shop in Mexico. Meanwhile he spoke to the press about becoming one with God.

Seed may or may not be able to fulfill his promise, but he certainly revived debate about the issue. President Clinton responded with an immediate call for a five-year ban (which his bioethics commission had already requested). UNESCO, the United Nations' science branch, also appealed to nations to ban cloning.

Boston medical ethicist George Annas, who is almost always quoted on such occasions, was dubious about the importance of the latest flap. The "demand" for cloning that Seed intends to serve does not exist, he said. "This is an overly enthusiastic marketer who doesn't understand either science or ethics," he added.

If nothing else, Seed is a vivid example of the exquisite dilemma in reproductive research that troubled the Human Embryo Research Panel and that will continue to frustrate American society. We cannot agree on effective means to regulate the progress of researchers in this emotive field without tying their hands completely. Meanwhile the enterprise of mastering our own reproduction lurches onward, taking us even farther into unexplored territory without a road map.

CHAPTER 6

The New Paradigm

I didn't want to be a guinea pig. You never know who might
have access to the DNA.

— Marine corporal John Mayfield, facing a court-martial for refusing
to allow the Department of Defense to test his DNA

CONSIDER FOR A MOMENT AN ENDEARING IMAGE THAT
appeared on page twenty-six of the *Rocky Mountain News* on Wednes-
day, March 10, 1993. Vatahan Goolsby, age four, and his three-year-old
brother, Dante Williams, fidget on their grandmother's lap. A research
technician gives Vatahan a small glass of Gatorade. He is meant to spit
it back out for science.

Instead, he swallows. The article quotes young Vatahan: "Yum," he
said, and "deelishus."

The setting is a special education center near Denver. Although the
article doesn't exactly say this, Vatahan and Dante are two of fifteen children being analyzed for the most common inherited cause of mental
retardation—a condition known as the Fragile X syndrome, which
causes a particular kind of break in the X chromosome. Girls, who have
two X chromosomes, can be carriers and are sometimes mildly affected;
boys, who inherit only one X, usually develop the syndrome and some
mental deficits if the X passed down to them is fragile. (One in 1,500
males and one in 2,500 females are known to be affected by Fragile X
syndrome, which often involves autismlike symptoms or hyperactivity
as well as varying degrees of mental retardation.)

The article tells us that the research team from the University of Colorado has already collected forty-seven cell samples in two nearby special education schools and intends to collect thousands more. Genetic
advances allow the team to detect the Fragile X mutation in cells
swished from the inside of the mouth. "This is so much nicer than the

blood sample," remarked the executive director of the National Fragile X Foundation in Denver. "It tastes good, and they're cooperative."

If someone like Vatahan swallows the Gatorade, the article explains, a test administrator "gently scrapes their cheek linings with a wooden tongue depressor, then dunks the stick in Gatorade."

Written in the chatty style typical of a newspaper feature, the article spells out the exact consequences of Fragile X syndrome and adds that the director of the foundation would prefer that the genetic test be administered immediately before or immediately after birth. As a result of the current program, presumably, educators will know the reason behind some cases of retardation, and some families will be alerted to a need for caution about reproduction.

What could possibly be wrong with that? One answer appeared in the *Rocky Mountain News* itself, three days later. A correction: Vatahan and his brother were not known to *have* Fragile X syndrome, as the original article stated. The two boys were merely being *screened* for it; results of their tests were not yet available to announce.

Beyond the obvious concern about invading children's privacy, is there also something worthy of special caution about putting a name — a name that makes reference to the genes — alongside the fact of someone's presence in a special education program?

Those familiar with this question know that the answer is yes: The DNA implicates other family members and attaches to them a stigma. At the same time it adds an aura of special hopelessness to the situation, in much the same way someone will say about a spouse's foibles, with a roll of the eyes, "I guess it must be in the genes." If something is genetically caused, presumably, it is irrevocable and also, somehow, beyond help.

This is not only a story about children who are retarded, it is a cautionary tale about broad-based efforts to go on a hunt for genetic risks of any kind.

The Colorado screening program for Fragile X has earned some notoriety because of the vigor and enthusiasm with which its implementers have sought to ferret out and ultimately eradicate a hereditary problem, starting from the level of researchers and state government rather than within the affected community. In 1994, well after the program was under way, the American College of Medical Genetics issued a policy statement recommending *against* widespread screening for Fragile X syndrome. It advised targeted testing, especially for those people with mental retardation who are known to have characteristics or a family history of the syndrome itself. The policy statement speaks of the molecular nature of the genetic defect and the variability of its effects on behavior and intelligence; it states no actual goals for testing beyond "reproductive counseling." In other words, the medical geneticists' main goal for this testing is to help parents avoid repeating the experience, not to help the children who are having it.

The situation with Fragile X testing is like one of those flat medallions that children sometimes find in cereal boxes: They show two images, depending on how you slant them. Understandably, some families who know they have to deal with Fragile X are vociferous in their support for access to the test, so that they can discover which girls in the family carry a Fragile X chromosome to pass on to their own children, and which fetuses or little boys are at risk of retardation as a result of Fragile X. On the other hand, to the small percentage of children in special education classes who will be found to have a fragile X, the testing itself is of no obvious direct benefit.

If they are hyperactive (as many are), most likely they will either need medication or not, regardless of *why*. It is not clear that knowing this name for a particular child's developmental problem improves his own prospects for the future. It *could* help his parents define his educational goals, although the nature of the syndrome (one in five males with a fragile X appears normal) is highly variable; sometimes simply knowing a name for a problem can comfort parents and relieve their guilt. But these advantages of testing tend to come up in the context of individual affected families and their doctors. Documents about the subject speak only of "recurrence risk."

In 1995, two years after the Colorado screening program took place, a prospective study showed that knowing the nature and degree of the mutation affecting a particular child with Fragile X syndrome predicts absolutely nothing about his exact IQ or degree of behavioral abnormality. Another research team, from Pennsylvania, studied the ability of children with Fragile X syndrome to understand emotional cues in people's facial expressions—this is a common difficulty in behavior problems that are related to mental retardation. They found no difference between children with Fragile X and children of similar IQ whose problem had no genetic name. Training mentally retarded children to recognize facial cues, the researchers decided, is important whether or not they have Fragile X chromosome.

Besides companies wanting to market genetic tests and doctors with an interest in performing them, society at large has a definite economic

FRAGILE X SYNDROME

Fragile X syndrome is a case of genetic stuttering, in this case one that involves the X chromosome, of which females have two and males have only one. Inside the gene known as HMR1, people may have fifty or more repeats of the small DNA fragment and be perfectly normal, or they may have up to two hundred–odd repeats — a so-called "premutation" — and be perfectly normal, although at risk of bearing a child with the full mutation and serious mental retardation. About a third of girls with a full mutation, defined as more than two hundred repeats, and even some boys, are intellectually normal.

Next to Down syndrome, Fragile X is the most common known cause of mental retardation. But its inheritance is far more complex. (People rarely use the term *carrier* for this syndrome because the inheritance is so variable and passes only from mothers, not from both parents.) Thus, however accurate the DNA analysis itself, the predictive value of Fragile X testing is highly imperfect. It is important, urged the American College of Medical Genetics in a 1994 policy statement, "to ensure that effective means are in place to adequately inform tested populations of the meaning and implications of results."

According to science historian Dorothy Nelkin of New York University, in the Colorado screening program informed consent procedures did not take place until after the testing had begun.

incentive to help affected families learn their recurrence risk and act on the knowledge. In 1991 none other than James Watson, the first head of the Human Genome Project, cited the cost of Fragile X syndrome as one justification for the genome project, noting that every year 2,000 boys are born with Fragile X syndrome and will all require care for the rest of their lives at $100,000 a year each, putting the burden of the disease at $200 million annually. "The project will pay for itself if we can go beyond the discovery of this one gene to doing something about it," he said.

By "doing something about it," clearly Watson meant preventing all those expensive babies from coming to exist. In the case of the Colorado screening program, the same economic incentive was spelled out in exquisite detail. Just a year before the program began, a team of economics researchers and pediatricians at the University of Colorado had carried out a dollars-and-cents assessment of the cost of caring for a child with Fragile X syndrome. They presented the results at an international conference on the syndrome.

Drawing on a survey of 123 families with children who had Fragile X syndrome (less than half of whom responded), the researchers concluded that such a family could expect to spend $11,326.36 annually "over and above the 'normal and average' costs of childrearing" for costs of care related to the syndrome. They estimated the total lifetime cost of caring for one mentally retarded adult to be more than $2 million, and the combined annual cost of state-provided care for all Fragile X individuals at a staggering $73,665,663.87.

It's not the $73 million that gets to geneticists and families affected by Fragile X syndrome when they see that estimate. It's the 87 cents. How could an analysis based on so many broad assumptions about children with the syndrome come to a bottom line in ten figures — down to the cents?

"The difficulty in gathering accurate data for Fragile X syndrome cost analysis has been complicated tremendously by the lack of accurate identification of Fragile X patients," said the published report of the study. There is no cure as yet, it pointed out, but genetic counseling "can affect reproductive decisions and potentially decrease the incidence of this disorder." But before counseling can be given to the many people within their families at high risk of having more children with Fragile X syndrome, individuals with Fragile X syndrome must be identified.

The cost of diagnostic testing, it concluded, "will be orders of magnitude below the cost of caring for each individual Fragile X person. If a counseling and awareness program resulted in a 50 percent reduction of the number of Fragile X affected births, the savings to the state would be tremendous."

The study might have vanished into library stacks had not New Hampshire resident Jamie Stephenson, who is now director of the Fragile X Resource Center of Northern New England, run across it just as she was trying to argue for reinstatement of her health insurance. Her coverage had been rescinded after the insurance company learned that she had given birth to a son with Fragile X syndrome.

"These numbers were published at the same time I'm writing to the insurance company and having doctors and geneticists write and say that a kid with Fragile X doesn't cost any more than any other kid,"

Stephenson recalls, speaking with a good-natured chuckle in her voice now that it is all over. The figures stunned her.

Her own son David has been in regular school since first grade, she remarked in an address to a conference on cost-effectiveness analysis in genetics. He had some problems, perhaps, but they weren't *medical* costs at all, and there was no good reason to assume he could not grow up to support himself. At the age of ten he had schoolmates who were close friends and enjoyed his company.

Stephenson did an informal survey herself of the members of her own support group for Fragile X families. No one could fathom how the Colorado team had come up with the figure of more than $11,000 a year in extra costs. The $377 in extra dental care really stumped them. "My children with Fragile X don't have braces," Stephenson says. (She also has a mildly affected daughter.) "The other two do." And how do you reckon the cost of remedial reading against "normal and ordinary" costs? Where do the tennis and piano lessons she buys for the unaffected children enter the picture, and the summer camps, and the college educations?

If the figures stunned Stephenson, the assumptions behind them took her breath away. Fragile X is much closer to Down syndrome in its nature than to Tay-Sachs disease, yet the Colorado study began with the assumption that all affected children would be in the care of state institutions when they reached the age of eighteen.

Among its other special features, the study that was used to justify Colorado's screening program invariably referred to people with Fragile X as "sufferers," identified people with premutations who show a normal IQ as having "significant emotional problems," cited a prenatal screening rate of "only" 16 percent among the respondents (which assumed that everyone would or should want screening and, presumably, abortion), alluded to the hours of time spent with a child who has the syndrome as hours "lost to care," and referred to the current "burden" of costs of care for children with Fragile X.

This study has been called a "classic" that will be used until the end of time as an example of how *not* to conduct a cost-benefit analysis in medical care. "It used a worst-case logic which has no relationship to real life," says pediatrician Allen Crocker of Boston's Children's Hospital. "It leaves one with a set of feelings that are so troubled it is almost too difficult to deal with rationally."

"The study proposed an alternative to raising someone with Fragile X syndrome," Stephenson observes. "The alternative is prenatal testing." She could not avail herself of that alternative, however, because it did not exist when her children were born. Against the "burden" of caring for them, Jamie Stephenson can place a "value" and express it eloquently, describing her affection for the person that David is and recounting ways in which his mere presence helps his class to learn concern for others who are different.

Several recent studies of cost-effectiveness have also begun to try to quantify the issue of quality of life from the perspective of people who are themselves disabled, rather than (as usual) asking members of the general population who may have little or no contact with people with disabilities. A 1996 study comparing adolescents who were born extremely small (many of whom developed disabilities) with those who started out at normal weight showed virtually no difference in how they rated their *health-related* quality of life: 71 percent rated it as 95 on a scale of zero to 100; 79 percent of the control group felt the same way. Studies of self-worth among young people with congenital heart disease and spina bifida found little difference from that of nondisabled teenagers.

In the long run the discovery of genes such as the one that explains the Fragile X syndrome could in theory lead to a better understanding of diseases and ultimately to new treatments. In the meantime, what such discoveries offer without exception is the possibility to test for the existence of the gene, either on a private and individual basis, or in public and on a widespread scale.

The distinction can be terribly important. For instance, in its Fragile X article the Denver newspaper used the words *testing* and *screening* interchangeably. Tests tend to apply to individuals; screens apply to masses of individuals. In common parlance screens are used to keep undesirable things out: weapons, insects, and presumably people. Were the Denver researchers testing, or were they screening?

The question was not lost on someone who had been quoted in the *Rocky Mountain News* two years before the program, at the time when the gene involved in the syndrome was identified. Ted Brown, the chief of genetics at a teaching hospital on Long Island, said testing for the new mutation should be voluntary and anonymous "in case they test positive." He specifically cautioned against making a test for Fragile X mandatory or even routine, as in a screening program. "You need to consider the consequences if you find out you are a carrier," Brown said, such as how it would affect your self-esteem, your insurability, even your marriageability.

The researcher who began the Denver program had already been doing chromosome tests on retarded children for more than a decade,

TESTING CHILDREN

Two decades before the Colorado Fragile X screening program began, some prominent geneticists had concurred that it is "probably unethical" to mount such genetic screening programs, unless specific treatment alternatives exist for those who are found to have the genetic type that the program wants to detect. Putting a genetic label on their condition may not necessarily affect how developmental professionals interact with them, but it may have unforeseeable consequences, such as discrimination.

In 1993 an expert bioethics committee from the Institute of Medicine concluded that it is absolutely inappropriate to go hunting for disease genes in children unless there is a valid way to prevent or cure the problem. "Childhood testing is not appropriate for carrier status, untreatable childhood diseases, and late-onset diseases that cannot be prevented or forestalled by early treatment," they wrote in *Assessing Genetic Risks*.

At the time Vatahan was having his cheek swabbed, many members of the public (who, unlike the committee, did not have a year to learn and ponder the implications of such testing) did not agree. When Boston sociologist Dorothy Wertz surveyed visitors to genetic clinics, she found that six of ten felt that parents should be able to have their children tested for the gene associated with Alzheimer's disease, and 47 percent felt they should tell their children the results. Nine of ten said that if they themselves were found to have a breast cancer gene, they would have their thirteen-year-old daughters tested. The troubling question is why parents would want to test children for a condition such as Alzheimer's, when there is no active strategy to help a child (or the future adult) at genetic risk.

What should a responsible geneticist do when parents want their children tested? The question came to a head at a genetics conference in Montreal in 1994. The matter of testing children raises a conflict between two bioethical principles: patient autonomy and the doctrine "first, do no harm," said Louisiana State University geneticist and attorney Mary Kay Pelias.

Autonomy is "shaky" in children, she went on, because they are not considered fully autonomous. "Society allows parents considerable latitude," she observed, pointing out that geneticists are in a difficult legal position. They have to ask to whom they owe a fiduciary duty: the parents who solicit their help or the child who is the patient. A physician would be hard pressed to deny a parent's request for a genetic test on the basis that it might harm the child, given a solid history of Supreme Court decisions in favor of parents deciding what is in their children's interests.

"The issue is doing our best to help the family adjust to and deal with their genetic situation," Pelias concluded.

Nonsense, retorted Vanderbilt University pediatrician and law professor Ellen Wright Clayton. "Physicians routinely refuse to do what patients ask," she said, adding that parents would have "no conceivable claim" if a geneticist refused to test a child for, say, predisposition to Huntington's disease. "It's very important to educate the parents," she went on, "but no enforceable civil claim can follow from refusal to provide testing."

Loud applause greeted Clayton. But we have to be careful, Pelias responded, not to "tread on the rights of parents." (It is instructive that the debate turned so quickly from ethics to legalities. In many cases, when medical societies have laid out and defended policies with regard to genetic tests or other kinds of prenatal testing, they have alluded to the legal risks or interests of their members.)

A year later, there was evidence that the whole argument was moot: parents were bypassing the doctors completely. At the next annual conference, in Minneapolis, Wertz presented results of a survey of gene-testing laboratories. Some 44 percent of the labs said they provided tests directly to patients without a referring physician. More than half had received requests to test children under twelve for the Huntington's disease gene; about a quarter had done so.

"What this suggests," Wertz said, "is that parents are testing these children so they can make plans. It's healthy children, simply to find out if they have the gene."

No one, Clayton pointed out, had set standards to help either doctors or laboratories decide which of the new genetic tests were appropriate, or when. "While all of us think that they should not be testing children," she added, "the fact is if there are no standards, they can't be deviating from them." Could someone sue the lab, Wertz asked, if the child committed suicide as a result of the test? "I think that's unlikely," Clayton responded.

and was urging early testing, with the explanation that it would lead to the use of medications that could help children improve their behavior and concentration. Tilt the medallion still farther in that direction: finding a chromosomal explanation could relieve parents' guilt and could even help them pay for treatment because doctors would be able to put a diagnosis code on the insurance form.

On the other hand, such testing could allow the insurer to refuse to pay—as happened to Jamie Stephenson. She eventually did get health coverage after all, but only because New Hampshire passed a law that required insurers to cover anyone who could afford to pay the premiums. Does this mean that only those families affected by hereditary diseases who can afford to pay for health care, either through insurance or out of their own pockets, should have full diagnostic information about their own genes or their children's? The medallion tilts back again. What of those who cannot afford to pay? What of those not lucky enough to live in states where their health insurance is mandated by law?

Meanwhile, there are broader issues to consider, which are expressed eloquently by Ruth Hubbard and Elijah Wald in their book *Exploding the Gene Myth.* "It is all too easy for genes to take on a life of their own," they write. "Genetic 'learning disabilities' are a stigma not only for the child who has them but for all the relatives and descendants of the child. They can be used to show why poor children do not do well in school and to explain why their families got to be poor in the first place and will continue to be poor in the future. . . . The tests will serve as an explanation and an excuse, getting schools and society off the hook by placing the blame on the children's unchangeable genes."

The difficulty with genetic testing, according to the head of the Hereditary Diseases Foundation, Nancy Wexler, is that the tests are done on a captive audience. "We can use this as a back door, saying: We have recognized this problem, and wouldn't your sisters like to know about it?" she says. "This can be a great relief, but there can be a whole cascade of events the family wasn't prepared for."

Now that science knows about literally thousands of genes, who should be screened, for what, where, by whom, and how? The answers given are seldom straightforward.

Bioethicists sometimes say that genetics presents them with no new problems. That may or may not be true, but screening is certainly a case that supports their view. You don't need to know genes in order to screen. Population screening per se is nothing new, nor are the issues behind it. American society has already been debating these issues for several years in the context of AIDS. For instance, should we mandate neonatal screening for AIDS, or let newborns with AIDS suffer in the interest of their mothers' privacy?

Nationwide, newborns are tested routinely for PKU (phenylketonuria), an inborn metabolic problem that interferes with digestion and can cause severe retardation unless the affected child eats a special diet beginning within weeks of birth. (The technology tests for a protein, not for the gene behind it.) Children in many cities have their blood tested for lead levels, to guard against lead-induced brain damage. People have also long accepted the idea of having blood tests before marriage to rule out venereal disease.

Any proposal for widespread screening to rule out a *genetic* disease, however, raises unsavory associations that must be contended with. In the early 1970s screening efforts for sickle cell disease turned into an unfortunate debacle. It was the first attempt at molecular genetic screening in the history of American medicine, and by today's standards it was misguided.

There was no cure for the disease at the time (nor is there still, as this is written). The ailment can be mild or severe, and its intensity is impossible to predict for any particular child. Besides that, the question of testing for the disease was fraught with racial implications.

Sickle cell disease, an inherited disorder of red blood cells that can cause episodes of severe disseminated pain and can ultimately damage internal organs, affects primarily black individuals. Most of those who promoted genetic testing for sickle cell disease in the 1970s, like most medical and public health professionals at the time, were white.

Like cystic fibrosis, sickle cell disease is a recessive trait—a child must inherit one gene from each parent to develop the condition. The carrier state, known as sickle cell *trait*—the condition of having only one affected gene, not two—can be detected by looking at the blood itself, without any resort to genetic testing, because it causes some red blood cells to have an abnormal sickled shape. The controversy about screening for the trait began in 1970, after four of some 4,000 army recruits died during basic training at a high-altitude camp; researchers reported that all four had sickled red blood cells.

The Air Force Academy quickly introduced a policy of summary dismissal for any cadet found to have the trait. In the next few years most major airlines grounded or fired employees with the trait. Over half of

SCIENCE NEWS FRAMES THE DEBATE

What would you counsel in the following cases?

1. A couple who both have achondroplasia want genetic testing. They would abort a fetus that was destined for normal stature.

2. A couple who have had a child with cystic fibrosis return for carrier testing, to learn their risk of having another affected child. It turns out that Dad is not the biological father of the first child.

3. A thirty-year-old woman is diagnosed with a hereditary disorder that carries a high risk of colon cancer. Should her children and siblings be told, against her wishes?

4. A pregnant woman with a family history of Fragile X syndrome wants prenatal testing. She would abort a female fetus who is a carrier but would not be retarded.

In 1994, hoping to provoke thought, the weekly magazine *Science News* printed these vignettes and asked readers to fax back their responses. The magazine also solicited opinions from a few respected ethicists and geneticists. The results showed how differently we feel, depending on who we are. For instance:

- Nearly 2,000 readers responded; one-fourth were adults. In general, students were much more hard-nosed, while adults were more willing to let people decide as they wished. For instance, 84 percent of adult readers said the center should perform the

medical insurers raised their rates for carriers of the sickle cell gene, without any scientific evidence that possessing a single copy of the gene caused a physical problem. In 1971 the Massachusetts state legislature passed a law requiring blood tests for sickle cell trait before children could attend school. By the mid-1970s, six more states had followed suit.

These efforts angered many black professionals, as did a statement by the Nobel Prize–winning chemist Linus Pauling, who had detected the mutant form of the blood protein that causes sickling. Pauling sug-

test for the dwarf couple in example 1. About four in ten students would veto it.

- A geneticist and a genetic counselor favored giving the dwarf couple the test; two well-known ethicists said the test should not be provided. They argued that using genetic testing to help abort a healthy fetus runs counter to its purpose.

- Adult readers split almost fifty-fifty on whether to tell the family in example 3, going against the patient's wishes. The ethicists agreed that the family ought to be told; saving lives, they said, overrides the right of confidentiality.

- Nine of ten adult readers would provide the Fragile X test in example 4. Students split fifty-fifty. Ethicists and one geneticist agreed that there was a slippery slope here, but they disagreed about where it lay. This case left ethicist Thomas Murray "very uneasy" because it flirts with eugenics, but geneticist Eugene Pergament was reluctant to advise *against* the test because to do so would be entering "that slippery slope of telling her what to do."

- Some readers, in contrast, felt that the case was not a slippery slope but a clear path to the future. "This case is on the frontier of how we define health," wrote one, and "will be the norm in not many years." It is "a perfect example of how applied genetics can benefit society," wrote another. "By making this decision, the woman takes steps to remove a harmful gene from the gene pool . . . improving the overall health of society." Another called the fictitious mother-to-be a "fine and noble woman . . . worrying about the future." All three of these commentators, for whatever it's worth, were men.

gested — evidently in earnest — that all sickle cell carriers should have a special insignia tattooed on their foreheads so they would resist falling in love with each other. "It is my opinion," he wrote, "that legislation along this line, compulsory testing for defective genes before marriage, and some form of semi-public display of this possession, should be adopted."

The critical flaw in the logic behind policies discriminating against *carriers* of the sickle cell gene (those who have only one copy of the gene and thus have the trait but not the disease) is that there was no good evidence that they were unfit for anything. The boot camp discovery may well have been a coincidence; the cells may have sickled after the cadets died, not before.

The adverse attention given to carriers of the sickle cell gene began to drift away only in the early 1980s, after a champion hurdler and mountain climber was found to have the trait and was forced to resign from the Air Force Academy, whose policy on the matter had been unchanged for nearly a decade. He filed a lawsuit and won. Two months later the Air Force abolished its policy of disqualifying carriers of the sickle cell gene.

Sociologist Troy Duster points out an interesting discordance between early screening efforts for sickle cell disease, which failed, and for Tay-Sachs disease, which have been a resounding success. Tay-Sachs disease is uniformly and quickly fatal. Sickle cell anemia is not—in fact, its course is quite variable—but only the latter was subject to *mandatory* screening in the 1970s.

WHY RACE MATTERS

Ever since Hitler there has been a taboo of sorts against linking genes to race. But it is becoming ever clearer that the matter of race is critical to genetic testing. For instance, the BRCA1 breast cancer gene now joins the Tay-Sachs gene as an inordinately common concern among Ashkenazi Jews.

Geneticists now realize that *race* is a cultural term, not a biological one, and that two different factors are critical to genetic testing: geographic origins (for instance, Ashkenazi versus Sephardic Jews) and cultural attitudes about testing.

"It's going to be ever more important to ask people about their ethnic origin," says geneticist Iordanis Arzimanoglou of Cornell University Medical College, who ran up against what he calls the "Hispanic dilemma" as he contemplated counseling patients about their risk of being carriers for cystic fibrosis.

CF is not especially common among various so-called "Hispanic" populations, but the frequency of the CF gene varies in different popu-

What accounts for the difference? Just looking at the screening programs themselves, he writes, will never give us an answer. At the very least, he suggests, we would need to look at information about the income, educational, and occupational status of the two ethnic groups to explain "the way in which genetic screening programs were funded, administered and responded to by the respective communities."

The development of programs for Tay-Sachs screening has tended to involve the affected communities, even to be instituted at their request. The medical profession has acted, as it were, on a consultancy basis. But one gets the impression that sickle cell screening (like the later Fragile X effort in Colorado) was a top-down affair.

Only four years after the Air Force Academy changed its policy about sickle cell screening, the federal Biomedical Ethics Advisory Committee, impaneled in 1988, decided to mount a study of the potential issues surrounding genetic testing for cystic fibrosis. A test to determine a person's CF genetic status was being developed at the time.

lations, so the question "What *kind* of Hispanic?" is not trivial. The risk estimates for American Hispanics vary depending on the geographic origin of the person's ancestors. Just as someone with ancestors from Mexico may not find much in common culturally with someone whose ancestors come from the Caribbean or Spain, their genetic profiles may be very different in important ways as well.

"It's amazing for me to find out that in the U.S. 20 percent of people can be labeled as Hispanics," he adds, "when they're different populations: from Puerto Rico, from South America, from Mexico."

Just as critical is the cultural difference in perspectives about genetic testing. A comparative study of black, Caucasian, and Puerto Rican–American women in Camden, New Jersey, showed wide and ethnically linked disparities in attitudes about many aspects of testing for breast cancer genes: how frightening the prospect of testing was, how women felt about having blood drawn, whether they wanted to hear the results alone or as a family, whether they would want a mastectomy "just in case," and how much comfort they found in spiritual matters. The context in which the information is imparted and received, as any good genetic counselor knows, is critical.

The committee was specifically concerned that such testing could create serious problems for society and might even lead to similar discrimination against CF carriers. What actually happened is a fascinating case study in social history. If you know of no one who has undergone cystic fibrosis testing, you're not alone.

In 1989 the CF test came into existence, but the Biomedical Ethics Advisory Committee (which was then dissolving due to a lack of congressional support) and other policymakers were hesitant to endorse CF screening programs, concerned that profit incentives among the testing labs, combined with fear of malpractice among obstetricians, would lead to a massive demand for the CF test, overwhelming the medical system.

The American Society of Human Genetics took a precautionary step at its 1989 meeting, endorsing a statement that advised limiting the administration of the test. Only those who had a relative affected with CF should consider undergoing the test, it said; general population screening—attempts to test everyone—should wait until the test was more definitive.

The Cystic Fibrosis Foundation, which had supported the search for a CF gene and cheered loudly at its discovery, was almost mute on the subject of screening. The foundation was intent on searching for a cure, which was the safer course to take. "With sustained research the primary objective," notes Robert Cook-Deegan in his history of the Human Genome Project, "divisive debate about [prenatal] CF testing and abortion could only undermine political support."

When the National Institute of Diabetes, Digestive and Kidney Diseases put out applications for grants to prepare educational materials to help CF carriers interpret their test results, it added a caveat that was certain to hamstring such an effort: "The scope of this topic does not include materials related to reproductive decisions." Nonetheless, its parent agency, the National Institutes of Health, stated that an urgent need existed for "pilot programs investigating research questions in the delivery of population-based screening for cystic fibrosis carriers."

One of the first studies of prenatal screening for inherited disorders had already been mounted by medical geneticist Peter Rowley at the University of Rochester. Rochester was the right location for a screening program: the university had a strong genetics program even before World War II. Doctors in the community were accustomed to helping with university medical research and would be more willing than most to undertake the extra effort required to use a new test for a relatively common hereditary condition.

Rowley began his research in the mid-1980s, before prenatal testing for cystic fibrosis was available; his study focused on tests for hemoglobin disorders. He contacted all the obstetricians in the community personally, at staff meetings, and offered to provide them with brochures and test kits, completely without charge, as long as they would offer hemoglobin-disorder testing to their female patients and their partners. Rowley wanted to examine three questions: Would physicians offer the test? Would women accept? And how would they use the information?

Only half of the doctors agreed to offer the testing, even in Rochester and even though it was free. Most of them offered it only to pregnant women, in part because that was the only scenario in which the test fit easily into their office routine. Most of the 50 percent of doctors who declined to offer the test said they were simply too busy to bother with it.

About 7,000 women were offered the hemoglobin-disorder test, of whom only half accepted it. Most of the remainder refused, they said, because they would not terminate an affected pregnancy anyway. However, of the ninety-seven women found to be carriers through this screening, all but five returned for counseling, and eighty-one of their partners came in for testing.

After CF tests became widely available in 1990 (a few years into the genome project), those physicians who were prepared to offer them often found themselves spurned by their patients. By 1994, even among the relatively few patients who were aware that a test for CF risk status existed, for instance, a mere 4 percent took advantage of it. Even members of the medical profession weren't particularly interested. Perhaps none of this would have surprised Rabbi Ekstein, but geneticists—who had expected demand for the test to be very high—were clearly taken aback.

"One of our concerns at the beginning was that the [prenatal CF] test would be so utilized, it would embarrass the cost of having a baby," said Rowley in 1995, meaning that the test might add inordinately to prenatal costs nationwide. But when he extended his study to include cystic fibrosis testing, the outcomes were similar to his earlier findings: "only about 30 percent of providers [doctors and other health professionals] took advantage of it. They felt it would take up too much time. And only half of pregnant women took us up on the offer. Few providers offered it to nonpregnant women, and surveys of women show they would rather have this when they are not pregnant."

The experience of Virginia Corson, a genetic counselor in Baltimore, was much the same. "I'm having nobody requesting CF screening, to be honest," she noted at a press conference in 1994. "People are not knocking at my door." Corson went on to say that she thought CF screening would eventually catch on through obstetricians' offices — where the matter would be "more complicated."

In another pilot project, researchers at the University of North Carolina offered CF testing to close relatives of ninety-nine CF patients. Testing happened one of two ways (chosen at random): either people came into the clinic, where they received traditional genetic counseling, or else they tested themselves at home, swishing mouthwash and returning saliva samples, like the children in the Colorado Fragile X program. People who were tested from home received a brochure along with the kit and could come in for genetic counseling later if they chose.

The results were unsettling. In one sense, having people test themselves was more successful: eight in ten people were willing to send back a saliva sample taken at home, while only six of ten among the other group actually showed up at the lab for testing. Clearly, one could generate the desired information by long-distance screening. However, few subjects in either group returned afterward for counseling.

By and large, those who tested themselves at home had no contact whatever with a professional. (Remember, these were not members of the uninitiated public. They had an affected relative.) People were willing to cooperate in helping doctors get the results of an imperfect test — but what did they understand them to mean for themselves?

Another research team, at Vanderbilt University, tried true population screening, making on-the-spot CF testing available to an estimated 50,000 people at university clinics, private doctors' practices, and even at a public walkathon for cystic fibrosis. The response was underwhelming, to say the least: only 166 of 50,000 people accepted the offer of a CF test. Well under one percent of people who saw the promotion even requested further information about the disease.

Why was the response so poor? Among those people who did follow up with a request for further information, about half said they feared that if they took the CF test, they would lose their insurance if their status was revealed. Nearly half feared what their partner might think of the result, and four of ten ignored the offer of testing altogether because they opposed abortion or had no plans to have children. Of the people who did accept the test, one in three were health professionals, and one in four either knew or was related to someone who had cystic fibrosis.

"This raises questions about the higher levels of uptake seen in other settings," reported the Vanderbilt researchers, "particularly about possible provider-induced demand for testing, and about the priority this type of screening should receive in allocation of health care resources." Testing that is encouraged in a doctor's office, in other words, is far more likely to happen.

Psychologist Joanna Fanos, who attended the session at a genetics conference in Montreal where these results were announced, put it more plainly. "Geneticists represent medical authority to a lot of people still," she said, "and I think we in the profession or related to the profession kind of forget that: the enormity of the authority. . . . People will agree for a lot of reasons, and one of the reasons I can see people might agree to these kinds of situations is, I want to be nice, I want to be agreeable, I'm kind of cowed by the whole situation, why not do it?"

Fanos would know. She lost a sister to cystic fibrosis when she was fifteen. While the Harvard experts were trying to rescue her sister, they used Fanos as a "little guinea pig." She remembers constant finger pricks, without anyone telling her what was going on. She was not being screened; as the member of an affected family, she was being *tested*, and with good cause. But she can identify with the mixed emotions evoked by a white coat.

There is an "underlying tension" about the goals of the screening projects, remarked pediatrician Neil Holtzman of Johns Hopkins University at the same meeting. (He would later head a national task force on genetic testing.) Are medical geneticists out to maximize the amount of testing or merely to let people know about their options? Their conflict of interest is hard to deny, because they are trained to provide the tests and to care for those who are having them.

In the genetic literature the very language used about testing is loaded. Geneticists routinely talk about "accepting" or "refusing" tests, and allude to levels of "compliance," as if not to be tested were to break a rule. When efforts to promote genetic testing are spearheaded by those who stand to gain from it, whether financially or just professionally, it can be difficult to discern whose interests are truly being served.

A case in point is the interesting episode of a New Orleans media event for genetic testing, sponsored entirely by the American Society of Human Genetics (ASHG) and spearheaded by that pioneer in the field, Peter Rowley. At the time of the society's 1993 annual meeting in New Orleans, Rowley, an influential member, rallied human geneticists to conduct nothing less than a public relations campaign.

The National Society of Genetic Counselors (NSGC) had moved its annual meeting out of New Orleans that year, in protest against an antiabortion law that had been enacted in the state in 1991. The NSGC's decision posed something of a dilemma for the ASHG, the organization of medical geneticists, who work day by day with genetic counselors and need their support. A serious rift about the matter seemed imminent,

GENETIC SCREENING: A MORAL ANALYSIS

How do ethicists actually dissect such issues? Here is a summary of one analysis, from a 1994 article about screening in the *Journal of Medical Ethics:*

Screening is ethically complicated because it can do both harm and good, depending on whose interests (ethicists like the term *utilities*) you consider. For instance, does the benefit of detecting cystic fibrosis at birth in one child outweigh the harm done to a different family whose child gets a false-positive test result? And how many false positives morally outweigh one true positive?

The principle of *double effect* says that harm is morally excusable if it is indirect and unintended. However, this argument fails in the case of screening, because it applies equally to potential harms caused by providing and by withholding the screening test.

The principle of *acts and omissions* might apply — saying it is much worse to actively cause harm than to fail to avert it. Many people are uncomfortable with this idea, however, and object to it as a high-minded excuse. If you can help individuals by preventing them from getting hurt, many people feel, you have an obligation to do so that is as strong as your obligation to avoid hurting them intentionally.

The problem with the latter argument, with dismissing the principle of acts and omissions, is that doing so places tremendous demands on society to avoid preventing harm whatever the costs. There is therefore an impulse to place boundaries around what we are required to do.

One way out of this dilemma, in the context of genetic screening, might be to say that people who are harmed by screening are identifiable and therefore are worthy of moral consideration, while those *not*

Rowley recalls. People were waving their fists and yelling when the subject came up at meetings. Unlike the genetic counselors, however, the medical geneticists elected to stand their ground in Louisiana and make a point.

harmed by *not* being screened are anonymous and therefore are not worth worrying about. But some ethicists argue that it is morally irrelevant whether you know exactly whom you have harmed, as long as you know you are harming someone.

Ethicists sometimes try to prioritize the various harms or benefits involved in screening, and to judge each case on its merits, but basing moral argument on the merits of individual cases has a name—casuistry—and a negative connotation. It begs for relative morality. As the ethicist Peter Singer writes: "If we can prevent something bad without sacrificing anything of comparable moral significance, we ought to do it." This brings us back to the original question: Whose "moral significance" do we respect, and how do we define "comparable"?

This remarkable pretzel of logical discourse illustrates a fundamental principle that ethicists like to bring out at such moments: It is not the purpose of ethics to tell us what is right. It is the purpose of ethics to help us frame the questions.

In the 1994 analysis the authors concluded by offering some principles for screening programs. They are rather simple and similar to those espoused by professional societies that have considered the same issue: The condition subject to screening should be important, treatable, and well understood. Screening should be cost-effective. The public should find it to be acceptable.

By these standards (as every state in the union has concluded), PKU screening of newborns is justified. So is mammography for the purpose of detecting *existing* breast cancers in women beyond a certain age. But screening for a genetic predisposition to breast cancer at that time failed to meet the standard because the mutation causing the predisposition was neither treatable nor (yet) well understood, the test was not cost-effective, and many women would find it frightening. The same is true of genetic testing for Alzheimer's disease.

The ASHG appointed a seven-member Task Force for Public Awareness, whose stated mission was to explain the purpose behind genetic services to the public. The task force enlisted twenty volunteers to offer themselves as speakers to local groups, and it also contacted news organizations to explain its mission. Families with serious hereditary diseases appeared on local talk shows to explain how they had benefited from prenatal diagnosis.

The society "has been of two minds" about social policy, said Rowley. "We have an experience with families that makes us want to improve the environment." The best they could do, he added, was to increase awareness. For genetic specialists, who had spent decades keeping a low profile in order to avoid reminders of a most regrettable history of abuses in genetic testing, the New Orleans public relations campaign was a noteworthy departure.

"There is a tendency of pilot screening programs to become institutionalized, without objective review of their merits," wrote pediatrician Holtzman in *The New England Journal of Medicine* in 1991. "If it is the technological imperative that drives the adoption of these policies," he added (meaning the urge to carry out new tests simply because they exist and can make money), "the scenario of premature adoption of screening will be reenacted many times as the human genome is mapped and tests are developed as spin-offs of basic discoveries."

"Commercial and academic labs are making tests available and are not making it clear that ... the test is still investigational," Holtzman wrote, reacting to a survey that showed that four of ten laboratories run by biotechnology companies, and one in four run in academic centers, had no contact whatever with the FDA or institutional review boards about any of their tests. Of the academic labs, 71 percent said they intended to market their tests to physicians who were not geneticists. The only federal rules that might govern such labs were aimed at regulating such matters as their personnel and physical facilities, not at inspecting the quality of their genetic testing. Moreover, because labs usually did not test entire families, they often could not put a positive result into the proper context to give meaningful odds of risk.

"A bigger problem that concerns many of us is jumping the gun," Holtzman went on. "Will there be organizations out there eager to test without sufficient information about false positives and false negatives?"

One American study found that of 100,000 babies screened for CF, some 300 had a false-positive result. Other research has shown that one in five parents whose baby gets a false-positive result has lingering concerns that the child is actually at risk. Who actually has benefited from those particular tests?

By late 1994, as the pilot projects for CF screening were being completed, the company that first marketed the CF test, Vivigen, had been sold to a competitor. The test failed to take off as promised, perhaps largely because of the American Society of Human Genetics' statement urging caution.

"When the CF gene was discovered," Vivigen's founder told *Business Week*, "I thought we were going to roll. But [the ASHG] took me to the woodshed."

In April 1997 a consensus committee convened by the National Institutes of Health recommended that CF testing be "offered as an option" (although not promoted) to *all* couples expecting or planning a child and "as early as possible." It was the first time a DNA-based test had been officially recommended to individuals not known to be at risk for the relevant disease.

"This represents DNA testing coming of age," declared Peter Rowley. Some other experienced geneticists cringed, however. The panel had neglected many of the practical and ethical issues that had been scrutinized in recent pilot studies of CF testing. For example, should it be offered to all couples, regardless of ethnicity? What about situations where both partners aren't available?

"This is a statement of what ought to happen eventually, but it's going to take a time which might be substantially long," remarked the head of the Human Genome Project, Francis Collins. Ultimately the consensus committee came to agree with him. Its final published report contained a subtle but significant alteration from its original recommendation as published in draft form. It now emphasized that genetic testing should "be phased in over a period of time to ensure that adequate education and appropriate genetic testing and counseling services are available to all persons tested."

While the gene experts and the biomedical industry were working at the riddle of cystic fibrosis, a number of important discoveries began to reorient the public debate from the unborn to the adult, from prenatal testing to predictive testing. Inevitably, genetic researchers turned their attention to some of the most alarming ailments that threaten adults in the industrialized world. Also perhaps inevitably, they proceeded to discover some of the genes involved in these diseases, most notably certain forms of cancer and Alzheimer's disease. The result is a number of new genetic tests that can be carried out on adults to determine whether they themselves—not their offspring—are at risk of developing a dread genetic disease.

A preview of sorts came in the late 1980s, with the emergence of a test for Huntington's disease, that rare, fatal neurological ailment that can beset a person in midlife and gradually erode both his ability to reason and his ability to move. The test provided the occasion to examine whether predictive testing was a boon or a curse, offering members of affected families the opportunity to learn whether they had won the biological coin toss (the disease can be inherited from either parent, so the odds are fifty-fifty if one parent is affected) or faced a grim and inevitable decline. Would people even want the test? How could they be cushioned from the emotional blow that would accompany the result, whichever future it foretold—the fear if the news was bad, or perhaps the guilt if it was good?

The experience of Huntington's disease testing was instructive. Although early surveys suggested that three-fourths of people at risk would take a genetic test when it became available, only 13 percent of them actually took the chance when it was offered.

People with the rare hereditary Li-Fraumeni syndrome develop cancers almost as easily as some children get scrapes—cancers of all kinds and in many locations: the breast, the brain, the blood. They inherit a known mutation in the p53 gene, which in its unmutated form inhibits cells from turning malignant. Someone with the p53 mutation particular to this syndrome has fifty-fifty odds of developing cancer by middle age, and a 90 percent lifetime risk.

A study at Dana-Farber Cancer Institute in Boston found that 42 percent of people in families affected by Li-Fraumeni syndrome—nearly half of them—refused the opportunity to discover whether they were at risk. Four in ten of those who refused said they were not interested; more than one in ten said they would rather not know.

Today, despite some strong opposition within the medical community and a great deal of public debate, companies are beginning to market tests for hereditary ailments that are much more common than Huntington's disease or Li-Fraumeni syndrome. At least two companies now market a test for genes that endow a susceptibility to breast cancer, and even though specialist organizations disapprove, a test that could be used to indicate a predisposition to Alzheimer's disease is also on the market. For many years to come, the field will be too volatile—and too rich with potential—for anyone to predict the future scope of testing, or indeed screening, for hereditary disorders among adults.

As with screening for Fragile X syndrome, the ability to test for genes that contribute to these two late-onset diseases has two faces. It holds the scintillating prospect of new treatments and cures at some point in the future. Meanwhile it presents dilemmas.

The issues are parallel to those surrounding prenatal testing: a potentially immense market to be served by (and to serve) commercial interests; the problem of distinguishing risk from certainty (you may have a gene for something that might never express itself depending on what else happens to you); the conundrum about how to endure the period between genetic diagnosis and promised genetic cure; and the ever-present risk of discrimination—as well as the specter of uninformed use of the test by doctors who can order it without thinking about the consequences.

"So many doctors will say to patients: 'Gee, if you're worried, there's this test. Why don't you have it?'" says Nancy Wexler of the Hereditary Diseases Foundation. She alludes to a case she knows personally in which a geneticist ordered a test for the presence of the gene underlying Huntington's disease as a special favor for a friend, who was a doctor. When the result came in, the doctor telephoned the patient and said the DNA test was positive. He offered no further counseling whatever, and a few months later the patient committed suicide.

Obviously such difficulties are not entirely new, but the genetics profession is still trying to come to terms with them. "Over time, it's sort of like the introduction of antibiotics, which changed the face of medicine," said genetic counselor Barbara Biesecker of the National Center for Human Genome Research at a press conference about the first gene implicated in breast cancer, BRCA1. "It will present us with a new way of thinking about many, many aspects of medicine."

At the time she was speaking, specific mutations in the BRCA1 gene had been isolated in only a small proportion of women from families in which breast cancer seemed to be hereditary. These families account for only about five percent of breast cancers. Women of Ashkenazi Jewish ancestry were particularly likely to harbor the first known mutation in BRCA1, but for women of other ethnic backgrounds—let alone for the 95 percent of women who will develop breast cancer that is not clearly hereditary—testing for mutations in BRCA1 was more or less useless.

Within a few years the picture has changed considerably. It would not be unfair, however, to say that it has become more muddled rather than clearer. Researchers are very excited to have worked out the nature of the protein created by BRCA1. It appears to be secreted from cells inside the breast and to control cell growth, perhaps rendering breast cells dormant after a mother stops breast-feeding. It is still too soon to expect any exciting new treatments as a result of this finding.

There are now more than three hundred known mutations in BRCA1, as well as at least a hundred in a second gene, BRCA2, also found to be involved in breast cancer. Few women (other than Ashkenazi Jews and members of a handful of other ethnic groups) can have any inkling which mutation might run in their family, making genetic testing for breast cancer cumbersome and expensive if it is justified at all. In any case, the number of known mutations linked to breast cancer is still so small that no woman whose result from breast cancer gene testing seems favorable can be sure she is free of risk. Surely other cancer genes remain to be found. We cannot know how many.

It is far too soon to say what proportion of women who harbor mutations in the breast cancer genes will actually develop breast cancer as a result. Many such "mutations"—alterations in the sequence of those particular genes—appear to represent normal, innocuous variations, or perhaps even protective factors, not harbingers of disease.

Meanwhile, it remains unclear as to what would be the best course of action after someone is found to harbor a mutation linked to breast cancer. Repeated mammograms may actually induce the cancer, because of the radiation risk. A recent study shows that the chemotherapy agent tamoxifen has a protective effect in women at risk, but it also has serious side effects. Not even removing both breasts will guarantee that the cancer will not emerge in surrounding tissue. BRCA1 has also been linked to ovarian cancer, where the only effective strategy for prevention is removal of both ovaries. No good tests exist that can detect this cancer in its earliest stages.

The latest studies suggest that for women at the highest risk—specifically Ashkenazi women—surgery may be lifesaving. For others, it's too soon to say.

With predictive testing for Alzheimer's disease, the scenario is similar, and like Barbara Biesecker, the pioneer of this test views it as a harbinger of the future. "This is the beginning of a new paradigm in medicine," says Dr. Allen Roses, forecasting that within the next decade medical science will unearth the genetic basis for other common disorders such as glaucoma, hypertension, and diabetes. "It's a paradigm of how that information might be handled," he adds. "All diseases that have susceptibility genes are going to have this paradigm."

As it happens, information about Alzheimer's risk already exists for some of us, because it pertains to a protein, Apolipoprotein E or ApoE, that was originally discovered to be a factor in heart disease. It is routinely measured in people with coronary artery disease, leaving cardiologists in a curious position. Dr. Roses himself has had triple bypass surgery. He knows that his own ApoE result sits in a medical record somewhere. Someone else probably knows what it is.

"If we tell you what your genotype is, the only thing we can do is potentially depress you or elate you, with no substantive thing we can do as a result," says Dr. Roses, who developed the test while working as a professor of neurology at Duke University. Research about ways to prevent Alzheimer's is "desperately underfunded," he says. "Rather than having that test, you should send the money to your favorite Alzheimer's research lab. That would do far more good." The best purpose for the Alzheimer's test he has developed, in Dr. Roses's own view, is to clinch the diagnosis in an elderly person who is already showing signs of dementia.

The incidence of Alzheimer's is rising in the United States, largely because Americans are living much longer than ever before. It's a disease that comes with aging, and in most cases you probably have to survive to a ripe old age to get it. Moreover, even if the genetic dice show that your odds of developing Alzheimer's disease are high, you have two consolations. First, once the dice are thrown, what they show is only *odds*, not a certainty. Second, as the saying goes, you should live so long as to have to worry about it.

A good many people who are getting the ApoE test because of heart disease may know their ApoE subtype, Dr. Roses says: "It has caused a lot of anxiety." For a while, as the one who discovered the gene's importance in Alzheimer's, he took a lot of heat about it. He was fielding angry calls from relatives of people who were very distressed after learning their ApoE results. In at least one case, someone was suicidal about the verdict.

The irony, as Dr. Roses had to explain again and again, was that the verdict wasn't a verdict at all. Any number of things could transpire in the decades between learning the test result and losing one's memory — if that was, in fact, what the future held. The test result did tend to focus the mind powerfully, but it was merely a proportion, a number, a statement without a context.

Duke University, Dr. Roses's employer at the time the ApoE test for Alzheimer's was created, holds the patent for that test. It has licensed distribution of the test to a pharmaceutical company, Athena Diagnostics

ApoE TESTING AND
ALZHEIMER'S DISEASE

Memory loss with aging varies in frequency, severity, kind, and cause. Alzheimer's, though the most devastating of such causes, can be diagnosed definitively only on autopsy, when the brain is seen to have distinctive plaques and tangles of fibrils.

Allen Roses calls these indications the "tombstones" of the disease — probably the detritus of a destructive process, not its cause.

While studying whole populations of individuals, Dr. Roses discovered that the age at which Alzheimer's disease develops is strongly associated with the inheritance pattern of a protein called Apolipoprotein E, or ApoE. A fat-transporting molecule in the blood, ApoE first captured attention in medicine as a risk factor for heart disease. It now turns out to be a strong risk factor for Alzheimer's disease as well, for reasons that are still unknown.

As in Tay-Sachs disease or cystic fibrosis, everyone inherits two "chances" at ApoE, two variant genes, one from each parent. There are three known subtypes, designated 2, 3, and 4. Separating the various subtypes is a difference of about twenty years in the average age of onset of Alzheimer's disease.

Incidence charts portraying the fraction of a population without the disease at various ages look like descending staircases. For the population of people with the 4,4 genetic type for ApoE, the stairs are much steeper. By age eighty-five, nearly all (but please note, not *all*) people who have the subtype 4,4 will develop Alzheimer's. Fewer than half of those who have no type 4 ApoE gene will develop the disease by the age of ninety.

In the general population, between around one in four people develop it by age eighty-five. If everyone lived to 150, Roses says, we'd probably all get it. It should also be noted that recent studies scanning the entire genomes of families affected by late-onset Alzheimer's suggest that altogether as many as eight genes may be implicated in the disease.

of Worcester, Massachusetts, which began to market it for diagnosis. Knowing an ApoE subtype can be most useful in determining whether an elderly person with altered cognitive function actually has Alzheimer's, which can affect the treatment strategy.

To prevent abuses, Athena Diagnostics puts limits on the test's distribution. When ordering a test, a doctor has to certify that the patient in question is already showing symptoms suggestive of Alzheimer's disease.

That's fine as far as it goes, but as Dr. Roses himself says, there are ways to get around it. First of all, cardiologists routinely test for ApoE type. Consider Philadelphia cardiologist Daniel Rader, who in all good faith sent a vial of blood for ApoE testing on behalf of a middle-aged woman who had an extraordinarily high cholesterol level.

The test came back showing that she had two copies of the ApoE gene associated with high risk of Alzheimer's. As he was talking to the patient about her test results, she revealed to him that her memory had been failing. Suddenly Rader was in the position of deciding whether to try to counsel his patient about a problem that belonged in another specialty entirely. He did tell her about the Alzheimer's risk. By his report she has weathered the shock fairly well.

Not so, perhaps, Dr. Rader himself. A specialist in lipid testing for heart disease, he was quoted as saying that after this experience he no longer wanted to use the ApoE test.

What shall we do about the Alzheimer's test? It is clearly unsuitable for widespread population screening, Dr. Roses writes (and consensus statements from various medical groups concur). At least half of patients with the disease do not have the high-susceptibility ApoE type, and many who do have it never develop the disease. While for people with clear cognitive problems, it can be helpful for a diagnosis of *existing* Alzheimer's, "it does not provide sufficient information to be an adequate predictive test," says neurology professor Richard Mayeux of Columbia University. It doesn't take into account other risks a patient may face, or even other effects of the lipid-protein system itself. The patient may be at more risk of dying from something else than of living with Alzheimer's.

Even the invisible, physically harm-free status of being a carrier — or perhaps *especially* that status — can cast a nameless spell over an individual. "Cognitive issues are only part of the question," says psychologist Joanna Fanos, who has spent much of her career studying how siblings of CF patients react to the prospect of testing for carrier status: "There's an underlying emotional issue." It takes time to unravel this issue, she adds, and like a genetic disease itself it implicates the entire family.

MUTATIONS, VARIATIONS, AND "NORMALITY"

In general, as we have known for many generations, inbreeding is risky. Inbred animals do not survive well in the wild. Hereditary diseases that are ordinarily rare tend to turn up more often in groups that are genetically isolated. Put very simply, a creature with a lot of variability in its genes is more likely to be robust.

Now that it has become straightforward to detect this variability, surprising facts emerge. Some people who inherit a subtype usually associated with a hereditary disease live long lives without ever showing a problem. Gaucher disease is a good example. There is also a wide range of variability in the severity of some mutations in sickle cell disease and cystic fibrosis. The explanation for this diversity may appear only slowly, if ever.

In many cases a genetic type is nothing more than a physical linkage. An identifiable gene lies very close on the chromosome to the as-yet-undiscovered gene that actually confers an illness, and both of them tend to be inherited together, so that someone with the identifiable gene is likely—but not certain—to possess the affected gene as well. The two genes may become unlinked from each other during the course of conception, because chromosomes can break and reattach in unpredictable ways.

Even if the gene actually implicated in the disease has been discovered and is detectable, for any number of reasons the disease may never

Fanos interviewed fifty-four siblings of CF patients at home, plumbing the depths of their imaginings about what it meant to them—or might mean, if they had not yet been tested—to be a carrier. Many of their responses were both misinformed and poignant, often revealing guilt and a certain alienation. Siblings assumed mistakenly that if they were found to be a carrier, other siblings would not be—although each child's chances are independent, like rolls of the dice—or that being a carrier meant being "a little bit sick" and therefore perhaps spiritually closer to the affected sister or brother.

develop in certain individuals. Other physical disorders may prove more troublesome. (For example, prostate cancer develops so slowly that many men die of something else before the cancer proves a problem.) People may possess unrecognized protective factors that prevent the disease from developing. We cannot know for certain beforehand who will escape a genetic susceptibility, or why.

A good case is the subtype DD of the gene that encodes angiotensin converting enzyme (ACE), a substance involved in the regulation of blood pressure. About a third of the population is homozygous for (has two gene copies of) the DD subtype, which is associated with a range of vascular conditions from high blood pressure to cardiac hypertrophy, pulmonary hypertension, diabetes, and a form of kidney disease. But this genetic subtype is far more common than the disorders with which it is associated.

Long before the Human Genome Project got under way, population scientists recognized that to confirm an association between a risk factor and a disease requires long study involving many thousands of individuals, including an appropriate control group that lacks the risk factor in question. Meanwhile, each association with a genetic variant leaves us with many questions: What is a "mutation," and what is a normal variation? What constitutes a "disease gene"? As some critics argue, is talk about such tenuous links between genetic variants and diseases just a molecular version of circumstantial evidence?

It's a question worth bearing in mind. As gene research continues, many such links will be sought and found. Many of them will be proven innocent. They will intrigue the scientists—and confuse the rest of us.

It can also alienate the carrier from others. "It is one thing already to bring with me when I enter a relationship," said one of her subjects, "or that I would have to bring up with somebody and say, 'This is who I am.'" Not surprisingly, Fanos feels that siblings may need counseling as deeply and as soon as the affected child does—and that siblings are often overlooked. It can be as difficult to convince some people that they are healthy as to educate some others about their illness, two doctors noted in 1978, speaking about sickle cell trait.

Gene testing has the clear potential to create a new population of "healthy sick": adults who live with the unwelcome knowledge that something in their genes gives them a distinct predisposition to a serious health problem—Alzheimer's disease or breast cancer this year, perhaps next year aggression or addiction. Beyond disease, we will need to acknowledge *dis-ease*: the state of expectation of a disorder that has yet to materialize.

It is sobering enough for someone to learn in the usual way that he already has a cancer growing inside his body. That knowledge alone deals his own psyche a severe blow and has immediate consequences for his family. But for an individual to learn, at a time when he is still quite healthy, that the seeds of cancer may have been sprinkled across the genes of his entire family—and can be unearthed on demand— may have effects that are at once subtle and far-reaching.

What should he do as a result of the revelation? Who else should be tested? Whose job is it to tell the relatives they may be at risk? Should he do it? Will his relatives be angry at him for bearing unwelcome information? How can he conceal this information, above all from his own brooding mind, in the desolate hours before dawn?

Research in the wake of the isolation of the breast cancer genes shows that when individuals are faced with the opportunity for testing, many of them choose not to know. A pivotal study reported in 1996 examined the preferences and decisions about genetic testing among 279 members of families known to be at risk for the breast and ovarian cancers linked to BRCA1. The study offered education sessions along with testing, then gave subjects the opportunity either to learn or to decline to learn the test results. Only six of ten subjects completed the education sessions, and nearly 60 percent declined to learn their results. More than 30 percent refused even to complete the baseline interview that preceded the testing.

The most common benefit the respondents associated with breast cancer gene testing (95 percent mentioned it) was the chance to learn about their children's risk of cancer. But four of ten mentioned concerns about the test's accuracy, and another third were concerned about losing their health insurance as a result.

"The results of the present study underscore the importance of conveying information, not only about the benefits of testing, but particularly about the limitations and results of these tests," wrote psychologist Caryn Lerman and her coauthors in the *Journal of the American Medical Association*. "Individuals who elect to receive these test results should be counseled extensively about the implications of these results, as well as about the limitations and results of available surgical and prevention options."

But Robert Wachbroit of the University of Maryland's Institute for Philosophy and Public Policy argues that, in this scenario, "the advent of genetic testing appears to have provoked a resurgence of paternalistic thinking." Some advocacy groups seek to protect test recipients from their own fear and panic, he says, "inadvertently ced[ing] the high ground to the for-profit laboratories that have rushed in to provide those tests."

The American Society of Clinical Oncologists, for example, recommended that cancer predisposition testing be offered only in the presence of a very strong family history or very early onset of breast cancer. The head of the Genetics and IVF Institute in Fairfax, Virginia, Joseph Schulman, disagreed. In early 1996, when he announced that his facility would offer breast cancer gene testing directly to patients who wanted it, whatever their reasons, he billed it as a patients' rights issue.

Both OncorMed and Myriad Genetics, the first two firms to market breast cancer gene tests, have made extensive efforts to educate doctors about the test and to ensure that those who sought the testing for their patients also enrolled them in long-term clinical trials, so the firms could clarify how often the test's predictions came true, one way or the other. Myriad set up a confidential, voluntary registry in collaboration with the Dana-Farber Cancer Institute to follow up on the various medical and surgical strategies that women and their doctors adopt after a positive test result for BRCA1 or BRCA2.

At the same time that the University of Pennsylvania's genetics lab offered the test, its Center for Bioethics began a follow-up study on how the decision to be tested would affect patients' lives. The National Cancer Institute set up a network for breast cancer genetic testing in which both counseling and research would be provided from the outset. This may be a model for the future.

Besides the deeply personal impact of genetic testing, we cannot ignore all of its adverse social consequences. Without adequate legal protections there is the risk that if such results are not kept secret, especially from employers and insurance companies, they could easily lead to discrimination.

In theory, the people who take samples of our blood could learn things about us and act to our disadvantage without even telling us what they have learned. Even if that Philadelphia cardiologist, for example, had ignored what his patient said about forgetfulness, her test result was

WHAT TO CONSIDER BEFORE YOU'RE TESTED

The National Society of Genetic Counselors has provided valuable guidance in its position paper on genetic testing for late-onset diseases. Although it was written for the benefit of doctors and counselors, the document also contains information about what patients can ask and expect as we consider genetic testing that might give us information about our own future. Here are the major issues to ponder before undergoing a gene-based test:

1. If something seems to "run in the family," are you sure that each relative actually had the condition you suspect? Many different disorders appear to be the same, and family histories may be inaccurate. The doctor should get as much written documentation as he or she can obtain about conditions relevant to the proposed genetic test in other family members.

2. It might help to have a support person who is not personally at risk of the same condition accompany you through counseling sessions and testing.

3. You need to understand how many people have the gene without ever developing the condition; the nature and variability of the disease in question; and nongenetic factors that may contribute to its development. What besides the gene may influence the onset and severity of the condition?

4. If the test is positive and you are at risk, what should you do to watch out for the emergence of the disease itself? What are the available treatments? Will you suffer anxiety or depression after learning the test result—and do you have unrelated emotional issues that you should sort out before undergoing testing? (For example, the position paper advises deferring testing if a relative has died recently.) What effect would a positive test result have on your relations with friends and relatives? Who will take

responsibility for letting your relatives know that they may be at risk? Would you be stigmatized? Or if the result is negative and you are not at risk, would you feel guilty? It is wise to decide beforehand who else you will tell about the results, and what impact that might have on their own actions, on your future, and on your relationships.

5. You should ask before testing how the results will be disclosed to you, exactly who else will learn about them, and where the results will be stored. Some physicians safeguard genetic information by using code numbers and keeping it separate from the general medical record. This protects patients against discrimination, but it also entails some risks: it shields the information from other medical professionals who might need it to make the best medical judgments, as well as from future generations.

6. Discuss beforehand who will pay for the test and how, and what will happen to the medical specimens afterward.

7. Take notes, or ask the doctor or counselor to take notes for you. You may want to refer to the information at a later date, possibly years in the future.

8. You should be asked for your informed consent, in writing, before you actually undergo the procedure. (Note that the word *informed* implies that you will be given all the information you need in order to understand what is happening.)

9. Inquire about how you can obtain follow-up information or counseling, in person or by telephone, from the doctor or counselor who has provided the test, as well as from other specialists and support organizations.

10. Most good gene-testing laboratories voluntarily seek accreditation from the College of American Pathologists/American College of Medical Genetics Molecular Pathology program. Inquire about the false-positive and false-negative rates for the test in question, and any other factors that may limit the validity of the result.

in her record. She might never have known what it meant, but if she filed a reimbursement claim for the test, her insurance company would. Without laws to stipulate what can and cannot be done with such information, individuals may be left totally in the dark, while others act on predictive information about them that is of dubious validity.

Allen Roses shares Richard Mayeux's concerns. "We strongly believe that insurance companies and employers should not be allowed to have access to such information that would have a major impact on patients' lives," he has said (immediately following a statement about the need to preserve the ability of researchers to "capitalize on the revolution in medicine").

Francis Collins told *The New York Times* in late 1995 that he found efforts to market the new cancer tests "alarming," because they were "treading into a territory which the genetics community has felt rather strongly is still research." Nonetheless, at least one network of oncology specialists had already signed up with OncorMed, the company that was then the leader in marketing predictive genetic tests for cancer (not only breast and colon cancer but also rarer malignancies such as retinoblastoma). "With time," predicted the CEO of the company, the option to test "will be available to every physician."

Probably the only thing that is certain about gene testing, two critics pointed out recently in *The New England Journal of Medicine*, is that it will make money for those who sell the tests. They warned doctors to recognize the limitations of the tests and the commercial pressures behind their speedy dissemination, as well as the many risks patients run by being tested. We cannot count on our own doctors actually to follow this advice.

Where the mutation involved in a familial disease is identified and well understood, and where a practical decision must be made based on a test result, genetic testing can certainly be helpful in a very concrete way. This is true not only of prenatal testing but also of tests for colon cancer, some other familial cancer syndromes, numerous rare diseases that can be treated by drugs or diet, and probably, before long, certain common disorders such as diabetes.

But for the majority of us at the moment, there is not much we *can* count on from most genetic tests, especially those designed to predict future disease in adults. Not yet, at least.

Their greatest promise is not for us but for our children or our grandchildren, as latchkeys to the information that may someday lead to cures.

CHAPTER 7

Missing Links

In a world where the actions and promises of the scientist are under increasing scrutiny, it is important for credibility ten years hence that this potential not be oversold now.

— James Neel, 1971

WE CANNOT PREPARE OURSELVES FOR AN UNCERTAIN future without an understanding of the events that brought us to this place. Throughout this century the genetic and reproductive sciences have been intertwined with social issues. Perhaps no one today understands this better than a population geneticist by the name of James Neel.

In 1939 Neel, who was then a young graduate student from Ohio, decided to devote his career to studying genetics in human beings. It was an eccentric decision, a most peculiar time to develop a fascination with the mechanics of human heredity. Writing about it decades later, Neel would refer to the decision as a gamble. Even before World War II the study of human genetics in the United States had gone through a decades-long slide, propelled by what he now calls "the incredibly sloppy and biased studies of the 1920s and 1930s."

The study of genes at the time was focused on nonhuman entities: small flies, worms, and rodents. There it flourished. Neel's mentors responded with disfavor to his intention to study humans. In 1939, to show too strong an interest in the mechanisms of human heredity was just cause for suspicion.

"Many of the senior geneticists with whom I had discussed a move into human genetics, geneticists for the most part studying [fruit flies], had almost perceptibly recoiled" at his stated intention, Neel writes in his autobiography. It had been only a few years since the German government legalized euthanasia for the "hereditarily defective," and most geneticists in America knew about it.

The United States and Britain had also flirted promiscuously with eugenics. In the early years of the century, many American states had passed laws mandating the sterilization of "feebleminded" individuals, and immigration laws had been tightened, largely on the assumption that fundamentally inferior immigrants were polluting the "American stock." Even before Germany's murderous excesses in eugenics became common knowledge, the field had been gaining disfavor among the American scientists who wanted to study "pure" genetics — the nature and influence of genes.

Neel finished his graduate studies, spent some time teaching biology at Dartmouth, and won a postdoctoral research fellowship. He applied to medical school and was accepted at the University of Rochester, still intending to pursue human genetics. But before venturing into the now-dishonored field, he felt a strong impulse to gain some firsthand knowledge of the best information on human genetics that was available at the time. He decided to delve into the massive archives stored — and by then, neglected — at the Eugenics Record Office at Cold Spring Harbor, about an hour east of New York City on Long Island.

For the previous four decades the office had been the nation's central repository of genetic information about American families and the wellspring of expertise about eugenics. Neel went to Cold Spring Harbor in 1942, hoping to find a wealth of good information gathering dust in those files.

By 1942 the place was abandoned and dusty — still crammed with paper but devoid of human presence. Its founder, Charles Davenport, perhaps America's most fervent proponent of eugenics, had retired and would die two years later.

The term *eugenics* was coined in 1883 by the English mathematician Francis Galton, a cousin of Charles Darwin. He defined it as the science of improving humanity by enhancing the chances that the "fittest" would produce more offspring than the "less fit." The eugenicists felt a mandate to help human evolution along. It may be impossible for us to understand this impulse fully, separated as we are from those people by a century of history including two world wars. "People were more confident of values and standards," writes historian Barbara Tuchman, "more innocent in the sense of retaining more hope of mankind, than they are today."

Galton pondered whether it might not be "quite practicable to produce a highly gifted race of men by judicious marriages during several consecutive generations." Put simply, eugenics was the concept of defining fitness in human beings and engineering its survival.

The Eugenics Record Office on Long Island was the brainchild of a patrician scientist and received its first support from wealthy business magnates. Like many other eugenicists, Charles Davenport, the man who brought this idea to America and made it sell, was an affluent Protestant. His father, a real estate broker in upper-class Brooklyn Heights, was a founder and ruling elder of the local Congregational parish.

Davenport had become intrigued by the quantitative aspects of genetics during his training as a mathematician, and grew devoted to the subject when he visited England and met Galton. In 1910 Davenport persuaded the widow of railroad magnate E. H. Harriman to provide startup funding for the Eugenics Record Office. He later won further support from John D. Rockefeller, Jr., and from the Carnegie Institution in Washington, recently founded by steel baron Andrew Carnegie.

"Davenport deplored the fact that the government had to support tens of thousands of insane, mentally deficient, epileptic and otherwise handicapped wards, not to mention prisoners and paupers," writes science historian Daniel Kevles in his detailed account of the movement, *In the Name of Eugenics.* "In part, his negative eugenics simply expressed in biological language the native white Protestant's hostility to immigrants and the conservative's bile over taxes and welfare."

From the benefactors' viewpoint, backing such an establishment as the Eugenics Record Office was doubtless the socially responsible thing to do—every bit as laudable as endowing a scholarship fund or supporting a home for foundlings. To be against eugenics early in this century "was to be perceived as being against modernity, progress, and science," writes anthropologist Jonathan Marks. "The ideas were inaccurate and insensitive—but they were modern science" at the time.

The Eugenics Record Office provided training in human heredity and field research to make extensive surveys and create genealogies of families across the country that had histories of supposedly hereditary problems, including insanity, juvenile delinquency, and various diseases. The field workers returned this information to the Record Office, where it was compiled, analyzed, and stored.

The office also issued publications and sponsored conferences for these field workers, and its officials and trainees traveled regularly, both to Washington and to state capitals, to consult about issues of heredity and eugenics. Davenport's right-hand man, Harry H. Laughlin, spoke before congressional committees and almost single-handedly won the House Committee on Immigration and Naturalization over to eugenic ideals.

Over the years people trained at the Eugenics Record Office got jobs at various institutions around the nation, where they used their skills to gather more genealogical information and to advise local government bodies about matters relating to eugenics. But their efforts and their training did not originate with the governmental agencies. As in Germany, American geneticists were influential in government in the early twentieth century, and their work was useful to some politicians, but they did not actually act for the government. The driving force behind American eugenics was not totalitarian or even federal. If anything, it was capitalist.

In his 1911 book *Heredity in Relation to Eugenics*, Davenport argued that there were clear signs that numerous undesirable traits, including insanity, "feeblemindedness," alcoholism, poverty, and criminality, were transmitted by heredity. Certain of these traits, he continued, had become uncommonly prevalent among members of particular ethnic groups — shiftlessness among Poles, for instance, and volatile temper among Italians. He favored selective immigration specifically on the grounds that it had been demonstrated scientifically that important traits "are inherited as units and do not readily break up."

Unless immigration was limited, he warned, the American population would become "darker in pigmentation, smaller in stature, more mercurial."

The problem in hindsight is that science had demonstrated no such thing, and that those traits were not well enough defined at the time to be the subject of rigorous analysis. Davenport lumped diverse behavioral and intellectual phenomena together, tended to ignore the influence of environment, and thought too simply of genes as single elements acting alone. He constructed extensive pedigrees without making rigorous attempts to substantiate what people said about the individuals in a family. Much of his edifice of statistics was built on shifting sand.

The Bible of the popular eugenics movement was *The Passing of the Great Race*, published in 1916. "The laws of nature require the obliteration of the unfit," wrote its author, Madison Grant, "and human life is valuable only when it is of use to the community or race."

The eugenics fad quickly became a nationwide movement. By 1923, when Davenport and others founded the American Eugenics Society, its membership included not only scientists but prominent educators, lawyers, and ministers — many of them also Anglo-Saxon Protestants. Like Galton's followers in England, they tended to identify as qualities of "fitness" the characteristics they ascribed to themselves: intelligence, industry, and moderation in personal habits.

The most visible eugenics efforts in the United States were the Fitter Families contests at state fairs, which put "human husbandry" in the same setting as the products of animal breeding. Contestants provided the judges with their family's "eugenic history," and the winners were chosen based on the results of medical, psychiatric, and intelligence tests.

The chief concern of the movement was the deterioration of the quality of American breeding stock through immigration and through overpopulation with undesirables. Teddy Roosevelt lambasted the middle and upper classes for committing "race suicide" by having too few children. He was among the proponents of enforced sterilization in the interest of eugenics, according to Kevles. So were H. G. Wells in England and Margaret Sanger, the founder of Planned Parenthood, in the United States.

It was eugenics, in fact, that transformed birth control from a movement of social disruption to a respectable social cause. Advocates such as Sanger noted that the middle class already had access to birth control and an inclination to use it. It was the poor and foreign-born who needed reliable contraception, to reduce births among paupers and criminals. "Feeblemindedness" ("the fertile parent of degeneracy, crime and pauperism"), Sanger argued, was on the rise, and meeting the "emergency" was "the immediate and peremptory duty of every State." The mission statement of the American Birth Control League, which she founded in 1921, lamented that "those least fit to carry on the race are increasing more rapidly" and that "funds that should be used to raise the standard of our civilization are diverted to the maintenance of those who should never have been born."

State governments responded in force. By 1914 some thirty states had enacted new marriage laws or amended old ones to limit the marriage of various types of "unfit" individuals, notably the "feebleminded." Many also enacted laws to enforce the sterilization of certain undesirables. By 1917 sixteen states had passed laws allowing the sterilization of certain criminals and, in many cases, epileptics and the mentally ill or "feebleminded" kept in state institutions. By the end of the 1920s, sterilization laws were on the books in twenty-four states, and nearly 9,000 Americans had been sterilized for eugenic reasons.

"FEEBLEMINDEDNESS"

Feebleminded, an ill-defined term from the outset, was used to refer to a wide range of mental deficiencies and deviant behaviors. Charles Davenport made the heritability of feeblemindedness a high priority at the Eugenics Record Office, and some of his field workers felt they could identify it on sight, without resorting to any testing whatever.

Psychologist Henry Goddard, who imported new intelligence tests to the United States from France in 1908 and tried them out at a training school for "feebleminded" children in Vineland, New Jersey, endeavored to codify feeblemindedness according to comparisons with the mean performance of people he categorized as "average" and classified by age. His terminology still colors our language.

Adults who were "idiots," Goddard said, had a mental age of one or two, and "imbeciles" were mentally ranked with children of three to seven. Those with a mental age of eight to twelve were "morons." He surmised that the feebleminded were a lower form of humanity, "a vigorous animal organism of low intellect." His intelligence tests showed high degrees of feeblemindedness among prison inmates and residents of homes for wayward girls. Truants, paupers, and prostitutes, he believed, were

Davenport's Eugenics Records Office played a pivotal role in the most notorious case of enforced sterilization in American history, the matter of Carrie Buck. In 1924 Carrie was committed to the Virginia Colony for Epileptics and Feebleminded, the same institution where her mother had already lived for four years. Carrie was seventeen and pregnant at the time she was committed (reportedly she had been raped by her employer's son) and gave birth shortly afterward to a daughter, Vivian. As a result of an intelligence test, Carrie was said to have a mental age of nine.

Information about the Bucks was submitted to the Eugenics Records Office, which decreed without examining any of the three generations that their feeblemindedness was primarily hereditary, describing them as members of the "shiftless, ignorant and worthless class of antisocial whites of the south." A Red Cross worker who placed the in-

doomed to their condition because of mental insufficiencies. He was certain that feeblemindedness was a Mendelian trait, like hair or eye color.

After seeing the results of the new intelligence tests, American eugenicists of the early 1920s, like Davenport before them, quickly fixed on immigrants as the root cause of the "menace of feeblemindedness," and they warned of a rapid decline in the quality of the nation's genetic stock. Few people remarked at the time that immigrants' low test scores could be the result of a poor command of English and ignorance of the purely cultural information asked on the tests, such as the names of automobile manufacturers and of famous individuals.

Around the time of World War II, standardized tests, introduced to the United States by California psychologist Lewis Terman, replaced Goddard's earlier version of intelligence testing. They were used at first to rank American military recruits—at which time some of their weaknesses began to emerge. Recruits who had had more schooling generally did better on IQ tests, yet many draftees who did not score high still performed creditably as soldiers. What exactly did the tests measure that was worthy of attention? We are still grappling with that question today.

"Feeblemindedness" was the true Achilles' heel of prewar American eugenics, because it was so ill defined that attempts to track it were corrupt from the start. One British geneticist referred to America's fascination with its purported heredity as "Mendelism run mad."

fant Vivian in a foster home judged her to be feebleminded because at the age of seven months she had "a look" that was "not quite normal."

The State of Virginia wanted to sterilize Carrie Buck. The order was challenged in state court and ultimately reached the Supreme Court, which ruled in favor of sterilization in 1924. Justice Oliver Wendell Holmes's opinion on the point has probably been quoted more often than any other single statement in the entire history of American eugenics.

"The principle that sustains compulsory vaccination is broad enough to cover the fallopian tubes," he argued. "Three generations of imbeciles are enough."

To judge from the subsequent evidence, he had overstated the number of generations by at least one. Carrie's daughter Vivian lived with a foster family until she was in the second grade, when she died as the result of an intestinal disorder. Her teachers reported that she was very bright. That leaves unresolved one bedrock-deep question: If Vivian was not actually feebleminded by any definition, what was Carrie's intellectual status? We do not know—but we do know that the means used to define intelligence at the time were highly unreliable. In any case, there is reason to question whether—even if the Buck family *had* represented "three generations of imbeciles"—its intellectual deficits were influenced more by inheritance or by social circumstance.

The Supreme Court ruling with regard to the Bucks was never reversed, but sterilization laws began to fall out of favor in the United States around the time of World War II. The Germans, as one Virginia eugenicist put it, "beat us at our own game." Perhaps ten times as many people were forcibly sterilized in Germany as in America before the end of World War II, even before the Nazi leaders and doctors extended their eugenics to mass extermination.

NATURE AND NURTURE:
NO CONTEST

Seasoned geneticists say that the old debate about nature and nurture is long dead. It has been obvious for decades—in fact, even Darwin himself knew—that heredity does not act in a vacuum. It is always defined by an environment. Nature and nurture interact.

Many of the eugenicists of the early twentieth century were blind to this reality or ignored it, assuming that they themselves were the "fittest" and that they were affluent and powerful entirely because of their genes. They ignored their nutrition, their education, their health care, their upbringing, their physical comfort, their social status, and the many other factors that went into making them who they were.

Not only do whole organisms act within their environments, so do individual cells. They respond differently, depending on which biochemical signals are acting upon them at any particular moment in the bloodstream, the gut, or the brain.

It is easy to see why other geneticists might have been nervous to know that James Neel was disturbing the dust at the Eugenics Record Office, searching for useful information about human genetics. He entered the stuffy library, dusted off one of the chairs, and sat down where young trainees in long skirts had once bent over large stacks of index cards. He set about poring through the records, searching for anything of interest, anything worthwhile.

Not all of the documents were unfamiliar. In 1933, as a junior at the College of Wooster in Ohio, Neel had written the Eugenics Record Office about his newfound interest in genetics. The office had responded with a "very eugenically oriented packet," including a fourteen-page "Record of Family Traits." Recipients were asked to complete the questionnaire and return it after documenting their family's characteristics "in whatever way seemed appropriate," Neel recalls, adding: "A more uncritical approach is difficult to imagine."

Without any former staff to help him, Neel found that he had

Twenty years ago we were obsessed with the idea that pollutants cause cancer; now we focus on the role of genes in cancer. Already, to many scientists in the field, both of those views seem too limited.

Smoking contributes to heart attacks, yes. But how? A team of French researchers found that one variant of a gene for the enzyme fibrinogen was strongly associated with heart attack and severe atherosclerosis. (Fibrinogen affects the thickness of blood by making the platelets stickier, thus contributing to the risk of heart attack.)

The correlation between the gene variant and fibrinogen levels held only in smokers, and the correlation with heart attack only in patients who had severe occlusion of the arteries. A nonsmoker might escape the gene's effects, or even a smoker who escaped other risk factors for atherosclerosis.

Similar interactions between genes and the environment must govern the link between diet and heart disease or diabetes, between chemicals and cancer, perhaps even between experience and mental illness. Which is more important, nature or nurture? The answer seems to depend on where and when the question is asked, reflecting the subtle and intricate nature of reality.

REFORM EUGENICS

Beginning in the 1930s a small group of eugenicists began to criticize the most egregious flaws of the movement and set about to reform it. American geneticist H. J. Muller argued that economic inequalities make folly of efforts to classify the heredity of either feeblemindedness or genius. He was so concerned about the effects of economic injustice that he wrote to Stalin about it and moved to Russia in 1935. (He eventually returned to the United States.)

British scientist Lancelot Hogben also lambasted geneticists for overlooking the influence of environment, and for racism as well. He scorned the studies that called a trait genetic simply because it ran in families. (So do such traits as mother tongue and food preferences.)

Historian Diane Paul notes that some classic eugenicists understood the weaknesses of their arguments, and some reform eugenicists had their prejudices. Nonetheless, something of a reform movement did overtake eugenics during the 1930s, she writes, when the American Eugenics Society "began to chart a more moderate course." Its leader, Frederick Osborn, tried to distance the movement from racism and warned against ascribing superiority to any group or class.

His efforts were doomed by events in Europe. By the late 1940s, after public revelations about Nazi atrocities, the eugenics movement and even the word *eugenics* had fallen out of favor.

assigned himself a formidable task. One drawer after another was stuffed with Records of Family Traits indexed "more or less" on some 750,000 file cards.

In the previous two decades, German eugenicists (some of whom later killed in the name of eugenics) had lauded the achievements of the office and regarded them with envy. Field workers trained and dispatched by the office had amassed more than 65,000 sheets of field reports and a few thousand genealogies. Charles Davenport had used all this information to respond to inquiries about the genetic fitness of proposed marriages and the inheritance of various illnesses. It had been a very busy enterprise.

This feverish activity notwithstanding, some of Davenport's own contemporaries felt that the founder of American eugenics — the man responsible for all those cards — was "not a clear strong thinker." One critic wrote to Galton in 1913 that Davenport's data had been collected in an "unsatisfactory manner," tabulated in "a most slipshod fashion," and led to conclusions that "have no justification whatever." He also lamented that others were finding it equally easy to reach similar conclusions by "loose methods," conclusions that "await the same chorus of praise from an uninstructed press, and from those whose passion it is to tickle the taste of the moment."

Among all the different files Neel examined at Cold Spring Harbor, he found only one containing material that seemed objective enough to warrant genetic analysis. It concerned red hair color, whose mode of inheritance at that time was still uncertain. The accumulated data in the file suggested it was a recessively inherited trait — and the data became the basis for Neel's first published paper in human genetics.

As he sifted through the documents at the Eugenics Record Office, a more important revelation came to him: the magnitude of the task that faced him or anyone else in his disfavored field. It became "brutally apparent," he writes, "what had to be done before human genetics could be a respected discipline. . . . There was little in the way of a legacy from the past to be realized there." In 1942, he realized, the best-organized efforts of American eugenics appeared to be all but worthless.

Although American geneticists don't like to think about it, seldom talk about it, and in some instances may not even be aware of it, there are many disquieting ideological and personal links between their history and that of the early eugenicists. Social historian Ludger Wess traces these links in his book *Träume der Genetik* (Dreams of Genetics). From the very beginning, he maintains, "the paradigm of modern genetics has declared as its goal mastering the phenomena of life — not [merely] understanding them."

A brief genealogy of genetics, as it were, shows how little has changed over a century. "I see an extraordinary potential for human betterment ahead of us," said James Watson in a 1986 article in *Time*, heralding the birth of the Human Genome Project. "We can have at our disposal the ultimate tool for understanding ourselves at the molecular level."

Almost a century earlier, in 1899, the *Chicago Tribune* had cheered that science was approaching the secret of life, reporting that biologist Jacques Loeb of the University of Chicago was attempting to create life in a laboratory dish. Loeb had been trying to get unfertilized sea urchin eggs to develop to maturity. He announced that it would be possible to apply the same techniques to mammals and ultimately to humans. The announcement caused a sensation.

Loeb was born and studied medicine in Germany. Later he moved to Zurich, where he became part of an intellectual circle that included eugenicist Alfred Ploetz, one of the founders of the racial hygiene movement that was later adopted by the Nazis. Then he went to Naples, which at the time was the international center of embryology. While there, he succeeded in creating tiny seawater polyps that had heads at both ends. It will become possible to control nature, he wrote excitedly to a friend, and to pursue a "technology of living nature."

In 1891 Loeb received a visitor in Naples, an American scientist named Thomas Hunt Morgan. The two became fast friends. In 1910 Loeb moved to the Rockefeller Institute for Medical Research in New York, where he was just across town and south of his old friend Morgan, who now worked at Columbia University.

Today Loeb is a relatively obscure figure in science history. He examined the structure of proteins, hoping to arrive at a mechanistic understanding of the nature of life. Morgan, however, is seen as one of the pioneers of genetics, because of the landmark genetic studies he carried out in fruit flies in the first few decades of this century (for which he won the Nobel Prize in 1933).

Morgan worked tirelessly to understand the mechanisms of heredity in laboratory animals by cross-breeding worms, frogs, salamanders, mice, and rats. Finally he turned to fruit flies, which were maddeningly tiny but also far superior for his breeding experiments because their life spans are so short. Examining cells of the fruit flies under the microscope, Morgan formed the theory that the elements of heredity must be contained in the long stringlike structures in the nucleus, called chromosomes. Luckily for Morgan, in fruit flies he had chosen a species whose chromosomes are unusually large and amenable to study under an ordinary light microscope.

Among Thomas Hunt Morgan's credits is the term *mutant*, which he used to signify an accident in heredity. He applied it to the chance discovery of unusual fruit flies with white eyes (the vast majority have red eyes). This discovery allowed him to pursue intensive breeding studies over many generations focusing on a particular, very well-defined

trait, and to reach important conclusions about the underlying mechanisms.

Morgan, who was in a sense the founder of American genetics, saw
fruit flies as a means to approach an understanding of human evolution.
He liked to read and think about the broader implications of the field,
and he especially appreciated a lecture in which Loeb spoke about the
possibilities of controlling evolution and society. In the same year that
Loeb moved to New York, Morgan espoused his own ideas in a manifesto he presented to the Pithologian Society of Columbia University,
entitled "Revolutions of Biology and Their Significance."

Mankind must take evolution into its own hands, he argued, and
must efficiently steward both individual and societal progress. Biology
must be used to improve human society. The forced sterilization of the
"feebleminded," he felt, was a step in the right direction, although he
also argued that eugenics should not be used to discriminate against the
lower classes and should be applied, by and large, voluntarily. Later he
explicitly disavowed organized eugenics and argued that meaningful
conclusions linking genes to race or behavior would be nearly impossible to reach. Meanwhile, he played an important role in sharpening
the focus of genetic research, drawing it inward, into the depths of the
cell nucleus.

One of Morgan's brightest doctoral students at Columbia, and an
important member of the group that carried out the groundbreaking
work on fruit flies, was Hermann J. Muller, a son of German immigrants
who had come to New York. Muller became one of America's most
prominent eugenicists and, for many years after others found the topic
distasteful, wrote in favor of voluntary efforts to improve the human
gene pool.

In 1933, during a research sabbatical to Berlin, he met the physicist
Max Delbrück and engaged his interest in the physical aspects of genetics. Delbrück became part of a group of scientists in Berlin who were
obsessed with working out the molecular details that defined the nature
of life. He began systematic studies of the effects of radioactivity in inducing mutations. It was perhaps the first work in the history of biology
to study biological phenomena at the level of atoms and molecules.

Some years later, a young American biologist named James Watson
became a student of Delbrück's. Delbrück persuaded him to move to
England in 1951, where a group of scientists were active in using X rays
to study genes and mutations. There Watson met a British biophysicist,
Francis Crick, and in 1953 they worked out together how genetic

information is stored in the molecule known as DNA. They won the Nobel Prize for their efforts.

Watson has been a prime mover in the course of molecular genetics in the United States. He championed the Human Genome Project before Congress and became its first director.

"We used to think our fate was in our stars," Watson mused shortly after the genome project was launched. "Now we know, in large measure, our fate is in our genes." Not surprisingly for someone trained just after the war, Watson has often spoken of the risks that genetic research could go ethically astray. As we will see, he took care to subsume the ethical analysis of genetic research within the genome project, ensuring that a small proportion of its budget was mandated for scrutinizing the social and legal issues related to the project.

Inevitably, many other intellectual pathways lead from the early proponents of eugenics to the leading lights of modern molecular genetics. Scientists stand on the shoulders of their forebears. What is worth marking is the deliberate amnesia as to some unsavory aspects of its history that has pervaded this particular field until very recently.

Once it was our mood as a culture to focus on genetics as the cause of our triumphs and our woes. Then we gradually drifted to the other extreme and fixated on the environment as both our cause célèbre (conservation) and our bête noire (pollution). Now we appear to have swung back again. There is determinism at both ends of the spectrum.

There are elements of truth in both extremes, of course. Reality, as we have discussed, lies somewhere in the middle. Those too enamored of the extremes serve neither science nor public policy very well.

Sociologist Troy Duster notes that in 1978, when he served as a member of a task force of the President's Commission on Mental Health, the shift of focus away from environmental and social causes of such problems was well under way.

Another member of the task force stated that the mission of the National Institutes of Mental Health had been "perverted" in recent years by studies that sought to explain mental illness in terms of poverty and other environmental stresses, at the expense of research into the genetic or biological roots of mental illness. "At several meetings," Duster writes, "I was astonished to learn how passionately several of my colleagues were committed to a biological or genetic interpretation of the causes of mental illness."

Such realities belie the assertion, especially common among researchers, that science has to be value-neutral. It cannot be. Scientists earn their livings, like the rest of us, by doing things that society finds valuable.

"Scientists are the ultimate prostitutes," admitted French geneticist Jacques Cohen a few years ago. "We have to go wherever we can to get the money we need to put our ideas into effect."

Naturally the questions they pursue will depend largely upon which issues their culture has decided are worth funding. Or they will campaign to win funding for the studies they want to do, for whatever reasons. They will probably want to do what their mentors have encouraged, based on the scientific paradigms in vogue at the time they are in training.

Thus the dominant social forces—whatever they are at any given moment—determine what will be studied and how. Then society takes the results of the studies it has supported and uses them where possible to bolster its decisions and actions. When we read that a new gene has been found to "cause" something or other, it is well to remember that nongenetic influences may also be involved—and that due to the fashion of the day, no one may have been paid to look for them.

Researchers like Davenport, or Morgan, or Watson, may sometimes work hard to shift the focus of social attention to a certain sector of science. However lofty their goals (or esoteric their methods), a scientist describes for us only one rational scenario about how things work. As to the definitions of concepts such as reality, importance, and merit— whether individual or collective—the lay perspective is worth every bit as much as theirs. We forget this at our peril.

CHAPTER 8

Otmar von Verschuer: A Gentleman and a Scholar

Let us hope that in seventy years we can reap the harvest
of this wonderful time.

— Charles Davenport, addressing the 1927 International
Congress of Human Genetics in Berlin

WHEN THE MOMENT FINALLY CAME IN 1946, WHEN THE
two American officials appeared at the door, Herr Professor Doktor Otmar Freiherr von Verschuer was not at home. It's easy to imagine his wife Erika, ever a faithful companion and defender of the eminent scientist, as she opened that door and saw two men, one of them in a U.S. Army uniform.

Major Vaughn Delong, an officer assigned to oversight of the University of Frankfurt, and Edward Yarnall Hartshorn, a civilian who was in charge of all the German universities under the occupation, had traveled all the way from Wiesbaden, only to learn that they had passed Herr von Verschuer going the opposite direction. He was back in Wiesbaden, trying to clear his name and smooth the way toward the creation of a new genetics institute in Frankfurt. But if the officials couldn't see the man himself, at least they could look at his archives.

Verschuer had fled Berlin as the Russian troops rolled westward, rescuing truckloads of papers from the huge institute of racial hygiene he had headed. Initially he had stored the papers in a number of inns surrounding his family estate in Bebra, a village not far from Frankfurt. For many months he had gone from one inn to another, sifting through the mountains of papers, filing this, burning that. All the human tissue samples that remained from the research had been destroyed in Berlin months earlier.

At the beginning of 1946 the president of the scientific research authority responsible for institutes like the one in Berlin, the Kaiser Wilhelm Society, learned of Verschuer's act and complained to occupation officials. Verschuer "is politically incriminated," wrote Robert Havemann, and it would be "impossible for him to responsibly be the leader of a Kaiser Wilhelm Institute." Verschuer had unfortunate political connections, Havemann went on, and "is to be counted with the prominent and activist representatives of fascism in science." Delong and Hartshorn had traveled to Bebra to see what they could discern.

There was nothing for Frau Verschuer to do but motion the two officials inside and watch as they began to pull documents and books from the shelves. The library indeed was full of works on genetics, but they would later describe much of it as "pseudoscientific."

The Americans examined a picture that hung on the wall of Verschuer's study. It was the image of Francis Galton. It was curious that Verschuer had chosen to hang the portrait of an English eugenicist. Why not a German eugenicist? Why not, for instance, Alfred Ploetz?

During their visit, Frau Verschuer volunteered that her husband had many friends among American and British geneticists. She tried her best to present him in a good light, but she could not have changed Hartshorn's mind about him. Still, neither could Hartshorn and Delong resolve whether Verschuer had actually ever done anything *wrong*.

"On the face of it," they concluded in a report about him, "Verschuer appears to be unusable [in a high position in a German university] under present directives, although he may be able to put up a strong defense on the ground that he has simply been applying standard eugenics, and not specifically Nazi 'race' procedures."

This conclusion was much gentler than what fellow Germans were writing about him in that same year, after he returned to the Frankfurt area following the collapse of the Third Reich. A local weekly newspaper referred to Verschuer as a "racial fanatic." He had been fined six hundred marks as a *"Mitläufer,"* a "fellow traveler" with the Nazis, someone who had turned.

A few months later Havemann urged that the new German government "should prevent this man ever again from serving as a teacher to German youths or as a scientist in his specialty of hereditary science and anthropology." Of course Havemann himself may have had a vested interest in frustrating Verschuer's ambitions: as a Berliner, he would have felt that the nation's premier institute in the field — it would be called "human genetics" now, not "racial hygiene" — should be in Berlin. But Verschuer intended to reestablish the great genetics institute in Frank-

furt, the first German institute of racial hygiene, where he had made his
start and which he had headed until 1942.

Now the books and documents from Berlin were not far from Frankfurt. He had always been a scientist of the highest professional standing,
and all the volumes he had published contained not a shred of evidence
that he had endorsed the gruesome acts of extermination that were now
coming to light. To his mind, there was no good reason why he should
not continue to pursue the rigorous science he had always practiced.

Other German scientists in his shoes had committed suicide on the
run. But not Verschuer. He had come back west, prepared to begin
again.

A decade earlier, in the spring of 1935, Verschuer had stood at a podium
in Frankfurt full of pride and optimism, gazing at the audience of high
business and government officials who had gathered to celebrate the
opening of his new institute. "We stand at the beginning of a new development," he had said. "Our research shall be responsible for making
Germany the world leader in racial and hereditary protection."

"To enable the progress of the German people through biology," he
had concluded at the end of a long address, "that is the goal of our work."
There would have been loud applause.

This was a year after Anne Frank and her family had left Frankfurt
for Amsterdam. The Eugenics Record Office on Long Island was already a quarter of a century old.

Two years had passed since a new law had relieved Jews and Communists all over Germany of their government jobs, including professors. Verschuer's new Institute for Genetics and Racial Hygiene would
inherit all of the furnishings of the former Institute of Anthropology,
which had been established and funded by Jews. The city government
had ordered Frankfurt University to see that all of Verschuer's wishes
were fulfilled.

In 1934 the Prussian Ministry of Science and Art had decided that
Frankfurt would be an ideal location for a new racial hygiene institute.
The population of the Frankfurt area offered "an unusually interesting
racial mixture of northern, western, Westphalian and Frankish types
and a variety of other mixtures," it noted. The city government had already set in place the mechanisms for gathering records about hereditary conditions in every resident of the metropolitan area.

"The establishment of such a professor with a huge institute, unique
in the west, would be of extraordinary importance for the university,"

wrote a government official. The advantages to society would go without saying. The university made a show of examining other candidates to head the institute, but Verschuer was clearly the obvious choice.

"Understandably, through his entire work area, Verschuer stands on the foundations of the National Socialist [i.e., Nazi] worldview," wrote university officials. "He stems from a Protestant, landowning family, is 38 years old, and brings by nature all the qualifications to teach genetic research and racial hygiene in the Nazi sense."

He was not a member of the Nazi party, the document granted, but then, he was "not of a combative nature." Nonetheless, he had served with distinction as a lieutenant in World War I. And in his chosen profession he already had distinguished credentials, as head of the division of human genetics at the prestigious Kaiser Wilhelm Institute for Anthropology in Berlin, under his mentor, the institute's director, Eugen Fischer.

What Verschuer had already published in the young field of racial hygiene was groundbreaking, and thoroughly upheld the aims of the Nazi regime. "A good *Volksmaterial* is the greatest richness of the state," Verschuer wrote in an academic journal in 1922, even before he graduated from medical school. "The quality of this national material depends upon the composition of its genetic makeup. The entire population is, as much as single individuals, subject to laws. Among the foremost purposes of the state belongs the responsibility to research these natural laws."

Frankfurt University set about to fulfill this responsibility, through Verschuer, with the utmost haste. Verschuer moved his family from Berlin to Frankfurt in the new year, took occupancy of a fine three-story house on Eichendorfstrasse, and set out to find a suitable parish where the family could attend church. By the time of the opening ceremonies on June 19, a mere ten weeks after Verschuer's official appointment, alterations were complete on the new institute, which was outfitted with the best possible furnishings. It was located on the top floor of Public Health House—a long, squat four-story building on the south bank of the river Main, near the university clinic.

To accompany the publication of his inaugural address in the new journal *Der Erbarzt (The Medical Geneticist)*, Verschuer provided a floor plan of the fifty-eight-room institute and a number of photographs. They show examining tables and stools, empty lecture rooms furnished with blackboards and overhead projectors, shiny chrome lamps, empty corridors, laboratories, and waiting rooms that were truly waiting. As head of the university's largest institute, Verschuer had every reason to expect unparalleled support and success. But there would be problems.

Given a favorable political climate, German medical professionals had worked quickly to set eugenics in motion. Adolf Hitler was appointed Reich chancellor in January 1933. One year later, in January 1934, the German government passed the first of its "racial hygiene" laws. The Law for the Prevention of Genetically Ill Offspring mandated the sterilization of all people with any of nine broadly defined conditions that were thought to be hereditary.

The law, like all the high-minded academic literature behind the eugenics program (including Verschuer's own writings), spoke as if these sterilizations would be voluntary acts of a populace that fully supported its own improvement. (It also assumed that the nature of "heredity" and "feeblemindedness" were well understood.) The law was promoted to the public through articles, seminars, broadcasts, films, and a variety of other propaganda measures.

By 1935, when Verschuer arrived in Frankfurt, the city already possessed a genetic registry, unrivaled in all of Germany, that gave health officials the means to find those people who should be rendered permanently infertile under the new law. The city health department had amassed some 100,000 "heredity cards" from a network of health agencies, which documented information about individuals with mental illness, hereditary disorders, sexual abnormalities, and alcohol problems. By law, doctors or agencies that failed to report such matters were subject to punishment. People judged to be "inferior" were thereafter excluded from public support and health care. City health officials had also begun extensive research into the backgrounds of applicants for marriage licenses.

In the same week that Verschuer opened his new institute, an article by Dr. Werner Fischer-Defoy, a Frankfurt health official, appeared in a local weekly magazine. After the listings of current opera and film openings (*Lohengrin* and Greta Garbo) and political events (a speech by Goebbels), Dr. Fischer-Defoy held forth at length on "The Health Services of the City of Frankfurt-on-Main."

Verschuer's new genetics institute merited one sentence in eight pages. But Dr. Fischer-Defoy devoted several paragraphs to the heredity assessment division of the city health department, which had been established two years earlier. This division "performs important work in documenting the hereditarily inferior part of the population, who must absolutely be recognized if all our available force and resources are to

THE LAW FOR THE PREVENTION OF GENETICALLY ILL OFFSPRING

"The *völkisch* state must see to it that only the healthy beget children," wrote Hitler. "It must declare unfit for propagation all who are in any way visibly sick or who have inherited a disease and can therefore pass it on." It was up to the state, with the help of eugenics scientists, to decide who was "hereditarily sick."

Those who were to be surgically sterilized by order of "hereditary health courts" (to which doctors were legally required to refer the relevant patients) included the "feebleminded"; people with schizophrenia, manic depression, epilepsy, Huntington's disease, or grave bodily malformation; the deaf, the blind, and the alcoholic.

The 1933 Law for the Prevention of Genetically Ill Offspring ordered that people were to be sterilized when, "in great probability, in the experience of medical science," their descendants would suffer "severe bodily or psychological genetic defects."

Individuals could apply to be sterilized on their own behalf, or representatives could apply on behalf of the mentally ill or those under eighteen. Doctors and heads of hospitals could also apply for a sterilization order.

Judgments about sterilization were made by a special Genetic Court, consisting of a civil court judge and two doctors. Its proceedings were confidential. Complaints could be made to a Genetic Appeals Court, whose decisions were final. If an appeal was rejected, doctors could apply to the police to take "necessary measures" to ensure that the sterilization went ahead. Persons involved in the process were ordered to keep it secret, under penalty of a fine or a year's imprisonment.

help the superior part of the population," he explained straightforwardly.

Verschuer's arrival at the university presented the local government with a problem unique in Germany: how could it accommodate two institutions, each of which was intent on registering its citizens under the new laws? In a letter to the mayor, Dr. Fischer-Defoy complained that creating a second advice center for hereditary and racial hygiene would bring problems. Verschuer's institute should be nothing but a specialized scientific establishment, he argued.

Verschuer disagreed wholeheartedly. In the same month that the institute opened, he applied for a license to order sterilizations and grant marriage licenses. "Teaching shall only be an outgrowth of medical practice, which . . . is in a unique position to undertake hereditary and racial protection efforts," he wrote in the application. "I want my institute to take part in the practical achievement of racial hygiene," he added. *Practical* was the important word; he was not going to allow the Institute for Genetics and Racial Hygiene to be reduced at the outset to an ivory tower.

The head of the city's genetics registry, Dr. Kurt Gerum, had suggested to Verschuer that his institute should limit itself to studying relatives of people who had already been investigated or sterilized by the city. Verschuer shot back with a five-point proposal of his own:

(1) There shall be from now on only one establishment in Frankfurt that provides expert opinions on heredity. (2) All marriage allowances, all sterilizations, and all naturalizations will be researched at the university institute. (3) Customary activities such as naturalizations and marriage licenses will be prepared at the university institute. (4) A place will be provided in the institute where the city health department will be allowed to examine recently approved expert documents, under the supervision of Herr Professor von Verschuer. (5) The [city] Division of Hereditary Advice will be limited to the maintenance of its existing heredity records.

In the end, the city government made a Solomonic judgment. In August 1935 it granted Verschuer complete authority over the 90,000 inhabitants of Frankfurt south of the river Main, while the city division of hereditary advice would have responsibility for everyone north of the river.

The compromise was never very effective. Despite the city's well-documented desire to take a leading role in racial hygiene, relatively few sterilizations were carried out in Frankfurt. During the war years only 3,565 sterilizations took place there, compared with 4,500 in Cologne and 24,260 in Hamburg. Between 1936 and 1939 doctors at Verschuer's institute ordered 148 women to be surgically sterilized.

Even when Verschuer gave a sterilization his personal authorization, it was not always carried out. In February 1941 he wrote an order for a sterilization and immediate abortion in the case of a thirty-year-old woman, K.R., who had applied for a certificate of "marriage fitness." Verschuer denied her application, because from her "appearance . . . (black hair, yellow skin) one can distinctly recognize a foreign racial influence (Gypsy) and because feeblemindedness is present." The woman K.R., whom Verschuer also described as "small and delicate," already had a one-year-old son by her fiancé, who was serving at that time in the German army.

In his sterilization order Verschuer elaborated on her circumstances: "Although she has lived for twenty years in Frankfurt, she has never gone to school and cannot read or write. Her lack of knowledge about the war and about current events confirms that she cannot read or work. . . . About her life she says that she was always working at home, either for her parents or in-laws. No other cause for her feeblemindedness is evident. The clinical examination showed nothing special."

The woman appealed Verschuer's decision, and the Genetic Appeals Court heard her case the following month. It overruled Verschuer's order, noting that although the woman had only a small vocabulary and was not well spoken, "she has a definite and accurate understanding for matters of everyday life and for the practical application of her experiences" and was well able to understand the future consequences of her sterilization.

"She often showed in the examination of the court that she is capable of fine spiritual sensibilities," the written decision continues. "One could also gain the impression from the son whom she brought with her to the appointment that she well understood how to fulfill her duties as a mother."

Verschuer lodged a complaint against the decision and took the matter to a higher court, arguing that the lower court had not ruled on his opinion that the woman was a Gypsy. He sent as evidence a book by one Robert Ritter, a psychiatrist who had made his reputation writing about the racial inferiority of Gypsies. He argued that the woman in question belonged to the same racial type, which Ritter described as having "disguised feeblemindedness."

The higher court conducted extensive follow-up studies on K.R.'s family, seeking further information from the Gypsy division of the criminal police (which called her entire family "asocial to the highest degree") and from the neurology clinic at the university. The latter wrote that K.R. comported herself so "completely trouble-free and inconspicuously" during her examination that it could exclude any sign of feeblemindedness. "One can make only the exception that K.R., solely on the grounds of her limited life experience, could be judged feebleminded," the clinic argued. The higher court also ruled against the sterilization.

Three years earlier, in his now-influential journal *Der Erbarzt*, Verschuer had argued for a change in the sterilization laws. He had suggested that the conditions for sterilization be broadened to "severe hereditary disturbances, severe hereditary illness, and severe hereditary physical abnormalities." His main rationale was that his experience had shown him that "the number of genetic illnesses is so huge and diverse that in the current diagnostic system everything cannot be ordered sensibly." In other words, he wanted doctors to be free to order sterilizations without being obliged to explain their decisions based on specific diagnoses.

Verschuer's suggestion was never written into law. Nonetheless, his influence on the course of racial hygiene in Germany was unparalleled. He was the only professor who was seen by virtually every student at Frankfurt University, where he lectured at the medical school, the law school, the school of social science, and to all freshmen through a course on "Population, State and Politics."

At the Institute for Genetics and Racial Hygiene, his students took part not only in theoretical science but in practice — doing statistical work, translating documents about racial matters into lay language, assisting in Verschuer's studies. In all, each year, the institute performed about one thousand examinations and provided between one hundred and three hundred written opinions to support sterilizations, marriage approvals (or denials), and paternity.

The paternity testing was almost always done in the interests of racial hygiene — to "document" whether someone had Jewish roots. Frau Verschuer insisted, after her husband's death, that he had created the institute in order to rescue people from the racial laws, but judging from what he wrote, he was more intent on rescuing society from such people. Certainly a paternity judgment from the institute could be a matter of life and death. No records survive to tell us how many such judgments were death warrants.

As editor of *Der Erbarzt*, Verschuer's many articles reached almost every doctor in Germany. Nearly every month he published an advice column disseminating his expert opinion about a question of heredity in a particular case. For instance, in 1935 a reader inquired about an otherwise healthy twenty-six-year-old man who had been born with facial abnormalities, which were successfully corrected by surgery. The young man wanted to be married.

"The statement that there are no similar facial abnormalities in the parents and other relatives of your patient says nothing about the heredity of the condition," Verschuer responded. "Probably if we studied the family carefully we would find other abnormalities." He recommended that the young man be sterilized. "More than the ordinary doctor," he wrote in the next opinion, "the racial hygienist finds himself in conflict trying to define the right path between the interests of the individual and the interests of the state."

Verschuer's particular passion was hereditary studies on identical twins, in whom he claimed to have proven a hereditary factor in susceptibility to tuberculosis. But he distinguished himself among eugenicists as a practitioner, as one who not only wrote voluminously and published studies about eugenics but helped to achieve its goals.

The man who took these actions was no demented tyrant. His friends described him as distant, cold, and very proper, but in a photograph published in a history of the University of Frankfurt, his face appears gentle, almost kindly. (He is tall and slender, wearing a white coat as he measures the shoulder span of a twin girl.)

"Many a skeptic would shrink back from the difficulties standing in the way, above all in connection with the affected human beings," he had said to his elite audience on the day the Frankfurt institute opened. "These [difficulties] shall be overcome," he continued, "through perseverance and patience, through adaptability and empathy—and through a warm heart!"

Verschuer was a highly principled man, whose deepest principles, as it happened, dovetailed nicely with the politics of the era. "For him God's will manifested itself in world history," said the son of one of his colleagues, "and obedience always seemed to him to be the chief virtue. So he believed in God and in his national leader, the Führer."

"My father always said, 'Give to God what is God's and to Caesar what is Caesar's,'" said his own son Helmut, after his father's death. Verschuer seemed to have little difficulty keeping the two separate. Even under the Third Reich he went to church every Sunday as a member of the Bekennende Kirche (the Confessional Church), a new denomination that evolved out of a resistance movement against Hitler. When he returned to Berlin from Frankfurt in 1942 to take up his new appointment, the family joined the Bekennende Kirche there, although the pastor of that parish was in prison as a dissident.

We don't know why Verschuer chose the Bekennende Kirche, but he could tolerate the irony because he was, as many friends put it, apolitical. Verschuer was a close friend of Adam von Trott du Solz, another member of the nobility from the same county. At von Trott's urging, Verschuer had decided against taking part in a loyalty rally for Hitler in their hometown of Solz. But when von Trott was later executed for plotting to kill Hitler, according to Helmut von Verschuer, his father said that such an action during wartime was "highly irresponsible."

Verschuer was a member of the Nazi party but not an avid one. As Helmut remembered, after the family moved to Frankfurt, his father was impelled to join the party in order to keep his position, but he somehow delayed joining until 1940. Helmut says he never remembered seeing his father wear the party insignia. What Verschuer wore instead was a white coat.

"As a scientist," according to a recent history of Frankfurt University, "von Verschuer sought to create a certain distance from the regime. . . . He said that [until then] narrow middle-class principles of the nineteenth century had created the standards to decide who should be excluded from reproducing, as a pest within the population. Verschuer dared to say that such selections should not extend to murdering the individuals."

It also seems unlikely that Verschuer was notably anti-Semitic. Helmut remembered that when he was eight or nine, a soldier asked him to buy a packet of cigarettes. When he returned from the newsstand around the corner, the soldier remarked that he should not be buying things from a Jewish merchant. Helmut promptly went home to ask his father what "Jewish" meant. As time went on, he said, he realized that many of the friends who had visited their home in the earlier years in Berlin were Jewish. Many colleagues said that before 1933 Verschuer had worked with many Jews, and that they had never witnessed any sign of aversion or discrimination on his part. (Members of his research team ranged from SS officers to former socialists and Communists.)

"He never said, 'The Jews are bad,'" recalled the daughter of Verschuer's mentor, Eugen Fischer. "'The Jews are different,' he said."

Like many Germans before and after him, Verschuer had nothing in particular against Jews except the fact that they were not, as he saw it, "real Germans" and therefore threatened to "pollute" the German race. A recollection in his own words describes his position best:

"In the spring of 1924," he wrote, "in a training camp established by a students' group, I gave a speech about racial hygiene. During the discussion one of the student leaders gave me the following opinion. He had noticed that anthropological science had as yet not proved the racial inferiority of the Jews. Such a proof, he said, was necessary for the foundation of anti-Semitism.

"I answered him that anti-Semitism is, in the first instance, a national political war, whose justification and necessity—independent of any evaluation of the worth of the Jewish race—established itself because of the threat to our population from the Jews. . . . The German national war is justified in the first instance against the Jews, because the German population was particularly threatened in this manner from Jewish infiltration."

For Verschuer, it was not by any means only the Jews who threatened Germany; there were Gypsies, and a wide assortment of people with hereditary "defects." He wrote in 1928, just after completing his doctoral dissertation, that "the users of today's unemployment insurance are to a man 'work shy' and are spiritually and genetically inferior people." Extending social insurance to the entire population, he argued, "leads therefore to severe racial hygienic damage."

In 1942 Verschuer's mentor Eugen Fischer retired as director of the Kaiser Wilhelm Institute for Anthropology in Berlin. Verschuer was appointed to succeed him. It was the most influential post a geneticist could have in Germany.

Several of Verschuer's colleagues chose to transfer to Berlin with him, rather than stay behind in Frankfurt and work under his successor, an avid Nazi. Besides, Verschuer was clearly a rising star, and as such he was the one to follow.

One of those who wanted to follow Verschuer was his chief protégé, a young anthropologist who had collaborated in Verschuer's extensive twin studies in Frankfurt. His name was Josef Mengele. Mengele had come to Frankfurt in 1938, where he carried out some respectable studies on the heredity of the cleft lip and palate. Later Mengele became notorious for his cruelty, but what he had always wished for himself was to become eminent like his mentor. The inspiration for his line of experiments, the role model for his career, and his constant supporter and coworker, was Otmar von Verschuer.

No job was open for Mengele at the Kaiser Wilhelm Institute in Berlin in 1942, but he soon found what both he and Verschuer viewed as a better opportunity. In 1943 he took up a new post as chief physician at the Auschwitz concentration camp.

For Verschuer (who probably never saw Auschwitz), Mengele's Auschwitz appointment was a marvelous research opportunity. In wartime conditions it was becoming ever more difficult for him to keep in touch with the subjects for his twin studies. They were dispersed all over Germany, and he could no longer travel freely to carry out his follow-up studies on their families.

The chief doctor at Auschwitz, however, was in the ideal position to screen a large population in search of twins. Verschuer applied to the German Research Society, on Mengele's behalf, for funds to support two studies. One was entitled "Specific Albumin" and the other was a study of the inheritance of eye color. Both applications were approved. The necessary equipment—incubators, centrifuges—arrived at Auschwitz soon afterward.

Since the end of the war, and after countless articles and some postwar court proceedings conducted in his absence, Mengele's image has become familiar. Survivors remember him as the embodiment of cruelty, a man who could give candy to children one moment and stamp a woman to death the next. He was the straight-backed man with white coat and riding whip who stood at the top of the selection ramp, whistling Wagner and smiling as he scrutinized the incoming mass of people and flicked his thumb to the left or right, death or slave labor. Often Mengele would plunge into the mass of humanity, shouting "Twins! Twins! All twins step forward!" When he located a pair of identical twins, he would beam with pleasure.

Mengele needed a variety of twins for his "experiments." He would inject their eyes with dye to see if they changed color. One woman who was spared death for Mengele's purposes recalls that she and her identical twin sister were given injections of blood from unrelated male twins. They endured severe fever from immune reactions, but they survived. They knew that Mengele intended to inseminate them with sperm from the male twins, but they were spared this fate by the ending of the war. Meanwhile Mengele gave them treats such as white bread and a tour of the Gypsy camp. He ordered the band to play for them, and it did. The next day the Gypsy camp was emptied, and the crematoria worked overtime, spewing ash into the air.

Mengele gave the twins special treatment because of their research value. He fed them well and often even coddled them—until he decided a particular experiment had come to its end, and it was time for dissection. Then he would personally inject cyanide into their arms or even directly into their hearts, which was even quicker. Afterward his slave pathologist, Dr. Miklos Nyiszli, would extract the eyes or any other tissues that might be of interest.

Nyiszli packed these tissue samples carefully, labeled them "Urgent War Materials," and shipped them off to Berlin. A letter of acknowledgment always followed, in which the directors of the Kaiser Wilhelm Institute "thanked Dr. Mengele heartily for this rare and valuable material."

Mengele's research on twins had at least the appearance of being systematic. He searched for twins who had one blue and one brown eye, killed them, and again sent the tissues to Berlin. He infected identical and fraternal twins with the same dose of typhus bacterium, withdrew blood at various times, sent the specimens to Berlin for chemical studies, and followed the course of the illness. Whether Verschuer ever knew that the twins had been intentionally injected and later killed, or assumed without asking that they had died during the frequent epidemics at Auschwitz, we will never know. As the war drew to a close, he destroyed all his correspondence with Mengele.

Mengele did come to Berlin several times to report on his progress. "My assistant Dr. Mengele has entered this project as a coworker," Verschuer wrote to the German Research Society in an interim report. ". . . With permission of the Reichsführer we have carried out anthropological experiments on the various racial groups of this concentration camp, and the blood samples have been sent to my laboratory for testing."

During one such visit, over dinner in their Berlin house, Frau Verschuer asked Mengele if his work at Auschwitz was difficult. "It is horrible," he replied. "I can't talk about it."

Afterward the laboratory workers in Berlin insisted that they had had no idea about the ghastly origins of their research materials. "We had no doubt," said Verschuer's former lab assistant Irmgard Haase. "This was decidedly science. We had extracted the blood ourselves, and blood extractions are not [harmful]. During the war we never once talked about it. I absolutely only learned about the atrocities after the war."

Did Verschuer himself know what was going on? No one has ever been able to answer the question conclusively. We have only hints as to his train of thought. In 1943 he gave a speech before the Prussian Academy of Science that he entitled "Genetic Endowment as Fate and Responsibility." It was perhaps the most definitive statement of German racial hygiene.

Protection of its own race is the prime responsibility of a state, he argued, and for every person "fateful borders for his development are laid down by his heredity." (Negroes don't have white babies, he argued, the "feebleminded" have primarily "feebleminded" children, and so on.)

Are human beings acceptable subjects for scientific research into these phenomena? Verschuer addressed the question as he drew to a close. "If we are placed by scientific understanding before a really new purpose," he concluded, "then we must freely and earnestly reorder the question, after a revision of our ethical views." Did he revise his own ethical views when his protégé was using human beings as laboratory animals? We cannot know for sure. At the time, recalled his son Helmut, it seemed a "comparatively courageous speech."

Until close to the end of the Reich, Verschuer apparently had no idea that it was about to fall, ending his research. One colleague saved a letter Verschuer wrote him in October 1944: "Plasma substrates have been extracted from over 200 individuals of various races, twin pairs and individual kindreds," he wrote. "So we can actually begin with our research in the near future. The goal of our various efforts is now no more to establish *that* the various hereditary influences are meaningful in some infectious illnesses, but rather in which manner they operate."

In January 1945 Verschuer wrote to the same friend, "It will interest you, meanwhile, that at last my research about albumin is in a decisive stage." A few days later he fled toward Bebra with his family. Mengele left Auschwitz. They never completed their projects.

After the war Verschuer never succeeded in reestablishing the Frankfurt genetics institute. Despite all his efforts to clear his name, the government of the county of Hessen finally ruled in February 1947 just what the current administrator of the Berlin Institute had recommended: Verschuer could never teach or practice genetics in Frankfurt again.

But grumblings were heard in Germany that this treatment was unfair, that the U.S. authorities had been conducting a private vendetta against Verschuer after the war. In 1949 a commission of German professors delivered its own judgment about Verschuer's culpability.

"However much Dr. Mengcle himself was oriented to the cruelty and death in Auschwitz . . . cannot be determined from the existing documents," it said. But "it would appear pharisaical if we were . . . to reckon an inexcusable moral burden against [Verschuer], who otherwise nobly and courageously pursued his difficult road and often confirmed his noble convictions. We unanimously underscore the belief that Professor von Verschuer possesses all the qualities that destine him to the role of scientist and teacher."

In the same year Verschuer was elected a member of the German Academy of Sciences and Letters. A flurry of appointments to other scientific societies, in Japan, Italy, Austria, and Germany, followed. In 1951 Verschuer was invited to create a new institute of human genetics in the city of Münster.

That year, beginning in a barracks, Verschuer proceeded to create Germany's largest institute of human genetics. The name would be different, but the procedures would be the same. Verschuer established a large genetic registry of the inhabitants of the surrounding area and continued his research on twins. Of his postwar research, he once said that others would live to gather the fruits. In 1956 he was invited as the leader of the German delegation to attend the first International Congress of Human Genetics in Copenhagen.

His publications continued in the same vein as before; just as they had never truly been incriminating in a legal sense (proving that Verschuer condoned Mengele's murders for science), they did not now need much revision to be socially correct in the postwar era. Professional embarrassment would only arise if someone chose to look back into the documents of the 1930s and 1940s to unearth his advisories for the sterilization of individuals such as the "asocial" without any evidence that such traits were inherited. The odds were slim that anyone outside Germany would have any interest in one comparatively inconspicuous geneticist. The German biomedical community, like the rest of the society, was in a state of reconstruction and denial.

In 1961, however, Verschuer suddenly received some notoriety in the United States, when L. C. Dunn, the president of the American Society of Human Genetics, in an inaugural speech in Atlantic City, dredged up a statement from an old eugenics text Verschuer had authored. The theme of Dunn's address was how long it had taken the study of human genetics to prosper, and Nazi policies naturally got some of the blame.

"The history of our science is most intimately connected with German history of the most recent past," Verschuer had written in 1941. "The leader of the German state is the first statesman who has wrought the results of genetics and race hygiene into a directing principle of public policy."

"The author has not to my knowledge publicly altered his position on enforced race hygiene," Dunn observed. Verschuer, wounded, forced himself to respond from Münster in writing. He cited some of Dunn's accusations in quotation marks.

"Whenever such statements of my earlier publications are taken out of context and quoted they do shock me today," he wrote. "I now realize the errors on which such premature formulations were based, and I recognize the possible sources of misunderstanding which I have caused for the reader as well as for myself. . . .

"I never was a politician," he added. "I endeavored to serve only science and I was not an adherent of 'enforced race hygiene.' It is today obvious and clear for myself that 'I underrated the dangers of the movement,' perhaps because I was not politically minded." Among other defenses, he quoted a statement he made in his contribution to an obstetrics and gynecology textbook published in 1953: "The past has given a horrifying example of misused eugenics."

On September 29, 1968, while on vacation, Verschuer was struck by a car while going to mail a letter. He fell into a coma from which he never recovered. Frau Verschuer stayed with her husband almost daily until he died on August 8, 1969.

His longtime colleague and friend Heinrich Schade, who had been chief physician at Verschuer's Frankfurt institute, wrote a long and glowing eulogy in a German medical magazine. Verschuer had "huge scientific charisma," he said. The eulogy contained nothing with a hint of criticism in it, but recounted Verschuer's extensive studies in medical genetics. "Countless students grieve for him," Schade wrote.

Perhaps Verschuer had written an even better eulogy for himself thirty years earlier, in Der Erbarzt. "The circumstances of human genetics are very much more difficult than in experimental genetics," he wrote. But "even if we human geneticists could never come as far as, for example, the geneticists who specialize in fruit flies, we would be rightly compensated by the satisfaction of being able to research the noblest object: mankind itself."

CHAPTER 9

What's Wrong?

The first step to being moral is to realize how thoroughly we aren't.
— Robert Wright, author of *The Moral Animal*

IT IS EASY TO CATEGORIZE JOSEF MENGELE, WHO murdered, maimed, and tortured in the name of science, as cruel and sadistic. A correct and dispassionate man like Otmar von Verschuer, however, is more puzzling for us, just as he must have been for the postwar authorities who were responsible for bringing to justice those who so ravaged human beings in their experiments.

For reasons that will never be entirely clear, Verschuer escaped justice. At least, that is how one might put it if one could be certain what would have constituted justice in his case—if there were general agreement about exactly which rules he had transgressed and how he should have been punished. Even fifty years later few people know enough about both the history and the science to say where the Nazi eugenicists—or eugenicists outside Germany, and there were plenty of them—went wrong. Those answers do exist, but many people, especially specialists in genetics, don't like to look too closely at them. The answers tend to lead to a mirror.

The judgments were more immediate and more troubling right after the war, when the atrocities that occurred in the concentration camps were fresh revelations and the perpetrators were at hand. Some of them were brought swiftly to court in 1946 in the German city of Nuremberg. The Nuremberg medical trials (which immediately followed the more prominent trials of Nazi political leaders) lasted two and a half years, generated transcripts exceeding 330,000 pages, pondered the fate of twenty-three defendants, and led to the executions of seven German scientists and doctors—including Karl Brandt, Hitler's personal physician.

The "medical experiments" that were considered during the trials and judged to be crimes against humanity eclipse such repellent matters as judging a couple's fitness for marriage or even enforced sterilization. Most of these experiments were intended to test treatments for illness or injury by deliberately inflicting the illness or injury on human subjects, or to test the limits of human endurance. The defendants exposed people to very high altitudes and very cold temperatures, to diseases such as typhus, and to toxins such as mustard gas, just to see what would happen.

Among the crimes that came under scrutiny was the Nazi "euthanasia" program, which was intended to rid society of thousands of "useless eaters," including the aged, insane, incurably ill, and deformed.

THE NUREMBERG PRINCIPLES

In his opening statement at the outset of the Nuremberg trials, the chief prosecutor, U.S. Brigadier General Telford Taylor, dwelt very lightly on the subject of medical ethics. "No refined questions confront us here," he said. The crimes were too egregious for that.

Nonetheless, lest there be any doubt, the tribunal set forth ten principles of ethics that applied to the use of human beings in medical experimentation. They are fundamental to modern biomedical ethics.

1. The voluntary consent of the subject is "absolutely essential." Subjects must have legal capacity to give consent and must "be able to exercise free power of choice, without the intervention of any element of force, fraud, deceit, duress, over-reaching or other ulterior form of constraint or coercion." They should also be informed about the purpose, nature, and duration of the experiment, as well as possible "inconveniences or hazards."

2. The experiment should be able to yield results that will be fruitful for society and cannot be gained by any other method of research.

Mengele was not tried at Nuremberg. He was not even sought until years later, and all the evidence points to his escape to South America, where he appears to have died in Brazil at an advanced age. But from the Nuremberg process of justice arose a clear set of principles for the ethical conduct of experiments involving human beings. These principles were set out in the court proceedings, and they underlie most of biomedical ethics today.

What did the Nazi doctors and scientists do that no one should do? The Nuremberg process provides an answer that can be summed up in one sentence: They did things to human beings, painful and often fatal, without gaining the subjects' informed consent—without explaining what would happen, and without getting their permission for the experiments.

Today this principle seems a self-evident tenet of basic morality. But

3. The experiment should be based on previous animal experiments and sufficient knowledge of natural science.

4. The experiment should be designed to avoid all unnecessary suffering.

5. The experiment should not be conducted if death or disabling injury is possible, with the possible exception of a study in which the doctors themselves are willing to serve as subjects.

6. The risks should never exceed the humanitarian benefits.

7. Precautions should be taken to protect subjects against "even remote possibilities of injury, disability, or death."

8. The experiment should be conducted only by qualified scientists using "the highest degree of skill and care."

9. Subjects should always be free to bring the experiment to an end.

10. Doctors must always be prepared to terminate the experiment at any point if it appears likely to result in injury, disability, or death.

some of the defendants went to their deaths unrepentant, despairing that society would ever understand the rectitude of their acts and their intentions. They hewed to a different moral line that put the interests of the common good above those of the individual. Here is what Hitler's doctor, Karl Brandt, argued in his final statement:

"It is immaterial for the experiment whether it is done with or against the will of the person concerned. For the individual, the event seems senseless, just as senseless as my actions as a doctor seem when isolated. The sense lies much deeper than that. Can I, as an individual, detach myself from the community? Can I remain outside and do without it? . . . The meaning is the motive—devotion to the community."

Nazi scientists in the dock at Nuremberg made several moral arguments in defense of their experiments, biomedical ethicist Arthur Caplan points out. Some said they used only people who were doomed to die anyway, and some even argued that participation offered the doomed a purpose for their lives. Some of the prisoners were really volunteers, they contended, because participation offered them a chance of freedom if they survived.

A fourth argument is "especially astounding even by the standards of self-delusion in evidence throughout the trial proceedings," Caplan notes. This was the rationale that it is not the responsibility of scientists and physicians to make ethical judgments; therefore they are obligated only to act in a value-neutral manner and make sure their experiments are designed and carried out as well as possible.

Beyond the question "Should they have done it?" lies one that is deeper and more troubling: "How *could* they have done it?" The massive eugenics and euthanasia programs carried out in Nazi Germany required the collusion of an entire generation of German doctors, enlisting them in a mass violation of the simple principle that underlies the Hippocratic oath, "First, do no harm." How did the Nazis pull it off?

Psychiatrist Robert Jay Lifton set out to answer this question in his book *The Nazi Doctors*. After years of difficult and painstaking efforts to locate and interview those doctors who were implicated in Nazi medicine but had not been brought to trial, convicted, or executed, he arrived at an explanation.

"The dominant tendency among these Nazi doctors was to present themselves to me as decent people who tried to make the best of a bad situation," writes Lifton. ". . . None of them—not a single former Nazi doctor I spoke to—arrived at a clear ethical evaluation of what he had done, and what he had been part of."

Lifton himself, however, did make an evaluation: that Nazi philosophy destroyed the boundaries between healing and killing, that it erased commonly accepted principles of medical ethics and replaced them (often forcibly, using law and police power) with a whole new philosophy of public health. The philosophy meshed perfectly with certain principles of science that had been gaining in popularity for many years, most notably natural selection and survival of the fittest. National Socialism, said Nazi party leader Rudolf Hess at a mass meeting in 1934, "is nothing but applied biology."

To salve the conscience of doctors whose minds were divided about human experimentation, Lifton says, Nazi science elevated their job description. An influential manual for doctors at the time said that the modern physician was no longer considered a mere caretaker of the sick. Instead he was a "cultivator of the genes," a "caretaker of the race." The concept had not originated with the Nazis but with the founders of eugenics who predated them.

To the turn-of-the-century pioneers of eugenics in Germany, Alfred Ploetz and William Schallmeyer, racial hygiene was a logical extension of personal hygiene. For a society already riddled by crime, ignorance, and severe economic problems, it provided preventive medicine by countering the overbreeding of "inferiors" and the threat allegedly posed by immigrants and the tendency of educated upper-class people to have small families. The new job title was "genetics doctor," *Erbarzt*, the name Verschuer gave his journal. The "gene doctor" was a figure responsible for the national goal of "keeping our blood pure."

This lofty rationale allowed the state to extend the definition of hereditary illness to include whole ethnic groups, including Jews and Gypsies. "The Jew," said one Nazi doctor confronted with the chimneys at Auschwitz, "is a gangrenous appendix in the body of mankind." He was expressing the biomedical orthodoxy of his own culture. As Lifton notes, Mengele "exemplified the Nazi biological revolutionary." His cynicism and criminality were "bound up with what all too many people in Germany and elsewhere at the time experienced as a compelling, even ennobling vision of the future."

The Nazi scientists, in other words, may have been *im*moral, but they were not *a*moral. "Bioethics has been speechless in the face of the crimes of Nazi doctors and biomedical scientists," writes Caplan, "precisely because so many of these doctors and scientists believed they were doing what was morally right to do." Today, we disagree. In 1948, their conquerors also disagreed — and decreed that some of them were worthy of execution because they had violated moral laws that the conquerors held to be inarguable.

Some of the moral laws they violated, however, are open to interpretation. As the American sociologist Troy Duster points out, "informed consent" takes on many different shadings and meanings, depending on the setting and the relationship between the person who holds the consent form and the person asked to sign it. The client who wants to please her husband and family or even her family doctor may be unwilling to question what a doctor or medical scientist says would be best for herself or her fetus. The man who cannot afford the best medical care may submit to an experimental procedure that a more affluent man would not even consider. The discomfiting question "How could they have done it?" evokes an even more unpleasant one: "Could *we* do it?"

At the outset that second question hardly seems to deserve an answer. Almost anyone would resist the idea that he or she is part of a culture that is inherently brutal or immoral. That was as true of good Germans at the start of World War II as it was of good Americans at the end, when we bombed Hiroshima. And it is true of doctors and scientists in general, who share their professions with the defendants at Nuremberg.

Historians point out that modern scientists use three arguments to distance themselves from Nazi doctors and scientists, and from the early eugenicists in general: (1) They were all mad. (2) The scientists weren't behind it in the first place — it was all the fault of the politicians (which was also, we remember, Verschuer's self-defense). (3) Their science was fundamentally flawed anyway; we would never make the same kind of mistakes today, because we know better.

The first argument is a knee-jerk response, and most people who bother to think critically soon abandon it, because it doesn't make sense. How could an entire generation of doctors and scientists have been completely mad? What of their students? Did the war's end miraculously jolt them back to good sense?

No one who was on trial at Nuremberg pleaded insanity, observes Caplan. "Among those who did their research in Auschwitz, Dachau, and other camps," he notes, "a considerable number had obvious psychological problems, were lesser scientific lights, or both. But there were also well-trained, reputable and competent physicians and scientists who were ardent Nazis. Some conducted experiments in the camps. Others decided who ought to be put to death. Human experimentation in the camps was not conducted only by those who were mentally unstable or on the periphery of science."

Lifton dismisses the rationale as well. "Neither brilliant nor stupid, neither inherently evil nor particularly ethically sensitive," he writes of the Nazi doctors he interviewed several decades after the war, "they were by no means the demonic figures—sadistic, fanatic, lusting to kill— people have often thought them to be." After having met and inter- viewed some of them, Lifton wrote about them with rather more pity (for their inability to comprehend and resolve their conflicts) than scorn.

As to the second argument, the one that lays all the biomedical abuses of the Nazi era at the feet of politicians, the evidence clearly re- futes it. Like Verschuer's Frankfurt institute, most of the various insti- tutes for racial hygiene in Germany were established in the early 1930s, before Hitler's rise to power. Long before the Hitler era, a reading of the medical literature makes clear, it had become professional dogma that the number of "inferiors" should be drastically reduced by measures such as sterilization. This was true not only in Germany but elsewhere. It was obviously convenient for Hitler that these policies were orthodox by the time he came to power, and he certainly embraced and exploited them with enthusiasm, but neither he nor National Socialism invented them.

The senior scholar in residence at the United States Holocaust Mu- seum in Washington, Robert Proctor, has pointed out that the gas cham- bers installed at Auschwitz and Treblinka were used equipment. They had been dismantled and moved there from psychiatric hospitals, where they had been tried out in euthanasia efforts aimed at eradicat- ing the mentally and physically "unfit" who were pursuing "lives not worth living." Many of the doctors and nurses who worked at the con- centration camps had taken their earlier training in these euthanasia programs. With racial hygiene, the Nazis merely extended and broad- ened what were already accepted practices in German medical culture.

"It has taken a long time to realize that psychiatric 'selections' fore- shadowed selections on the ramp at Auschwitz," Proctor writes, ". . . and that white coats can hide a capacity for great cruelty. But those are some of the more sobering lessons of this ugly side of history."

The third contention, that racial hygiene was bad science, has con- siderable merit as a *fact* of scientific reasoning—but none whatever as an ethical argument. As you can see in the box on page 175, the most enthusiastic supporters of eugenics were blind to a number of logical flaws and were unaware of certain things we know today about genes and evolution. But this argument implies that if your science is valid, it is impossible to be immoral — just as some defendants at Nuremberg argued that their only obligation was to carry out the experiments competently. It does not address the question of whether eugenic efforts *backed by valid science* ought to be considered worthwhile.

As it happens, some of the experiments conducted at concentration camps *were* good experiments from a purely scientific point of view, or would have been seen as such if they had involved mice instead of humans. In fact, some of them were so "good," scientifically speaking, that there has been considerable debate afterward about whether we should profit from the knowledge they provided. (In general, the consensus is that we should not. For one thing, to do so would dishonor the memory of those who suffered and died in the process. For another, modern-day critics are wary of results reported by scientists whose morality was so badly skewed, and who may themselves have been coerced in conducting and reporting on the experiments.)

All of this aside, it is comforting to think that no one in modern times, and certainly no *American*, would be involved in or even stand by and watch an experiment carried out under the convenient assumption that some individuals are less worthy than others. But while this thought may be comforting, as anyone who follows the newspapers knows, it is a fallacy — as is borne out by examples from our own recent history.

One of the most blatant such experiments began in 1932 and continued until the 1970s, under the auspices of the U.S. Public Health Service and under the gaze of peer reviewers of medical articles on the study. The now-infamous Tuskegee "experiment" involved some four hundred African-American men, many of them sharecroppers and day laborers living in the area of Macon County, Alabama. Its object was to study the natural progression of syphilis.

In 1932, when it authorized the study, the Public Health Service had been apprised of an unusual fact about this population: of those men known to have venereal disease, some 99 percent had never received treatment, although medical articles at the time called for treating symptomless or "latent" venereal disease aggressively, with mercury or arsenic compounds or, later, with penicillin.

This fact, together with the anticipated cooperation of local hospitals, "offers unparalleled opportunity for carrying on this piece of scientific research, which probably cannot be duplicated anywhere in the

THE SKEWED LOGIC OF POPULAR EUGENICS

Even in the early twentieth century, many good scientists knew that mainstream eugenics had gone astray. Eugenicists had many blind spots. Among them:

1. Their evidence linking traits such as "shiftlessness" and "feeble-mindedness" with the lower classes had an intrinsic bias. Most of that "evidence" came from institutions, whose inmates came largely from these strata. Upper-class people then, as now, could afford to keep their less intelligent and unemployed relatives away from institutions.

2. They defined *race* as a biological term based on physical appearance. In fact, it is a social construct based on elements of culture. Genetic studies show that people we identify as belonging to the same race are no more similar in their biochemistry than total strangers or even bitter enemies. Racial "cleansing" is nonsense. Not only are the races not clean; genetically, in a sense they do not exist.

3. They ignored evidence, available even in the 1920s, that all individuals harbor disadvantageous recessive genes of some kind. The selective breeding of healthy individuals would never eliminate these genes.

4. Heredity is a largely random process, in which genes are shuffled much like playing cards in a deck. There is no guarantee that two "superior" people, however this word is defined, will produce a genetically "superior" child.

5. Whatever selective breeding *might* be accomplished in humans would work very slowly. Based on eugenicists' estimates for the prevalence of "feeblemindedness" (whatever that is), one analysis estimates that it would take 8,000 years of totally restricted breeding to reduce that prevalence by two-thirds.

world," wrote the U.S. surgeon general at the time. And so the study proceeded. Each man was given a thorough physical, was told that the U.S. government was going to treat his disease, and then received a mercurial ointment that the doctors in the study knew to be absolutely ineffectual against syphilis and gonorrhea.

World War II came and went, the medical abuses in Nazi concentration camps flourished and were legally avenged, and for four decades the black men in Tuskegee, Alabama, were subjects of an experiment in the natural history of untreated venereal disease. In 1955, fully eight years after the Nuremberg principles were published and publicized, a medical article reported that more than 30 percent of the test group had died from advanced syphilis.

In 1972 someone finally blew a whistle. The study came to the attention of the Associated Press, and a major scandal ensued. As Troy Duster points out, it can be assumed that as late as 1971 the best-trained and informed of American scientists and physicians, including researchers, scholars, officials of the Public Health Service, and editors of medical journals, "never found it in their collective wisdom" to notice that several hundred aging black men in Alabama were the subjects of a violation of the Nuremberg Code. The experiments even violated a policy statement that had been issued in 1966 by the Public Health Service itself.

The Tuskegee experiment is now renowned as an infamous example of blatant disregard for informed consent, but it is far from an isolated case. In the 1950s and 1960s (to cite just one of numerous examples) the U.S. Army quietly released a chemical into the air over cities and rural areas of the United States and Canada—with little knowledge of its effect on animals and none on humans—in order to test the possible dispersion of biological weapons. Recent studies suggest that those who were exposed to zinc cadmium sulfide suffered no harm as a result, but the army did not inquire at the time, and certainly no members of the public were asked for their consent.

Jay Katz, a professor of law, medicine, and psychology at Yale University, was a member of the panel that advised the government after the 1972 scandal about the Tuskegee syphilis trials. Recently he reflected on the broader issue of informed consent. "During this century and particularly since World War II," he wrote, "biomedical research has increased in magnitude unprecedented in the millennia of medical history. Medical practice has become radically transformed, often obliterating the vital distinction between therapy and scientific research.

This problem is compounded by physician-investigators' proclivities to view subjects as if they were patients, treating the latter with the discretion and authority doctors have customarily enjoyed when making decisions *for* rather than *with* patients.

"Physician-investigators, in their understandable scientific pursuit of alleviating the suffering of mankind, have been reluctant to think deeply about the philosopher Hans Jonas's observations that '[medical] progress is an optional goal, not an uncompromising commitment' and that 'too ruthless a pursuit of scientific progress' could threaten 'the erosion of moral values . . . that would make its most dazzling triumphs not worth having.'"

We can assume that all of the educated people who endorsed or failed to curtail the Tuskegee experiments were not mad. We can assume they were not themselves the victims of political coercion or of flawed scientific reasoning. What we can also assume is that on this issue it is neither safe nor wise to place ourselves, and our own society, beyond the bounds of suspicion.

Evidently many African-Americans harbor such suspicions. When the University of North Carolina surveyed more than a thousand black churchgoers in five cities, they found that one-third believed that the HIV virus, which causes AIDS, was created by whites as a form of genocide, while another 30 percent said they were not sure. Public health workers who treat many African-Americans say that a deep distrust of the mainstream medical system pervades this segment of our society, and that it traces back to the Tuskegee study.

CHAPTER 10

Genes and the Bomb

The possibilities recently opened up by biological research in this area
have been likened to the sudden thrusting of the atomic bomb upon a
world not ready for it . . . Their social meanings will likely dawn upon us
piecemeal and unheralded if we are not watchful.

— Biologist Rollin D. Hotchkiss, August 16, 1965,
speaking at the University of Illinois

WHEN THE WAR ENDED IN 1945, JAMES NEEL, HIS EF-
forts at the Eugenics Record Office concluded, was working as a medical resident in Rochester, New York. He lived with his wife and infant
daughter over a grocery store, on a busy street just across the river from
the medical center.

Still wondering how to bring the rigors of fruit fly genetics to the
study of human genes, Neel knew that the end of the war might also
bring an end to these aspirations—or at least a long interruption. As a
medical student, he had not been drafted. Now he owed the government some service, presumably in a hospital in an occupied area.

The atomic bombings of Hiroshima and Nagasaki in August had not
come as a total surprise to him. Neel had known during the war that
some professors in Rochester were involved in top-secret activities, including some of his own mentors. Immediately after the bombs were
dropped, he noticed speculations in the popular press about the implications of all that radiation for public health. Surely, he told himself,
someone else somewhere was also pondering what was on his mind: the
effects of the bomb fallout on human genes.

The bomb's developers themselves had paid hardly any attention to
these risks, the records show, but geneticists had been using radiation
for many years to induce mutations intentionally, and well knew what
it could do to microorganisms, fruit flies, and larger animals such as laboratory mice. As little as 25 to 50 roentgens (the international unit of radiation exposure) was sufficient to cause genetic damage in a fruit fly.

(The bomb had exposed some residents of Hiroshima to ten times that level of radiation.) The damage could persist for generations.

One genetics expert of the time, J.B.S. Haldane, had proposed that as little as 3 roentgens of radiation would double the present mutation rate in human beings. What had happened, Neel wondered, to the genes of survivors in Japan?

It was fairly easy for Neel to identify a doctor who had contacts with the Manhattan Project, and simple to ask whether any efforts were being made to inquire into the genetic effects of that radiation. Then barely three months later his military orders arrived. Neel had become a member of a research team charged with designing the very study he had in mind: to probe the effects of atomic radiation on the only human beings who had experienced it in massive amounts and survived.

Little more than a year after the bombs hit their targets, Neel found himself on a military transport plane with two civilian experts on radiobiology, sent to survey Hiroshima and Nagasaki and report on delayed effects of the bombings. Human genetics, so recently viewed as despicable, had become important again at the highest of levels.

What stunned Neel, on reading the top-secret documents to which he now had access, was how little attention had been paid, before the bombings, to the possible risks of radiation for the survivors. Evidently no one had contemplated that there *would* be survivors. "Any person with radiation damage would have been killed with a brick first," stated one report. What little existed by way of estimates had focused on the possible radiation hazards to those who were building the bombs.

Agencies such as the Department of Defense and the Atomic Energy Commission had little official wisdom to impart. Based on limited evidence from the literature, their estimates of the radiation dose needed to double the background human mutation rate varied by factors of 100, from as little as 3 roentgens to as much as 300.

On average, those at the center of the blast site who nonetheless survived the impact might have received radiation dosages somewhere in between these extremes, Neel estimated later. But radiation doses to individuals could also have ranged widely, some as high as the maximum compatible with survival, 500 roentgens. In 1956 a National Academy of Sciences committee would estimate the safe maximum limit for human radiation exposure at 50 roentgens over thirty years of life span. (For comparison: An ordinary medical X ray of the abdomen exposes unshielded internal organs to about 1 or 2 roentgens. Over thirty years natural background radiation from sources such as cosmic rays delivers a total of about 4.3 roentgens to a person's reproductive organs.)

Some critics, most notably the geneticist Hermann Muller, argued that the human genome was so fragile, so delicately balanced between beneficial genes and deleterious ones, that a relatively minor change in the mutation rate could spell genetic disaster for a population. Muller predicted that if the survivors of Hiroshima could foresee the future one

GENES AND MUTATIONS

The time-honored analogy is this: A gene is like a word in a message, and a mutation is like a typographical error. But a value judgment is implicit in the comparison. We think mutations are bad because the ones we have been able to detect most easily are those that cause bad diseases.

Countless genetic accidents—mutations—happen, countless such variations occur that are meaningless. Some are even beneficial. Mutation is the mechanism by which, according to classical evolutionary theory, Nature "tries out" a variety of responses to an environment.

Scientists focus on the mutations that follow exposure to radiation and chemicals because those are the ones that they know how to induce and to study. But genetic accidents happen spontaneously all the time, as cells recopy their DNA in the normal process of cell division. It has been estimated that every time a single cell divides, whether to continue growing fingernails or to replace cells that are damaged or sloughed away, the genetic machinery makes three errors.

Given that every cell division recopies some three billion DNA sub-units, that's an enviable quality control record. The credit goes to a new-found class of molecules known as DNA repair enzymes, which monitor the genome for breakages and scan the DNA for misprints, slicing out damaged sections and repairing the gaps.

Once thought to be important only in cases of radiation damage, DNA repair enzymes are now known to be on patrol constantly. When errors arise in the genes that specify those enzymes, inactivating the repair system, the result can be cancer. Three-fourths of us live and die without developing a cancer—or at least without ever knowing about it—in part because of a DNA repair system that never goes off duty.

thousand years hence, "they might consider themselves more fortunate if the bomb had killed them."

If a dose of as little as 25 or 50 roentgens could cause mutations in a fruit fly, what would a dose of hundreds do to human beings? Hiroshima and Nagasaki suddenly presented a living laboratory to address the question. Neel would be the principal investigator.

In the United States the word *holocaust* has one popular implication, beyond its dictionary definition of mass destruction by fire. It stands for what Hitler and his followers did to six million Jews. Americans tend to forget what their own government did, for better or worse, to innocent citizens of Hiroshima and Nagasaki, also en masse, and also (metaphorically speaking) by fire.

The case of the atomic bomb deserves some attention here on two counts. First, it provided the circumstance by which genetic studies of human beings became respectable again, even perhaps laudable. Second and less obviously, it illustrates how wide of the mark people can be when they try to predict the impact of a new technology.

Hindsight is useful here, because we can see easily the blind spots of those prophets who saw fit to make pronouncements just after Hiroshima. It took some time for people to grasp the then-strange fact that they had gained the power to destroy everything on the planet. (Now we must confront the unsettling fact that we are gaining the power to bring about permanent and fundamental changes in our own blueprint. How wide of the mark are we, now, as we try to predict the implications of our exploding knowledge of the genome?)

"In an instant, without warning, the present had become the unthinkable future," *Time* magazine intoned shortly after the atomic bombs were dropped. Atom Year I, as *Business Week* called it in July 1946, was marked by "more debate on a single subject than any twelve months in the world's history."

But almost no one that year, and certainly not in any popular forum, focused on the peril that atomic weapons now represent to most of us: the threat of irrevocable, total destruction. Apparently seven of ten Americans in 1946 thought it was a good thing we had unleashed the bomb.

One year after the bombings, John Hersey laid out dispassionately in the pages of *The New Yorker* precisely what horror we had visited upon ordinary human beings in Japan, awakening Americans from their postwar euphoria to an unwelcome angst. Former president Herbert Hoover did point out to a group of newspaper editors that "despite any sophistries," America had introduced to the world a weapon whose purpose was to kill innocent civilians.

But what the public read about most often was not the dangers of atomic weapons but the prospect of a new world made safe, peaceful, and fulfilling through atomic energy. *Coronet* magazine predicted that countries would no longer have an incentive to invade each other because of the "unlimited wealth" made available by atomic energy. An article in *Time* speculated that atomic energy would release vast amounts of free time, giving birth to new cultural and spiritual advances, and would free humanity from disease, famine, and early death.

If any concern was raised about all of this, as Paul Boyer notes in *By the Bomb's Early Light,* it was that the human race could not tolerate so much free time. It might lead to class conflict and social unrest, some feared, or corporate or political forces would somehow use it for unsavory ends, or individuality would be lost in some brave new technocratic world.

Some religious leaders did express deep concern and contrition about the loss of life. (A blue-ribbon report to the Federal Council of Churches called the surprise bombings "morally indefensible.") One New York minister wrote about the "ghastly" fact that the bomb was released "not by Hitler in some mad mania of lust" but by "sane and good men" who were "the self-appointed custodians of civilization." Still, hardly a single harmonious voice from organized religion spoke out against the fact that the bomb had been used.

There also was a certain disquiet about the fact that scientists could actually have conspired to create such a thing in the first place. One commentator noted with some horror that the bomb had been produced by scientists "who only dimly grasped its long-range implications," acting as one-dimensional specialists rather than as complete and moral human beings. His words echoed a statement by nuclear physicist J. Robert Oppenheimer, director of the Los Alamos laboratory that designed and built the bomb, that has become famous in the years since. Having seen that it could be done, Oppenheimer said, "one had at least to make the thing."

Most of the American press may have been otherwise engaged, but James Neel was disturbed to find that "lurid and feckless speculations" had been made in both the United States and Japan about the effects of radiation without any evidence whatever to support them. Within the bombed cities themselves, rumors ran rampant that survivors had been giving birth to human monsters. This fantasy lived on for years, in popular movies about creatures such as Godzilla or Mothra, supposedly unleashed by the force of radiation.

In a society where arranged marriages were common, survivors could all too easily be stigmatized. The need to replace fiction with fact was urgent. Neel and his team of Japanese and American assistants set out immediately to learn whether infants born shortly after the blast suffered any obvious radiation damage.

Neel realized quickly that if he failed to be sensitive to cultural and social issues, he would ruin his chances of gaining the information required. As both a scientist and a conqueror, identified with the use of a weapon that had led to a degree of human devastation that Neel himself has never found the right words to convey, he was in a difficult position. How would Americans have reacted, he wondered, if the Japanese had won the war and then sent medical teams to study the survivors?

He soon discovered, however, that the Japanese were if anything too cooperative. Given the abuses of genetics on the other side of the world, how could he possibly gain truly informed consent to study the effects of the genetic damage that his own people had inflicted upon the Japanese? Was there any valid way for a conqueror to ask for permission to obtain medical information? Was not coercion implicit in the situation? This problem haunted the project continuously.

Furthermore, it became clear that the research team could not necessarily rely on existing Japanese birth records for accurate information. In order to ascertain whether the atomic bombs had caused an increase in birth defects, the critical question they had to answer was how many babies had been born with birth defects under ordinary conditions. But upon posing the simple question, Neel learned that it was unanswerable. Many babies were delivered at home by midwives, who "in olden (and not so olden) times," he writes, might discreetly smother a malformed infant—concerned only for the family's reputation—then register it as stillborn.

The simple but brilliant solution to this problem came from the head of Hiroshima's health department, who had been trying to study the bomb's effects on his own, almost since the devastation began to clear. He pointed out that the Japanese government had instituted a rationing program to ensure that pregnant women had adequate nutrition. The supplements were available only to women who registered as soon as they recognized they were pregnant and again at the end of their fifth month. Neel could now use these records to gain information about who was pregnant and when she was expected to deliver. (The researchers also wanted to study miscarriage rates but were forced to abandon the effort. Because the government was actively encouraging abortions as a means of population control at the time, it proved too cumbersome to distinguish the elective abortions from the miscarriages.)

The research program hired eight to ten Japanese physicians in each of the two cities to examine all newborns, alive or dead. The team completed exhaustive questionnaires about all babies born abnormal and about every tenth baby whatever its condition at birth. In addition, all pregnant women who registered for prenatal care had to fill out a questionnaire about their radiation history and that of the prospective father. Shortly after the baby's birth, a clerk completed another form about the infant itself. In 1950 Neel and his associates initiated a nine-month examination of all children in Hiroshima and Nagasaki.

Three years later, there was good information for some 70,000 newborns. Based on the demographic structure of the two cities, it could be presumed that about 70 percent of the children who would ever be born to survivors who had been living within the radiation zone at the time of the bombing were already born.

The results of the genetic studies were startling to all the genetic Cassandras of the previous decades. They showed "very little if any difference" between children born to survivors of the bombings and those born to otherwise similar Japanese parents who had not been in Hiroshima or Nagasaki at the time. There was very little statistical likelihood that even the most severe evidence of first-generation radiation damage—stillbirth or neonatal death—had even so much as doubled in the offspring of people exposed to the blast.

"Ionizing radiation is perhaps the worst kind of damage a cell can receive," wrote Neel in his autobiography. "But whereas Muller, a generation ago, could view radiation as uniquely disruptive, now it appears rather as the extreme in a spectrum of disruptive forces for which evolution has prepared the DNA....

"Since we found little in the way of a genetic effect of the A-bombs," he went on, "the principal tangible result of our study has been to dispel the nasty rumors, to provide reassurance." It was comforting to think, after all the eugenic evil in Germany, that genetics could actually provide reassurance, that it might do good as well as evil.

After he completed his service, Neel became the head of a new human genetics program at the University of Michigan, which remains one of the most respected such programs in the United States. Now interested in the effects of background radiation, he went off to South America to begin genetic studies in Amerindian tribes.

The Atomic Energy Commission (AEC), a predecessor of the Nuclear Regulatory Agency and the current U.S. Department of Energy, also retained an interest in genetics. It supported fundamental studies of the effects of both radiation and chemicals on the genes of humans and other organisms. Some of its early funding went to the studies of Francis Crick and James Watson, who worked out how DNA functions as the bearer of the genetic code.

In the years immediately after the war, the AEC's support for genetics dwarfed that from other sources. Much later the Department of Energy became (as it is today) one of the two major sources of funding for the Human Genome Project—but its role is often neglected in the press in favor of the more obvious home for studies on human genetics, the National Institutes of Health. In 1984, when a scientific meeting in Hiroshima called for an effort to preserve indefinitely cells from all remaining survivors of the bombing and to develop ways to study their DNA, it was the Department of Energy that agreed to provide the funding.

In the late 1980s, when the Human Genome Project was poised to start, many press reports referred to it as the "Manhattan Project of biology." It was a relevant analogy, although many who used it certainly could not have realized the full implications. Mapping the genome was a big collaborative project, as they recognized, and it promised to have an important impact on our views of the future. But also like the Manhattan Project, the genome project's origins were secret.

"It has been called the Manhattan Project of biology, yet it has a benevolent goal," said the newsletter of the Cold Spring Harbor Laboratory, a major genetics research center, in 1988. Certainly those who touted the genome project were not proposing to destroy innocent lives by the thousands, and they often promised that it would lead to new cures for intractable disease.

But in a letter to the journal *Nature* in 1986, four years before the project officially started, three scientists had come closer to identifying the project's real motivation: "Man's feeling of self-importance will probably not be satisfied until the last bit of his genome has been sequenced and filed somewhere."

Most writers on the subject date the origins of the genome project to a conceptual breakthrough in 1980 and a public conference in 1985. MIT historian of science Charles Weiner traces its history considerably farther back, to a small private meeting of biologists held at Rockefeller University in October 1966. Nobel Prize-winners Salvador Luria and James Watson were present, as was biologist Norton Zinder, who would become not only head of the university but in the late 1980s head of the working group assigned to sort out the logistics of a government-sponsored project to map and then decipher the human genome.

The invitation to the 1966 meeting at Rockefeller University reviewed work that at the time seemed to hold out the promise for genetic engineering. "The problem is obviously immense," it noted, "and almost fantastic in implication." Without a "massive frontal assault," it went on, no progress would be achieved in the "foreseeable future."

All that remains of the meeting are Zinder's archived notes, which Weiner reviews in *Are Genes Us?* The notes document how the vision for the project coalesced, largely because it seemed inevitable that the technologies would come into existence and be used. "What can be done, is done," Zinder noted in his summary of the discussion, "and what can be used, is used." The main issue of the discussion was whether the meeting participants would prod development of the technology to decode the genes. The general conclusion was that if those present did not do so, others would.

"Can we really discuss the feasibility of such endeavors without discussing the desirability?" Zinder noted. "Some feel yes, others no." One scientist noted that although society generally resisted eugenic measures, individuals tended to have mostly positive responses toward genetic interventions and that as such they have "qualities analogous to those which sell soap."

Its marketing potential notwithstanding, participants decided not to make any publication or official report of the meeting, in part because the subject was so controversial that anything they said was likely to be "overplayed and over-interpreted."

"Considerations of desirability rarely govern the transition from 'it can be done' to 'it has been done,'" biologist Leon Kass argued in a letter to *The Washington Post* in November 1967, a year later. "Biologists today are under strong obligation to raise just such questions publicly so that we may deliberate *before* the new biomedical technology is an accomplished fact, a technology whose consequences will probably dwarf those which resulted from the development of the atomic bomb."

Unfortunately, the future leaders of the genome project had already decided that the project was inevitable and that therefore they should undertake it. Having seen that a human gene map could be accomplished, they at least had to make the thing.

The benevolent impulse to study the genetic hazards of radiation had given the Atomic Energy Commission a long-standing interest in studies of genes. It also left an influential body of geneticists eager to continue their work after they had answered the first questions about radiation.

CHAPTER 11

The Atlas of Ourselves

Don't learn too much. You'll just delude yourselves.

— James Watson, 1993, speaking to honors biology students

MORE THAN TWENTY-FIVE YEARS AGO, IN *FUTURE SHOCK*, Alvin Toffler observed that technology was changing more swiftly than people could adapt to it. Not surprisingly, among many other topics, he included genetics. "The nature of what can and will be done [with human genes] exceeds anything that man is as yet psychologically or morally prepared to live with," Toffler wrote.

Among the lengthiest quotations in *Future Shock* on the topic of genetics came from a speech delivered by California biophysicist Robert Sinsheimer during an anniversary celebration at Caltech.

"How will you choose to intervene in the ancient designs of nature for men?" Sinsheimer had asked. "Would you like to control the sex of your offspring? It will be as you wish. Would you like your son to be six feet tall—seven feet? Eight feet? What troubles you—allergy, obesity, arthritic pain? These will be easily handled. For cancer, diabetes, phenylketonuria, there will be genetic therapy. The appropriate DNA will be provided in the appropriate dose.... Even the timeless patterns of growth and maturity and aging will be subject to our design.... None transcends the potential of what we now know. They may not be developed in the way one might now anticipate, but they are feasible, they can be brought to reality, and sooner rather than later."

Fifteen years afterward Sinsheimer tried to take concrete steps to move things along. By then he was chancellor of the University of California at Santa Cruz—and as short of funds for his institution as most university heads. In 1985 he seized on a remarkable proposal to attract big money to UC–Santa Cruz: the university should establish an Institute to Sequence the Human Genome, with a goal of reading out the entire human genetic message, base by base.

"It was . . . evident to me that physicists and astronomers were not hesitant to ask for large sums of money to support programs they believed to be essential to advance their science," explained Sinsheimer. "Biology had always been 'small science,' and it occurred to me to wonder if there were scientific opportunities in biology that were being overlooked simply because we were not thinking on an adequate scale."

In hindsight, it's difficult to judge whether the idea was endearing or laughable. The project Sinsheimer envisioned exists now—massively huge, involving countless researchers around the world, at a cost in the hundreds of millions of dollars per year in the United States alone. No one had proposed it in public before Sinsheimer did; he could not have known how ludicrously audacious the suggestion would later seem—to carry out the grand project at a single university.

After conferring with biologists on his faculty, Sinsheimer sought foundation and government funding to back a genome project, and he also sponsored a workshop in May 1985 to explore the idea. Mapping and sequencing the genome would be "a noble and inspiring enterprise," agreed biologists at Santa Cruz in a document supporting Sinsheimer's proposal. An account of the meeting in the magazine *California* dubbed the proposed project "Genesis: The Sequel."

That fundraising effort was as far as Sinsheimer himself got with the idea. He was among the first to publicize the fact that it would soon be possible to catalog all the chromosomes, and the first to gain some serious theoretical support. But no one was willing to ante up and the project languished. In retrospect Russell Dolittle, a Nobel Prize–winning biologist who was involved in promoting the idea much later, sees Sinsheimer's initiative as more significant than a mere moneymaking proposition for his institution. "What it did," he says, "was start people thinking."

Since the 1950s scientists had known that the factors of heredity first proposed by Austrian monk Gregor Mendel in 1865 were encoded within the long helical molecule called DNA. In the 1960s they learned the meaning of the code in which the genes operated, and how the molecular subunits of DNA (known as bases) could be read off by machinery inside cells, then chemically translated into the building blocks of proteins to create all the molecules needed to operate a human being.

A ROUGH HISTORY OF GENETICS

1860s: Austrian monk Gregor Mendel studies plants and suggests some basic rules of heredity, proposing it travels as particles.

1870s: Charles Darwin has expounded in full his theory of evolution. *The Origin of the Species* and *The Descent of Man* are both in print, both hot sellers.

1910s: Eugenic movements gain force.

1920s: Studying fruit flies and other small creatures, Thomas Hunt Morgan clarifies the roles of chromosomes and genes in heredity.

1930s: Heredity patterns are worked out for two sex-linked conditions, hemophilia and color-blindness.

1950s: Watson and Crick describe the structure of DNA and how it acts as genetic material. The phenomenon of genetic linkage between hereditary traits is discovered.

1960s: Biologists learn how to make genetic hybrid cells that contain some human and some animal DNA.

1970s: For the first time the complete DNA sequence of a gene (for the outer coat of a virus) is elaborated. Scientists learn how to use enzymes to cut DNA at predictable locations, and how to insert the fragments into bacteria.

1980s: An international repository for human gene fragments is founded in Paris. A project is proposed to map the human genome, based in part on comparing sizes of specific genetic fragments among members of thousands of families worldwide. In 1988 the Human Genome Project is established in the United States.

1990s: Genome mapping begins. The first human gene therapy trial is approved. Wisconsin passes legislation forbidding insurance discrimination based on genes. The NIH first submits, then withdraws, an application for a patent on thousands of human gene fragments. First the Equal Employment Opportunity Commission, and then a federal health-reform law governing employer health insurance, prohibit discrimination on the basis of genetic risk.

In the 1970s the molecular biologists stumbled upon the first good tool that would give them access to that huge DNA text: molecular scissors. They discovered enzymes made by bacteria that would slice DNA at specified points, between certain sets of DNA bases. Because DNA fragments were of different sizes, they traveled to different locations if they were placed on a slab of gel and then exposed to an electric field. Even if no one yet knew what the fragments meant, they could be separated and sorted.

Just as important, it was now possible, using nonspecific enzymes that broke down DNA strands, to create hybrid cells that contained mostly rodent DNA but a fragment of human DNA as well, and to maintain them in the laboratory. If a hybrid cell culture suddenly produced a protein that its all-rodent parent could not, it was a likely bet that the message coding for that particular substance originated in the human cell.

Molecular scissors provided a way to create small snippets of DNA whose loose ends were identifiable. The gels made it possible to recognize fragments by their size. The hybrid cells provided a way to identify something about the genetic message within such a DNA fragment. Marrying the three techniques allowed researchers to isolate and identify specified DNA fragments, cultivate them, and look for their function.

This molecular science began and matured not with human subjects but with bacteria and yeast. For about three decades, however, researchers had been using heredity studies of human families to puzzle out the genetic basis of hereditary conditions such as hemophilia and color-blindness, which are passed most often from mothers to their sons. (Based on rules of heredity that go almost as far back as Gregor Mendel, they could deduce that these genes had to lie on the X chromosome, of which women have two but men have only one.) More recently, they had begun to work out the heredity of some conditions that had nothing to do with gender. Suddenly, now, the molecular tools made it possible to deduce where on the chromosomes some of these genes must be located.

"Suddenly we had these tools to look at genes," recalled James Watson, explaining the advances to a congressional hearing. "We could find the general rules. . . . If you said, 'Well, how far are you getting toward understanding humans?' we weren't very far. But suddenly we had the tools."

During a 1978 meeting at the Alta ski resort in Utah, a conceptual leap set geneticists on a clear path toward the goal of localizing human genes. A graduate student from the University of Utah was describing experiments in which he had found a difference in DNA patterns between people affected with a hereditary condition known as hemochromatosis

MENDEL'S LAW

Studying pea plants in his garden in the 1860s, the Austrian monk Gregor Mendel came up with some basic ideas about how traits can be inherited. (The traits he focused on were the height and color of the plants.)

These principles (which are valid in many cases but which we now know are extremely simplistic) are often called Mendel's laws:

1. Traits are inherited as units, as if they are particles. They are inherited in pairs.

2. Some traits are dominant, or overpowering, while others recede, are recessive.

3. If each parent has one dominant and one recessive particle, three-fourths of the offspring will show the dominant trait and one-fourth will show the recessive trait.

4. Many traits are inherited independently of each other. Thus, plants may be of similar height, but the color of their blossoms may vary. Some traits are unvarying within a certain hereditary line, but other traits vary independently.

We now refer to these "units" or "particles" as genes. We also know that traits are inherited independently if the genes that determine them are located on different chromosomes. Not surprisingly, inheritance is far more complicated than Mendel envisioned—but he was the pioneer, the first to come up with a theory based on rigorous research.

and their close relatives who were unaffected. Certain unique-sized DNA fragments almost always appeared in blood samples from family members who had the disease, and almost never in those who did not.

These fragments did not necessarily contain the genes involved in hemochromatosis, but because they coincided with the condition so closely, it seemed likely that they must at the least be located very near those genes. Much as the corner grocery store is not your house but can help people to find your house, these DNA fragments were a strong clue to the location of interesting genes within the human chromosomes.

Hearing about the hemochromatosis research at the Alta meeting, molecular biologists Ronald Davis of Stanford University and David Botstein of MIT glanced at each other and had a shock of recognition. This technique could actually make it possible to generate a map of the human chromosomes — similar to the way both of them had been working to map the much smaller genome of yeast by inducing and studying mutations, then locating the genes that allowed yeast organisms to survive under conditions of stress. The two scientists realized that if enough gene fragments could be found that were linked to recognizable human variations such as hereditary diseases, they could be used as genetic landmarks along the chromosomes.

The result of their brainstorm was a 1980 paper in the *American Journal of Human Genetics* (coauthored by Botstein, Davis, and the two organizers of the meeting) that proposed a "systematic approach to finding and organizing markers on the human chromosomes." The authors admitted that finding enough landmark fragments to span all the DNA across twenty-three human chromosome pairs would be an enormous challenge, but they concluded that "it should theoretically work."

In retrospect, it is remarkable that it took another five years before anyone, let alone Robert Sinsheimer, was bold enough to pick up the gauntlet thrown down in that paper. In March 1986, a year after Sinsheimer's bold proposal, Charles DeLisi of the health research department within the Department of Energy sponsored another meeting with the same intent, in Santa Fe, New Mexico. Like their fellows at Santa Cruz a year earlier, the scientists in Santa Fe concluded in the strongest terms that a genome project was feasible.

In the same month the geneticist Renato Dulbecco wrote an editorial in the journal *Science* promoting a project to discover the molecular sequence of the genome, noting that it would speed progress in cancer research.

Two months later he repeated the point during a speech dedicating a building at Cold Spring Harbor Laboratories, the site of the institution once known as the Eugenics Record Office — and still a world-renowned center for genetic research. One of the listeners was James Watson, the laboratory's director.

Until he heard Dulbecco's appeal, Watson says, he was skeptical that the time had come to go for the details of the genome. "But I listened to my friend Renato Dulbecco . . . and he was right," Watson admitted. "Within a couple of months I had ceased being a skeptic and I thought, gee, we have to do it. Because when you really look at

ATLAS, MAP, SEQUENCE

The Atlas

In the olden days, in the 1970s, just about the best gene map available was the chromosome spread of an amniocentesis test, the chromosomes stained with dyes that gave them identifiable stripes. Interesting though it was, it had about the same level of detail as a photograph of Earth taken from the moon.

The Map

In the 1980s the Human Genome Project set itself a goal of narrowing the focus dramatically by placing recognizable landmarks along all the chromosomes at a distance of 100,000 bases apart. Mapping involves slicing chromosomes into small fragments that can be duplicated and analyzed, then putting the fragments in the same order they occupy on the chromosome. This can be done in two ways: by comparing patterns of fragments as they are inherited within families (linkage mapping), or by molecular analysis of the DNA itself (physical mapping). Results from the two strategies are constantly integrated into a single map.

This mapping has been achieved ahead of schedule, both within and outside the official project, through worldwide collaboration of research teams that search for the genes involved in human diseases (genetic mapping) with those who try to fit small segments of DNA together in order, like a massive invisible jigsaw puzzle (physical mapping).

The Sequence

The task beyond the genome project is to narrow the focus yet further: to work out the exact molecular sequence of human DNA, one base after another. For a substantial proportion of human genes—half, perhaps—this is already complete. By and large, the effort is automated.

Knowing the precise sequence of a gene provides, by deduction, the identity of its protein product. Databased genetic information from studies of other species, such as mice, worms, and fruit flies, has also provided useful clues, because many genes have similar functions throughout the animal kingdom. Because many known animal proteins already exist in available databases, finding a gene sequence often leads to a quick and astute guess about its function.

it, besides cancer (which is due to changes in the genes which occur over a lifetime) there are so many diseases which have genetic components — diabetes, Alzheimer's, asthma, arthritis, atherosclerosis — that to really understand why some of us come down with one disease and not another, we're going to really have to look at our genes."

By 1987 a number of high-profile organizations were exploring the merits and drawbacks of using public funds to create a map of the human genes. That September, on the very same day, two independent advisory bodies to Congress — the U.S. Office of Technology Assessment (OTA) and the National Research Council (NRC), an arm of the independent expert body known as the National Academy of Sciences — decided to embark on studies of the feasibility of a genome project.

By that time, the concept had gained a certain cachet; people had the feeling that simply by talking about it, they were part of making history. The atmosphere was energizing even to people who were already eminent.

The National Research Council's committee on the genome project featured "a very large number of towering figures in science," recalled Russell Dolittle, who himself had won a Nobel Prize. "It was a room you went into on the morning of the meeting, and the air exuded power and ego."

Their agenda was to decide whether the project should be undertaken at all. (But Dolittle says that, like the secret committee at Rockefeller University two decades earlier, the NRC committee spent "a tremendous amount of time discussing how quickly the data should be released to the public.")

Dolittle also recalls many debates about whether the committee should be a "big science" project to map and sequence the genome, or whether biologists should wait until the technology had evolved more fully. "The story was told at this meeting about the homesteading of America," he recalls, "whether instead of traveling fourteen miles per day in a wagon train we should have had everyone wait in New York until the day when they could all fly to L.A. by jet in five hours."

Not everyone was enthusiastic about plunging into the project. "A large-scale, massive effort to ascertain the sequence of the entire genome cannot be adequately justified at the present time," declared the council of the American Society for Biochemistry and Molecular Biology in 1987, clearly concerned that the esoteric research of many of its members would lose funding to a massive centralized genetics project more reminiscent of the moon mission than of basic biology. Three years later a group of biologists circulated a letter to government figures calling the project "mediocre science and terrible science policy."

The general tenor of debate about the project was thus not *whether* to survey the entire genetic landscape but how, and how quickly, and who should pay for it. Critical voices were heard within the scientific community, granted, but instead of raising Alvin Toffler's question — whether science was moving faster than society's expertise to deal with its consequences — they focused by and large on whether the time, energy, and money devoted to stripping the genome to its bare bones might better be spent in other areas of biology — in other words, on their own turf.

A subsidiary debate focused on whether there was any point in trying to read out the complete molecular *sequence* of the entire human genome, subunit by molecular subunit, all the way from the first to the 2.9 billionth, or whether it would suffice simply to map the genome, work out the general location of the landmark segments, and focus on the areas of interest surrounding them. From what scientists already knew about the DNA sequence, much of it seemed to be meaningless, with no evidence that it was converted to working protein molecules or served any useful purpose inside the body. Much of it, in other words, appeared to be genetic garble. Did it make sense to work out painstakingly the molecular sequence of all that "junk"?

For a time the idea of teasing out the complete sequence of the human genome "became the butt of jokes," writes Robert Cook-Deegan, who headed the OTA study looking into the idea of a genome project. An eminent cancer geneticist, Robert Weinberg, said he was surprised that "consenting adults have been caught in public talking about it . . . it makes no sense." It would be much more rational, many scientists argued, to devote the effort to regions of the genome already known to be important.

As the debate about the molecules swirled about them, many medical geneticists around the world quietly continued the research they had been pursuing for decades: looking for inheritance patterns in families affected by diseases that were obviously hereditary. The first association between a particular genetic fragment and the occurrence of a hereditary disease — sickle cell anemia — had been reported in 1978 and was quickly turned into a test that could be used for prenatal diagnosis as well as for detecting carrier status among prospective parents.

A decade later, when the genome project was about to be launched, teams of scientists were engaging large families all over the country —

JUNK DNA

When gene probers learned enough to compare "raw DNA" taken from chromosomes with the final genetic message translated into protein, they made an astounding discovery: The obviously meaningful bits of genome are interrupted, over and over, by long segments of genetic gibberish. In fact, the coding regions of the genome (comprising at most some 5 percent) appear to interrupt long, monotonous stretches of garble.

These sequences, known officially as "introns," quickly gained an unlovely nickname: junk DNA. What are they? Rubbish left over from previous stages of development? Litter left behind by viruses? Or important and meaningful processing signals that we're simply too unsophisticated to comprehend?

Some junk DNA has survived so much of evolution intact that it is reasonable to conclude it must have a purpose. One classic bit of junk DNA, known as the Alu sequence, is so typical in mammals that it is used as a laboratory trademark for identifying mammal cells.

Recent studies suggest that some so-called junk DNA may act as docking sites for proteins that regulate genes. Other "junk" regions apparently specify the shape that DNA takes as it coils and winds itself into chromosomes.

Some "junk," however, is not only meaningless but destructive. Disorders such as Huntington's disease are caused by the intrusion of genetic stutters, repetitions of DNA sequences that destroy the usual function of the gene they interrupt.

Another genetic mystery is the prevalence of "pseudogenes," stretches of DNA that are all but identical to coding regions except that they lack control elements. These pseudogenes may constitute as much as 10 percent of the genome, although it's difficult to know because no one has conducted a systematic search for them. It seems that most genes may have several corresponding pseudogenes — misguided ancestors, perhaps, who have lost their way in the genome and can't get back home.

indeed, around the world — in studies aimed at identifying DNA segments from their blood cells that would give clues to the heredity, and molecular origin, of the particular condition that affected them. By 1987 various research teams were hunting for the approximate location of the genes involved in scores of hereditary diseases both common and rare, including the eye cancer retinoblastoma, colon cancer, muscular dystrophy, and Huntington's disease. A particularly exhilarating race was under way among a number of teams all trying to unearth the genetic basis of cystic fibrosis.

Whatever its other potential, there could be no doubt that a detailed catalog of human genetic material would speed such work immensely and would lead to the isolation of genes involved in countless other human conditions. By the time the genome project was under serious debate, the raw material needed for the effort was already being amassed in a central location.

Thanks largely to an endowment from an admirer, French scientist Jean Dausset had been able to found a massive repository of cells from thousands of large families worldwide who showed interesting patterns of hereditary disease. Scientists could deposit in or withdraw from the cell bank at the Centre d'Étude du Polymorphisme Humain (Center for the Study of Human Genetic Variation) or CEPH — but only on the condition that they would share whatever they learned as a result.

Early in 1988 both the NRC and the OTA released reports largely favorable to the idea of a major project to map and then sequence the genome. James Watson had already appeared before Congress to request an annual budget of $30 million for the project. Congress, however, was not the first to ante up.

Partly because of infighting between the Department of Energy and the National Institutes of Health over which agency should be at the helm, the government was not involved in the Human Genome Project at its inception. The first seed money came from hundreds of unrelated government grants to individual researchers, from small but organized efforts through a few interested biotechnology companies, and from the Howard Hughes Medical Institute, a research foundation created by a legacy from the estate of the wealthy recluse.

It seemed likely that the biotechnology industry would benefit eventually from a genome project. In fact, surveys at the time revealed that industry figures were staunchly in support of the idea. (A UCLA survey in the late 1980s showed that government and industry figures were much more likely than academic scientists to consider the genome project "a worthwhile use of taxpayers' money and scientific resources.") But the fledgling biotechnology industry was engaged in a risky business, with little if any profit to show investors. There was no way such fragile firms could afford to lay out the massive amounts of money that would be needed for so speculative a venture as a genome project.

But should the government back the project if the most obvious beneficiaries were to be industry? Supporters could and quite persuasively did argue that the program was vital if only to keep America at the forefront of biotechnology worldwide — one of the few industries where it still had a clear preeminence.

Congress spent much of 1988 debating the project, weighing the august advice of the OTA and the NRC. It finally approved it in 1989, as a joint effort of the Department of Energy and the National Institutes of Health. The project officially began in October 1990, within an entity known as the National Center for Human Genome Research (NCHGR). One of the strongest proponents of placing the NIH at the helm was the president of Rockefeller University, Norton Zinder — the very person who thirty years earlier had recorded the proceedings of a clandestine meeting to discuss whether such a project should be undertaken. The head of the center was James Watson, the charismatic figure who had puzzled out the structure and function of DNA thirty-five years earlier.

As Robert Cook-Deegan points out in detail in *The Gene Wars*, the creation of the Human Genome Project was sold to the public as a way to make inroads against human diseases. But it was not *driven* by any organized lobby for the cure of human disease. It was driven primarily by the curiosity of scientists like Watson and Dulbecco, biologists and biophysicists who were passionate to develop a new technology that would help them answer interesting questions about genetics. It was only later that people outside science saw commercial and political advantages in the project.

These subsequent motivations came across transparently at a 1989 conference in Washington, cosponsored by the American Medical Association and the Alliance for Aging Research, under the bold title "Unlocking Potential: The Promise of the Human Genome." Congress was embroiled in that year's budget process at the time, and one item on the budget agenda was the recently approved genome project. At the conference, key figures lobbying for the genome project had a chance to state their case publicly before a broad audience including government officials, industry representatives, and journalists.

"There are many individuals who question whether we can afford this," said geneticist Thomas Caskey of Baylor College of Medicine. "But the cost savings in prenatal diagnosis has already saved the cost of research and development."

Leroy Hood of the California Institute of Technology, one of the leading lights in technology development to support the project, pointed out its advantages over another megaproject competing for funding: the superconducting supercollider. The genome project, he noted, would be closed-ended, with results that would "profoundly change medicine." New technologies could be certain to emerge from it, and it would be carried out in a "very dispersed fashion."

The Europeans, the Soviets, and the Japanese all would be involved, Hood said. Collaboration sounded good to some listeners, but others gave competition the clear advantage. "The pillars of our economy have fallen," remarked Representative Mike Andrews, who was present. "Biotechnology is one area where we can have a clear lead."

Republican Senator Pete Domenici of New Mexico, one of the staunchest supporters of the program in the federal government and a member of the Senate Budget Committee, prepared remarks that were shown on videotape. "Our competitors in this field," he warned, "are dancing a very fast tune." He was talking, unquestionably, about the Japanese.

To the general public, however, the talking point was clearly the potential that the new genetics would — speakers used the word again and again — "revolutionize" medical care. "Over the next ten-year period," predicted geneticist Walter Gilbert of Harvard University at the Washington conference, "science will change, in that molecular biology will move from the lab out to the service industries. . . . The most challenging point is not only to identify specific diseases — we'll do that in passing — but all aspects of our life. This will not only be a medicine of diagnosis or prognosis, but of tailoring to individuals."

That was what the scientists forecast, certainly, but it was not their deepest motivation. Sydney Brenner, head of the United Kingdom's vigorous effort in gene mapping, portrayed most clearly what was impelling prominent scientists to pull every string they could to get the project up and rolling. "For years," he said, "we've been trying to look into this area by looking through little cracks in the fence. Big doors will now open."

So they did. What surprised everyone most, in retrospect, was how quickly—after all the hand-wringing and debate—the project reached and even surpassed its stated goals. In the mid-1980s "the genome project was something people thought was a really bad idea that would never come to pass," says its current director, Francis Collins. "There were only two genes that had been found . . . at that point, or three: muscular dystrophy, chronic granulomatous disease, and retinoblastoma. People thought, you know, this isn't going to work except in rare circumstances where you have a chromosomal rearrangement. And now we're finding them every week."

A joint five-year plan released in 1990 by the DOE and NIH arms of the project called for the creation of a complete map of the human genome with at least six hundred molecular landmarks spaced at about 100,000 base pair intervals. Five years later, as Collins pointed out at every possible opportunity, the project was ahead of schedule and under budget and well on its way to completing the map, as projected, by the year 2005.

Several new high-tech strategies had streamlined the process of slicing the genome into workable pieces, mass-producing the segments quickly from vanishingly small amounts of material through a process known as PCR (for polymerase chain reaction), and separating them by size in order to distinguish them from one another.

The ability to store and share information about DNA in databases had also mushroomed, along with extensive amounts of sequence information from other species that were being mapped at the same time. This process could shorten from years to hours the time a researcher needed to confirm the nature of a particular DNA fragment, or even to gain important hints about its function within the body. For example, within days of the discovery of the cystic fibrosis gene, researchers could deduce from its structure and parts of its sequence the nature of the corresponding protein and, using knowledge gained from other species, also deduce its normal function.

Just as important, scientists had been working hard to devise statistical and analytical methods to tease apart the functions of individual genes that might work in concert to cause complex phenomena such as cancer and heart disease.

In 1995 Harold Varmus, the head of the National Institutes of Health, had predicted that the existing databases of DNA would allow the creation of a map of "more than half of the human genes" within a year. It happened only six months later: researchers from CEPH in Paris

POLYMERASE CHAIN REACTION

In theory (or in a movie about political intrigue), a barber could destroy the president's career by giving hair cuttings to a molecular geneticist who could search his genome for the portents of a disease. Polymerase chain reaction (PCR), the technique that makes it possible to get enough DNA to convict someone from a nail cutting or a blood spot on a glove, also revolutionized gene mapping in the last decade.

PCR borrows an enzyme, DNA polymerase, from a bacterium that is found in hot springs. DNA polymerase is an enzyme that copies DNA, making new strands of it using the old strands as a pattern. The enzyme from the hot-springs bacterium works at high heat, which is what biologists use to separate DNA strands and then to copy them.

Unlike polymerase from other sources, that from the hot-springs bacterium works despite the heat, so geneticists no longer need to interrupt the reaction and let the strands cool before copying them.

The strands keep separating, and new copies keep being made. From inconceivably small bits of DNA, you can derive enough to learn something useful.

For instance, one of the World Trade Center bombers was identified based on DNA taken from the back of a postage stamp on a letter containing a bomb threat. The DNA evidence also showed that someone else sealed the envelope. It's sometimes also possible to extract DNA from a fingerprint.

published a map that covered more than three-quarters of the genome with closely spaced molecular landmarks. All that remained was to fill in the gaps between the landmarks—and not a voice to be heard was pessimistic about that.

"The result will be a flood of information about disease and the genes that cause or predispose to it," announced a press release on the latest version of the gene map in September 1995. The more finely detailed the map to which they could refer, of course, the easier it was for scientists to pin down the location of a gene and take the steps necessary to identify and characterize it. "Current mapping projects have enough momentum to reduce average [DNA landmark] spacings to 100,000 base pairs throughout the genome within a year or two," announced molecular biologist Maynard Olson in an article in *Science* a month later.

The grueling process of turning chunks of DNA into symbols of molecular sequence that could be read off a chart or a database had been so thoroughly automated that what had ten years earlier generated hours and pages of debate—the prospect of obtaining a complete subunit-by-subunit catalog of human DNA, from one end to the other—was no longer speculative. It was just a matter of time, and not as much time as had been anticipated.

For about a year several molecular biologists had been arguing that the time had come to move ahead to sequencing in a big way. No unexpected breakthrough was likely to emerge, they argued, but existing technology could make the job feasible—if sponsors were willing to sacrifice a little accuracy (99.9 percent rather than 99.99 percent) in those regions of the genome not known to code for a functional protein.

In the autumn of 1995 the genome project's director, Francis Collins, stated a goal of completing the sequence within a decade. The following spring he announced that the NCHGR was ready to fund the final push toward reading out the sequence of the genome, base by base.

He had decided to provide more than $20 million that year and some $60 million over the next three years to researchers at six centers, to find the genetic sequence of, all together, about three percent of the chromosomes. The hope was that this first plunge into sequencing would provide the expertise and technology to finish the job. But the implication was obvious: not only could the sequence be accomplished, it was within reach.

Now and again some people at scientific conferences were beginning to raise an entirely new speculation. Where would the field turn its attention *after* the genome project? It was a mind-boggling question, and few people really took it seriously. The answer was rather self-evident: scientists would have plenty to do trying to figure out what all those genes were up to, once everyone knew what and where they were.

Meanwhile it was astounding how few people outside the world of science even realized and took note of the fact that a centralized and very expensive government project stood behind the genetic advances they were hearing about in the news every week. A 1994 survey of individuals contacted through genetics *clinics* revealed that only 61 percent of "consumers" and barely half of health professionals had even heard of the Human Genome Project. Among the latter group, barely two in ten medical doctors knew about it.

"It is nothing less than the first atlas of ourselves," crowed the journal *Nature* in 1995, heralding the publication of the newest version of the human gene map. The statement echoed the kind of hyperbole that had surrounded the triumphs of gene research for many years. The atlas might give us the nuts-and-bolts specifications of the human machine. The sequence would even give us a readout of the molecular text. But precisely what would *that* give us?

"The development of a human being is guided by just 750 megabytes of digital information," wrote molecular biologist Maynard Olson of the University of Washington at Seattle that same year in *Science*. "In vivo, this information is stored as DNA molecules in an egg or sperm cell. In a biologist's personal computer, it could be stored on a single CD-ROM."

What would all of that information really have to tell us—if anything—about what *Nature* had called "ourselves"? Through the shift from molecular to electronic information, would the contents of that CD-ROM (or simply its mere existence) begin to dictate to us in some unforeseen way how we should regard "ourselves"—perhaps more as products of a code than as personalities transformed by our own efforts and perceptions and our interactions with each other? Will what that CD-ROM tells us about ourselves come to mean more to us than, or merely something different from, old photographs, say, or visits to a psychiatrist, or long stares into a mirror? Learning the answer to this question, surely, is the project beyond the genome project.

CHAPTER 12

Days of Miracle
and Wonder

Don't cry, baby, don't cry. Don't cry. It's a turnaround jump shot. It's
everybody's jump start. . . . Medicine is magical and magical is art.

— Paul Simon, "The Boy in the Bubble," 1986

THE TERM *GENETICIST* INCLUDES A NUMBER OF DIFFER-
ent job descriptions. There are the mappers and the other molecular
biologists, who work with genes at their most elemental dimension —
take them apart, figure out how they're made, and fit the pieces back
together. Their tools are test tubes, biochemicals, and increasingly computer databases.

They are a different breed altogether from population geneticists like
James Neel, who view genes from a great distance. Using statistical
models, population geneticists inquire into properties of the genome as
a whole — how variations arise, and how the composition of the genome
shifts and drifts due to migrations, intermarriages, the vicissitudes of human history.

Medical geneticists and genetic counselors hold the middle ground,
focusing neither on molecules nor on masses but on individual human beings. They read the results of genetic tests, and to the best of
their ability, they explain to the individuals and families involved what
those results mean. Then they shake hands and smile farewell. Or else
they remain on call for months, to prop up the patients and their families when the news is inscrutable or downright bad.

In the month of October 1994, the mappers met at one conference
and the gene doctors at another. The discontinuity in mood between
the two big meetings was striking. Like the two men in Einstein's
thought experiment about the theory of relativity, one of whom was

on the train and the other on the platform, the mappers saw one situation and the doctors another. It was the year when the pace of gene-mapping began to accelerate, and what that meant depended entirely on where you stood.

The U.S. government-sponsored project to explore human DNA, the NIH's National Center for Human Genome Research, was now four years old. That October the journal *Science* hosted its annual conference on the human genome, coinciding with the publication of the latest genome map. The map was printed as a wall poster. The poster is dense with alphanumeric labels, many hundreds of different DNA fragments pinned to specific locations along the chromosomes. Molecular geneticists knew where the fragments were. In the molecular sense they often knew what the fragments meant as well.

The editor of *Science*, Daniel Koshland, opened the mappers' proceedings. Always a booster of genetic research, he portrayed its prospects in glowing terms. The genome project is a "great adventure," he told the scientists in the darkened ballroom. Like many others, he compared it to the moon shot. But this venture, he added, would have a practical payoff for humankind.

Genetic research was taking off, he said. Where a few years earlier it had been like a neighborhood full of mom-and-pop shops, now we had a superstore. It was an apt analogy. The sponsoring journal was called *Science;* much of what went on was really about business.

It was one of several human gene maps published that year, the previous year, and the year to come. The maps kept getting finer and finer in detail. "No longer will we have a situation where we can't place a gene because the map isn't good enough," said Francis Collins, the director of the genome center at the NIH, who was next to speak.

The sooner the road map was complete, Collins said, the faster the researchers could get where they were all going. Fifteen years earlier, as one geneticist put it, everyone working on a chromosome could get together in one room and talk about the genetic landmarks that had been identified along its length. That wasn't possible anymore. These days they needed databases to keep track of all the information.

"For the first time, in the last year there's beginning to be a consensus that we can see a way to get this thing done," he added. No longer were geneticists awaiting new technology for the way forward. The goals were within reach, and they were racing toward them.

That was the tone of the official meeting: exhilaration and pace. Donna Shalala, the head of the U.S. Department of Health and Human Services, addressed the gathering on the promise genetics held for conquering human disease. The elite in her audience listened attentively and respectfully. Then, during the applause, they slipped out a back door and ascended an interior escalator.

In a back room upstairs, scientists and representatives of biotechnology firms crowded into a small room where the Wellcome Trust, a British philanthropy, was hosting a very private meeting with a very specific agenda on behalf of the international Human Genome Organization. HUGO, a group of genome researchers formed in 1989 to foster international collaboration in the field, had issued a limited number of invitations six months earlier. The intention had been to discuss the prospects for a hot new strategy to speed the search for genes. In the meantime a deeper issue had arisen, a source of conflict that lurked beneath all the jubilation and mandated a change in the agenda: Who would control access to the identity of genetic sequences, which everyone needed in order to progress?

At that moment one scientist — Craig Venter, formerly of the National Institutes of Health, now head of a private genetics venture called The Institute for Genetic Research — had nearly a monopoly on the most abundant genetic tags that were being used as landmarks on the DNA map. While at the NIH, Venter had come up with a bold idea for mapping the genome, a way to generate thousands of DNA sequences that would at once be useful ID tags throughout the chromosomes and also sites of unusual interest for sequencing. Not surprisingly, some people suspected that Venter wanted to run away with the project single-handedly.

Craig Venter is a biochemist and, by his own description, an extremely impatient man. He began his career in a lab that spent a decade trying to purify human proteins from the heart. When the Human Genome Project began, he said, "I got very excited, because the idea of getting all the genes in ten or twenty years seemed a lot more efficient than what I had just spent ten years doing."

In the mid-1980s the time-honored way to find genes was to do a linkage study, to compare gene fragments from family members in search of the ones that coincided with the occurrence of a disease, and then pare away, painstakingly, at the region of whichever chromosome those fragments occupied. This process was too slow for Venter, especially after machines came along that automated the process of DNA sequencing. Still, once you had a gene sequence, how could you interpret what the sequence meant?

Venter proposed to seek out small segments of DNA while they were actually being processed inside cells, on their way to becoming proteins. Such fragments — caught in the act of being copied and read — must be of some current use to the body, because they were captured at the moment of *being* used. Clearly they were not "junk DNA."

Venter wanted to isolate thousands of these fragments, which molecular biologists call "expressed sequence tags" or ESTs, not only to locate the larger genes of which they were part, but also to use them as landmarks on the gene map. Trying out the strategy, he located eight new genes in two years — but that wasn't fast enough. "I didn't want to wait 20 or 240 years for the rest of the genes," he says.

He had a vision: ranks of sequencing machines, run by a small army of technicians, churning out the DNA sequence of thousands of these DNA tags and pinning them like molecular Post-its along the chromosome map. The problem was that the National Institutes of Health, where Venter worked, wasn't willing to share the vision by paying for the ranks of machines and armies of workers. Many scientists were offended by Venter's approach. They saw it as scattershot, crude, and inelegant, and some predicted it would come to naught.

When Venter published his first results in *Nature* in 1991, they "caused quite a stir," he said. "But we were actually embarrassed, because it had only 337 genes in it."

By February 1992 he had identified more than 2,000 of these DNA tags, many of which had no known purpose at the time but presumably were important for something. (Otherwise why would they be in use inside a cell?) He persuaded the NIH to apply for a patent on these tags — leading to a controversy not only worldwide but also within the U.S. government.

Others had gained patents on genetic information before, but only on defined genes that had been isolated in full and were well characterized. What was scary about the NIH application was that at that time no one knew what most of Venter's DNA tags *were*. They were simply thousands of undefined bits of human DNA, and the NIH patent application claimed rights for all possible future uses — not only for the fragments but for the larger genes that would eventually be found to encompass them, and also for the proteins those genes would be found to encode.

Was it acceptable for anyone — even a government, let *alone* a government — to patent so much of the human biochemical machine, without any idea what it was? The advisory body to the NIH branch of the genome project was unanimous in its opinion. The twelve-member committee issued a statement "deploring" the application, largely on the grounds that it would retard the free flow of information vital to scientific progress.

But the National Institutes of Health maintained that the patent application was necessary to ensure that the sequences were used properly, and that their commercial potential was applied to the best advantage—besides which, it said, the application was required by a new law promoting links between government agencies and private industry. Nonetheless, James Watson, head of the NIH genome project at the time, viewed the action as a land grab. He left the project in 1992, in part because of this dispute, and returned to Cold Spring Harbor.

Venter did little to dispel impressions like Watson's. At a press conference, in answer to the charge that "his" DNA tags were genetically meaningless, Venter responded, "There is so much information contained in the 300 to 500 base pairs [in each tag] that it is more specific than fingerprints at identifying you."

He too left the government, but in a quite different direction. With $70 million seed money from a private investor, he founded the nonprofit Institute for Genetic Research in order to pursue his vision. The institute was bound by complicated financial ties to a profit-making medical products development firm, Human Genome Sciences (HGS), and by a business agreement with the pharmaceutical firm SmithKline Beecham, to which it promised commercially useful results.

Venter's Institute for Genome Research soon assumed the acronym TIGR, which Venter pronounced "tiger." It was a fitting nickname, because the institute gained a fierce reputation. Venter said he aimed to "do the genome project" himself, using industrial-scale processes to sequence as many as 60 million bases—one-fiftieth of the entire genome—each year.

Within a short time TIGR and HGS had done what Venter had originally envisioned at NIH: TIGR had amassed thirty sequencing machines, which hummed quietly in a factorylike room, attended by robots that added the necessary dyes and by about twenty-five human technicians. Together, they worked hour after hour to generate genetic sequences.

By mid-1994 Venter and TIGR had left the Human Genome Project tasting their dust. They were claiming to sequence 750,000 DNA bases per day. The Human Genome Project had aimed at accomplishing

OWNERSHIP OF GENES

In May 1995 a group of American religious leaders held a press confer-
ence to announce their opposition to the patenting of human genes.
More than 180 religious figures—Protestant and Catholic Christians,
Jews, Muslims, Hindus, and Buddhists—had signed a petition to the
U.S. Patent and Trademark Office stating that they opposed "the patent-
ing of human and animal life forms."

The Patent Office had been granting patents of life-forms ever since
1980, when it allowed a General Electric scientist the rights to a genetically engineered microorganism that could clean up oil spills. Since
then it had awarded numerous patents on gene-altered animals and also
several patents on human cells—leading to new drugs for short stature,
heart attack, and bleeding disorders. Worldwide since 1981, a total of
1,175 patents had been granted for human DNA sequences.

Many press articles cast the issue as one of religion versus science, a
characterization that both sides disputed. "The motivation of biotechnology is not to play God," said a representative of one genetics-based
firm. "It is to play doctor." A Catholic bishop said he was most concerned
that decisions were being made without any public forum for debate.

A few months before the religious leaders issued their petition, the
head of a pharmaceutical industry organization argued that most of the

this in six months. By the time of the 1994 Washington conference,
Venter said he had sequence information for DNA fragments representing about half of the total in the human genome. HGS chairman
William Haseltine projected that the company would have a near-
complete set of human genes within two years.

"We've been sequencing about 1,000 human clones [of DNA frag-
ments] each day for quite some time," Venter said at the 1994 conference. Those fragments originated from every major organ and tissue in
the human body. He also had sufficient computer power to keep databases of similar sequences from other organisms, including plants,
which allowed almost instant insights into the possible function of any
DNA snippet that turned up. More than one eminent geneticist who

opponents simply misunderstand the meaning of patents, which do not confer "ownership" of anything—merely a seventeen-year (it's now twenty) monopoly on rights to make money on it. Without that short-term monopoly, he argued, new research by biotechnology firms would dry up. However, a statement by the head of the panel that signed the petition showed that the dispute cuts to the heart of the issue, which is the patentability of DNA segments.

"The issue is not science versus religion," said Methodist bishop Kenneth Carder. "It's the commodification of life and the reduction of life to its commercial value and marketability." The argument that patenting is necessary for research to proceed "assumes that anything profitable ought to be permissible," he added, calling it "a form of colonialism."

Whatever the convictions of their leaders, there was no subsequent evidence of a mass protest movement among the religious lay public. The following year a group of feminist leaders protested the patenting of DNA. On the other hand, many consumer groups with an interest in specific hereditary diseases are strongly in favor of patenting genes, which they see as a way to speed research toward a cure.

The U.S. Patent Office continues to grant patents for segments of human DNA. In 1996, for instance, it granted Myriad Genetics (a private company with ties to the University of Utah) a patent on a newfound gene that predisposes some women to breast cancer.

made arrangements to log into Venter's database to look up a sequence he was interested in had come away, minutes later, knowing almost exactly what it was used for.

"Think about the implications of this," Venter said. "People have been studying one gene at a time. Now we can study thousands of genes at a time." The prospects for the study of human disease were "tremendous," he pointed out at a press conference during the 1994 genome conference. And it was clear that he took them seriously.

"We have people coming to the institute all the time, representing disease foundations, organizations, themselves," he added, and then (with a catch in his voice), "young kids with devastating genetic disease depend on us to do something.

"This is urgent work," he went on. "We should do it in a very rational way to produce the best result possible. Every year, millions of people are dying without a cure. Any year we lose millions of people to die. This is not a game. I myself have family members with genetic diseases, so I know what I'm talking about. . . . Everything we can do to help society, we should do."

Perhaps the most breathtaking fact about Venter's tags was that they were *sequenced.* The information was not stored in snippets of actual human DNA preserved inside microorganisms in rack upon rack of tiny test tubes; it had been transformed into an alphabetical pattern of symbols for DNA subunits and stored as digital information in a computer database. Venter's genome tags were in a form that could easily be saved, copied, shared, and compared.

Unfortunately, whatever Venter's own intentions, there was no guarantee that this sharing would actually happen — and that caused a change of agenda at that clandestine meeting-during-the-meeting in Washington. SmithKline Beecham, with which his institute had a commercial affiliation, had placed certain important roadblocks in the way of releasing information about the genetic tags. It insisted that HGS and TIGR would have first commercial rights to applications of genes discovered as a result of the database, and it also insisted on being notified sixty days before any data derived from the database were published.

What was originally envisioned as a small intimate conversation among some of the scientists attending the Washington genome conference had swollen to several dozen participants, because Baylor College of Medicine geneticist Thomas Caskey, who was president of HUGO, had persuaded Wellcome that under the circumstances it was only fair to invite representatives of the major biotechnology firms to the private meeting. Word had gotten out that something interesting was happening, and the meeting would not have a useful outcome if it excluded some of the parties involved.

Would outside scientists agree — were they in fact at liberty to agree (since each of them worked at an institution that would probably want to establish its own policies on the subject) — to SmithKline's conditions, in exchange for information about any of Venter's DNA tags? "There was ferment in the community," recalls Caskey. "The NIH and the DOE had neglected this area, they had not focused on expressed sequences [those genes known to translate into identifiable proteins.] . . . It was a major screwup. Many of us tried to persuade them that it would be wrong to omit this important area. HGS and TIGR had come in and filled this void fantastically. They had this power and this database, but now they were making very unreasonable demands for accessing the database."

Baylor College of Medicine — Caskey's employer — and the NIH itself let it be known that they would not play along, as did some individual scientists. "I don't want to find that I've spent the last four years of my life building a map that I intend to have as openly available as possible," said one scientist at the NCHGR, "only to find that some of the key rivets in it have strings attached."

"The opposite of patent protection is trade secrecy," argued Venter, "and then we all lose." If the public NIH had not been willing to fund his ambitious venture, he felt, why not reward with patent protection the private companies that were willing to take that risk?

At the epicenter of the controversy were the scientists who wanted access to information about these thousands of DNA segments for their own research, although the shock would radiate much farther. Should one man, or one private institution, have exclusive control of so much information about human DNA?

For four hours, Collins and some forty other participants in the Wellcome meeting argued about what kind of arrangements should be allowed for control of DNA information. At the same time an unanticipated development was shifting the foundations of the debate. Caskey, who at the time was on the board of Merck, one of SmithKline Beecham's major competitors, had been making the same arguments in the boardroom that he and many others had made about the government's Human Genome Project, in favor of a public DNA database. Merck had seen the power of his arguments and had committed to contributing about $10 million to create its own database of similar DNA tags. It would fund a nearly identical effort at Washington University in St. Louis, starting from scratch. Merck proposed to offer full and unrestricted public access to the information.

Of course, like a Monopoly player who hoards one of the two blue properties on principle, Merck stood to gain by denying its competitors exclusive use to something valuable. But Caskey, who was so instrumental in creating it, says Merck's competing database would simply not be a profit-oriented activity. Perhaps it was more a matter of corporate style: while an increasing number of huge pharmaceutical firms contract out for basic research, Merck continues its long history of continuing research in-house.

"Merck just wanted the data," declares Caskey. "This was a cheap way to do it." It would be cheaper and more effective, in any case, than bowing to a competitor's strictures on the data.

All that was really left to discuss, it turned out, was recommendations for how the new public access database venture should proceed. It should be accomplished quickly, everyone agreed, and just as Venter had done it—but making the data freely available to all researchers.

Some of the participants, including Venter, appeared at a press conference afterward. Venter handed out the full text of TIGR's conditions for access to its database and defended the policy, but in public the scientists tried to present a face of equanimity. "There were heated discussions," said Caskey, "but we ended up friends."

"When we gathered yesterday, there was no major problem," said Jacques Cohen, head of the major French gene-mapping center known as Genethon. "We all agree that what has been done by Craig [Venter] is the most important work in twenty-five years. We all understand that private work has to be rewarded. It will all eventually be made public. Doing it privately is quicker. There is no controversy. Everybody agrees about that."

In retrospect, perhaps the problem of access to Venter's data was never as dire as the scientists feared. Eventually he released some 90 percent of the sequence on the World Wide Web, including the complete sequence of the bacterium that causes influenza. His goal had always been to keep the data as open as possible, he maintained.

In fact, TIGR later split from its commercial partners. Soon afterward, when Venter's team worked out the sequence of a bacterium found to cause human stomach ulcers, they published the sequence almost immediately.

In 1993 the Patent Office denied the NIH's application on all those DNA tags, holding that sequences could not be patented without having some idea about what they were. NIH director Harold Varmus declined to rewrite the application and reapply.

In 1996, while signing agreements to sequence the genome, six major genetic labs agreed to share new gene data almost immediately, and at a private meeting in Bermuda (again sponsored by the Wellcome Trust), a number of major gene labs agreed to release their sequence information within about three months of finding it—just long enough to confirm the results internally. The dispute flared again a year later, however, when an official of the Patent Office gave a speech favoring patents on DNA tags—which prompted hasty responses from Varmus and later from the president of the National Academy of Sciences. Because such patents might allow claims on discoveries not yet made, both of the responses argued that such patents would stifle research.

The patent dispute surrounding DNA tags is probably the most prominent source of contention among molecular geneticists, but it is only one of many rough spots along the road toward a future whose outlines are still barely visible. "We're living in a time period in medicine in which the speed of information transfer is greater than we have ever experienced," remarked Thomas Caskey, who would move in 1996 from Baylor to Merck, where among many other responsibilities he would oversee the new public access database. "Also," he added, "the speed of change of the rate of discovery is greater than anything we are used to."

Merck's database of DNA tags met its own target dates for completion. Caskey came to view Merck's venture as inevitable but disappointing, because (as he put it) events would always favor the person who withheld data. "I think what we have to do is stand back and say that we made a gift to the scientific community, and we should have no expectations from it," he muses. "But we find ourselves competing with ourselves," because other biotech firms could use the Merck/Washington database as a basis for learning more about specific genetic sequences they had discovered that Merck had not been focusing on. On all fronts, in any case, gene discovery would continue to accelerate.

By the autumn of 1997, no fewer than five genetics-based biotech companies were producing new proteins by back-translating the genetic tags from these databases to see what they encoded, in search of completely new kinds of medicines. The prospect was exhilarating.

The key competitive question by then was to learn which of these thousands of previously unknown proteins could become useful drugs. Some companies were purifying them and monitoring their actions at the cell level; others were pumping them straight into laboratory animals and watching what happened.

These proteins are totally new to human understanding. Our bodies have manufactured them for millennia; now we can learn what they do and adapt some of them to specific therapeutic purposes. It is indeed a frontier.

The space-travel metaphor that Koshland used to open the 1994 Washington conference has become a cliché—but it is compelling nonetheless. In the mid-1990s human genetic research did take off like a rocket. Tumbling along in its wake came those middlemen, the medical geneticists, who had the good sense to wonder where the wind was blowing them.

Two weeks after the gene mappers dispersed from Washington in 1994, the gene doctors and genetic counselors gathered in Montreal for the annual conference of the American Society of Human Genetics. In Washington their counterparts had debated who would control access to the genetic information itself. In Montreal the human geneticists worried about a companion issue: Who would control access to the *meaning* of that information — and would they be in a position to convey it clearly, and responsibly, and fairly?

Over the next five to ten years, warned medical geneticist Michael Kaback in an early session, his profession would quickly lose control of the diffusion of genetic information. It would be pediatricians and obstetricians, general practitioners and internists, he predicted, who would administer all the new diagnostic tests based on newfound genes.

Most of them would do so under some sort of compulsion, Kaback added, whether it be pressure from a company marketing a profitable test, fear of litigation from patients who want it, or simply the knowledge that the test is recommended by a managed-care guideline. "What I'm concerned about is that without major education, we are about to jump into genetic screening, and start walking before we can crawl," he said.

Kaback spoke at a workshop entitled "The Future Is Here." It was a scintillating title, with a hint of great promise. What chiefly emerged, however, was apprehensiveness: the impression that medical geneticists were being dragged by an undertow rather than swimming with a current.

A national directory of DNA diagnostic centers, called Helix, already listed 230 diseases that were amenable to DNA testing and 180 labs were prepared to provide it, noted geneticist Roberta Pagon of the University of Washington, as she opened the session. Some 1,700 users were purchasing these services, and Helix was answering thirty to forty inquiries each day about testing. Such "informal decision-making networks" would soon be overwhelmed by queries and requests.

Yet no standards were in existence to determine when DNA testing was appropriate, noted Pagon. The decision as to when testing was appropriate and which issues, if any, to raise with patients or their families were left to the individual physician.

It should not be left to individual doctors, she went on, to decide who should get which test for what. But the following speaker offered little hope that the situation would soon change. David Ledbetter of the National Center for Human Genome Research pointed out that, although testing became available in 1991 for Fragile X syndrome, it had taken three years for the American College of Medical Genetics to develop a policy statement on such testing. "The interval has been fairly slow," he admitted. "How do we speed this process?"

The speakers conveyed a sense that events were already out of control. When it came to prenatal testing, noted geneticist Arno Motulsky, "we say it should be done at thirty-five, but now people are starting it earlier and earlier. People say, well, there's a test for that—why don't we do it?"

Motulsky was head of a National Academy of Sciences expert panel that had just published a major report about genetic testing, entitled *Assessing Genetic Risks* (see next page). The panel had urged a great number of policy initiatives, from increased efforts to improve public education about gene tests to tighter regulation of laboratories that provide them. It was far too soon to say whether any of those advisories would bear fruit, but Motulsky did not sound optimistic. He sounded, at best, cautious.

"We are living at a time where things go so fast that as we are gathering information, things are shifting," he remarked to his fellow geneticists. "It's very difficult. We have widespread testing where the treatment is partial but not that good. Do people really know what they're getting into?"

Kaback broke back into the discussion. "Let's not talk about them versus us, guys," he said. "We're the entrepreneurs. We've got a conflict of interest. Our presentation of whether someone should take a test or not is influenced by our monthly heating bills—I see a number of nodding heads out there." Nearly everyone in this room, he went on, ran a laboratory for which they charged a fee, and that created "a difficult conflict of interest." The number of private labs ready to provide gene testing for a fee was burgeoning, but many tests were also being done by the academic labs that had found a genetic marker in the first place—also for a fee, and often without any oversight whatever. In a time of tight research funding, offering testing was a good way to make money. Now and again the academic labs turned commercial or undertook large-volume contract work. The lines of accountability and interest were vague indeed.

Kaback's statement provoked a barrage of responses from the audience. One geneticist from Utah rose to the microphone and opened up:

ASSESSING GENETIC RISKS

It was obvious from the outset that the Human Genome Project raised a large number of ethical and social issues. Throughout 1992 the Institute of Medicine (an advisory arm to the National Academy of Sciences) convened a number of public forums and meetings of an expert panel to discuss these issues and ponder ways to avert social problems arising from the huge new project.

The following ethical principles guided the panel's discussions: voluntariness, informed consent, and confidentiality, founded upon respect for autonomy, equity (fairness), and privacy. Much of the funding for the effort came from the genome project itself.

The result of these efforts was a large report, released in book form in 1994, entitled *Assessing Genetic Risks*. Many of the issues it raised became focal points for later research and policy debates, but its concerns and recommendations remain largely unresolved. They include the following:

1. "Entrepreneurial pressure" may lead to widespread genetic testing, unregulated by government bodies. The problems this may raise about informed consent, confidentiality, and discrimination "threaten to outrun current ethical and regulatory standards."

2. People who are offered prenatal diagnosis must be fully informed about the risks and possible outcomes, as well as about alternative options and about the "spectrum of severity" of the genetic disorders involved. "Reproductive genetic services should not be used to pursue eugenic goals [like reducing the prevalence of an inherited disease], but should be aimed at increasing individual control over reproductive options," says the report.

3. Long-term studies should prove the value of predictive genetic tests for adult-onset hereditary diseases before such tests reach the market, and population screening should be considered only if an effective therapy or preventive strategy exists. (Experience with gene-based tests to predict breast cancer and Alzheimer's disease suggest this plea is being heard.)

4. Existing quality control programs for laboratory testing are inadequate for the special issues raised by gene testing, and the government should consider stricter oversight. (It has considered it but has not yet acted.)

5. Primary care doctors should have more training for genetic counseling and decision making about genetic referrals. (The amount of medical school training in this subject area declined in recent decades. However, special new education initiatives are under way.)

6. Public and private health plans, geneticists, and consumers should "work together" to develop guidelines for reimbursement of genetic services. (An idealistic notion: although guidelines do exist for the *use* of some tests, guidelines for their reimbursement are not in place.)

7. Every entity that stores DNA should have procedures in place to protect the confidentiality of the donors. (Many don't; see page 225.)

8. Risk-based health insurance should be eliminated, and in particular eligibility for health insurance should not be based on genetic considerations. (Another idealistic notion: nationwide protections for insurance eligibility exist only for people who work for large employers, and there are no limits on the premium cost that insurers can charge people who are known to have genetic risks. State law protections are spotty. At this writing, no legislative proposals have been made to eliminate risk-based health insurance.)

9. Tests for untreatable genetic disorders should not be lumped together in the same procedure with tests for treatable conditions.

10. A national advisory committee should be created to oversee the release and wide-scale use of gene tests. (As yet no such committee exists.)

"What I see potentially happening is that once a test is accepted, any practitioner will decide they know how to use it. A pediatrician will do a smorgasbord of genetic tests for a child with developmental delays. These tests can be ordered by anyone, and fewer and fewer patients who have diagnosable conditions will end up going to geneticists."

Then what? Pagon, the chairman, provided the answer. "Often these doctors don't view the patient as part of a family, so they send only the patient to genetic counseling—or do none at all, which is too often the case."

Meanwhile, Kaback retorted, some labs were sending notices to obstetricians and gynecologists pointing out that carrier testing was now available from their facility, noting that such information "could be a help to families," and perhaps doctors should make patients aware of it. "That word *should* is a dangerous word," he added.

Several years earlier, Kaback had consulted for a bioethics institute on the subject of genetic engineering. The institute staff had raised a number of fanciful issues, he recalled, such as the specter that someone might do strange cloning experiments to create a modern Frankenstein. Kaback had been stunned. "You guys don't need to talk about science fiction," he told them. "There are very important issues going on right now!"

It is all too easy to find a mutation where there may not even be a disease—just a normal variation—so "you've got to be damn sure you know what you're talking about," Kaback said. But the laboratory scientists who unearthed such mutations often knew little if anything about the diseases that might be involved—and doctors, especially primary care doctors, almost certainly did not have the time to learn much about the intricacies of mutations, or the broad implications of testing.

In fact, given everything else they have to deal with, doctors were often not even very interested in talking about genetics. How to engage them in the process was a critical question, especially as the tests began to expand from very rare diseases to very common ones.

That year, 1994, counselors and medical geneticists had come face to face with a prospect that had been looming for years: widespread predictive testing. Only weeks before the Montreal conference, a team at Myriad Genetics had announced the discovery of BRCA1, the first gene linked to breast cancer. It also appeared to influence the development of ovarian cancer.

The discovery of BRCA1 had hit the popular press before the Montreal conference, but the news was still fresh enough to generate considerable interest and discussion. As yet, it was unclear how many other genes would also be linked to the risk of breast cancer, how many people had the same gene in their family but no unusual prevalence of breast cancer, how many women who had BRCA1 lived or died without developing either breast or ovarian cancer, or even how widespread the prevalence of BRCA1 was going to prove to be.

How different is the presence of BRCA1 from a high cholesterol reading, or high blood pressure—or even a breast lump? In any of those cases a condition already exists, as well as something that can be done to resolve it. In the case of the breast cancer gene, however, the reflexive responses to a positive test—more regular mammograms or even mastectomy to prevent cancer from emerging—bore their own risks and were not demonstrated to be effective in preventing the development of breast cancer for women found to be at risk.

Medical geneticists were forced to grapple in earnest with the implications of a test that could suggest (within a considerable range of uncertainty) that a living adult—someone sitting there right across the desk—might develop a particular cancer somewhere down the road. Yet they could offer neither a definitive solution to the dilemma nor much consolation.

The scenario itself was not entirely new: it had already been played out in the case of Huntington's disease, the incurable wasting neurological disorder that emerges sometime around age forty (see page 222). A genetic linkage had been found, allowing geneticists to predict whether someone would or would not develop Huntington's disease, but only if many members of his family would also agree to testing in order to identify exactly which mutation ran in that family. Later researchers had run the gene itself to ground. Now anyone, at least in theory, could be tested simply by giving a blood sample.

Inevitably, a press conference was held in Montreal during the medical geneticists' conference to give reporters the latest information about the new breast cancer gene. Mary Claire King of the University of California at Berkeley, an early researcher in the area, was present to field reporters' questions on the subject. They were tougher than she had anticipated.

Shortly before the press conference a curious figure materialized in the press room. Wearing a pinstripe suit and lugging a large videocamera, he looked out of place among the reporters in their baggy trousers and open collars. He chose a seat close to the front and turned on a bright light and his videocamera.

Most press conferences that take place during scientific meetings

HUNTINGTON'S DISEASE

A degenerative disorder of the brain, Huntington's disease (HD) is caused by a single dominant gene mutation. If you inherit one copy of the affected gene and live long enough, you get the disease. (Symptoms rarely emerge before the age of forty.) It leads to dementia, paralysis, and eventually death.

The gene behind Huntington's was one of the first to be mapped by new genetic methods, but it took an entire agonizing decade to locate the gene and begin to define the problem. In HD the gene is interrupted by a stutter: scores of repeats of the same simple three-base sequence. Evidently this stutter interferes with the brain's ability to make use of its major energy source, sugar.

HD has a long and troubled history in human genetics. Charles Davenport claimed to have traced all the HD cases in the United States back to six individuals and said "all these evils" might have been avoided "had these half-dozen individuals been kept out of this country." Not to sterilize anyone with HD, he wrote in 1916, would be "impotent, stupid, and blind."

Huntington's was one of the conditions listed in Germany's compulsory sterilization act of 1933, and people with HD were later vulnerable to government-sponsored "euthanasia." It is not clear how many were killed.

are rather formalized affairs, low-key and often quite boring. A panel of scientists discuss the findings in simple terms; the reporters, orderly and usually quite deferential, state their questions matter-of-factly. This time the interloper with the camera leaped in with the first question: How soon would the test be licensed?

King declined to make any prediction. A great many more studies needed to be done, she said, before the test would be ready to be used for routine diagnosis. A news reporter might have followed up with the question: What kind of studies? What was missing? But this questioner had different interests, and he kept after King: How soon did she think the test *would* be ready? Did she anticipate regulatory barriers to licensure of the test?

After the briefing the staff member in charge of the press room noticed that the man was not wearing a press badge. She asked who he was and why he was attending. He responded by handing her a card, which bore the name of a firm and the words "investment analyst." The man vanished as quickly as he had come. Officers of the American Society of Human Genetics surmised afterward that he must have been trying to coax a statement out of King that would persuade investors to back a client involved in genetic testing.

Facing the bright light and the videocamera, King had weathered the assault well and did not allow herself to be filmed saying anything substantive about when the test might be ready. But the man's presence endowed the press conference with an unspoken message: there were people with a powerful financial interest — an interest not closely allied to the Hippocratic oath — in seeing the breast cancer test come into regular use.

For a while the financially interested, like everyone else, suppressed their speculation. But not for long: in 1996 two labs put the BRCA1 test on the market — although many professionals felt it was too soon and guidelines for such testing had yet to be released.

Genetic counselor Barbara Biesecker of the National Center for Human Genome Research also faced the reporters at that Montreal press conference. Recently, she said, an oncologist had told her that perhaps ten times each day he had to tell someone the bad news that he had cancer. None of those people got counseling afterward. What was so special, he asked, about people with a cancer gene? What Biesecker said next might have been illuminating to the intruder, had he stayed until the end of the press conference.

"It's very, very difficult to persuade people that genetic testing is different" from other kinds of diagnostic tests, she said. But undeniably it is. There are many, many reasons to go slow.

For one thing, genetic testing immediately implicates other people. It has implications not only for reproduction but for the rest of the family. If I have the breast cancer gene, should I have more children? Should I have my five-year-old daughter tested? Should I tell my sisters and urge them to be tested? Would it anger them to face the unwelcome prospect of being able to learn whether they are at risk for breast cancer?

For another, the issue of how widely genetic tests should be applied is not at all clear. "Once we say the whole population should be tested, we're no longer making autonomous decisions," Biesecker pointed out. "But most of us feel these are decisions we should make for ourselves." Counselors were worried about all the potential harm a genetic test could cause if someone ordered it up before a woman or her family were ready. In fact, no one had even defined *ready* in such cases.

Biesecker harked back to the memory of two families she had counseled early in the studies that had eventually led to the discovery of the gene. One set of young women in a family riddled with breast cancer coped by having prophylactic mastectomies by the age of twenty-five, while they were still healthy. They chose that deadline because the youngest woman in the family to develop breast cancer had been twenty-six at the time she was diagnosed.

"They know this doesn't really eliminate the risk," Biesecker said. (Cancer could also be lurking in lymph nodes outside the breasts.) But "it's their way of coping with it."

By contrast, the women in the other family in the study would not consider having their breasts removed even for preventive reasons, she said. "They thought it was totally barbaric."

It wasn't clear to Biesecker or anyone else exactly how to counsel such patients, partly because there was no good medical evidence to guide such decisions, and partly because genetic counselors themselves were still feeling their way toward a consensus about their role and their obligations. "Clearly in the last few years the main theme in the hallway has been, 'How can we keep up?'" said Biesecker, who had spent years in a breast cancer program at the University of Michigan, counseling women in families with an unusually high prevalence of the disease. "How can we streamline what we do so others can do it? How can we figure out the essential elements of what we do? It's sort of overwhelming for us."

In reality, standard testing protocols exist for some genetic diseases. Anyone who provides the test for Huntington's disease, for instance, is supposed to ensure that the patient is emotionally ready for the verdict. But Huntington's disease is very rare, affecting only some 30,000 Americans. Breast cancer is not rare. More recently, the linkage of the ApoE subtype to a risk for Alzheimer's disease had come to light. There were no protocols, no assurances whatever that doctors who ordered the tests would take the psychic implications into account.

"I'm worried about the scenario where someone walks into her GP's office and says, 'I keep losing my keys and forgetting names,' and the doctor says, 'We have a test for that,'" Francis Collins, the head of the Human Genome Project, said at one point during the Montreal conference. "The doctor might say, 'This is familial. Maybe you ought to bring the kids in.' Then he could say, 'You have it, and you, and you, and someone might go out and blow his brains out.' What kind of protection is going on here? What kind of pilot projects?"

To judge from the evidence, the public with interest in such matters was disturbingly unaware of the implications. In her latest surveys about genetic testing, sociologist Dorothy Wertz of the Shriver Center in Boston had been asking people who had just been tested for the first time what they thought about the idea of collecting genetic information about individuals without their explicit consent. Whose DNA should be banked without his or her knowledge, and what others should have access to this information?

Perhaps not surprisingly, 98 percent of the respondents thought DNA should be collected from convicted sex offenders. But 88 percent felt the same about members of the armed forces, and fully 87 percent felt DNA should be collected and banked for all newborn infants. Who should have access to those DNA results without the express consent of the individual? Personal physicians, said 68 percent, and spouses, added 64 percent. Nearly half (46 percent) felt any blood relative deserved to have information from another family member's DNA, whether or not the person who had been tested wanted it released.

Meanwhile, who was actually in control of the samples used to generate those test results? Apparently no one. J. E. McEwen from the Boston College Law School reported a survey of all the DNA banks in the United States, the academic and commercial labs that store DNA samples for future retrieval and record the identities of those who gave the blood from which the DNA was extracted. McEwen contacted all of the labs in the Helix directory and asked how many had written policies designed to prevent misuse of the information in that banked DNA.

Ninety labs responded. About half of them said they kept DNA samples in live form, cultivated in cells living permanently in tissue culture. Thirty percent had no written policies about who could have access to DNA samples, or for what purposes.

Several members of the audience in Montreal pointed out circumstances they knew of personally that could weaken control of the samples still further. Testing labs were being gobbled up by corporate mergers. Sometimes the doctor or researcher who collected the samples left the university where they were stored without leaving behind instructions as to their disposal. There they sat, perhaps with name tags on them. Nobody had really made any rules.

At least those twenty-seven molecular biologists who had authored the report about the latest gene map, which was celebrated at the

Washington conference, were not oblivious to the implications of what they were doing. In the last paragraph of their report, they pointed out that our ability has "never been greater" to "identify genetic predispositions" and to characterize ("if present") the genetic nature of normal variations such as height, intelligence, and sexual preference.

But while it might be technically feasible, they added, "whether these maps should be used for these ends should be resolved after open dialogue" to review the implications and devise policies.

In May 1998, Craig Venter upped the ante. He announced that he was stepping down from TIGR to start a joint venture with Perkin-Elmer, a scientific instrument maker, with a goal of completing the human genome sequence within three years. As ever, Venter felt he had a better way—and other scientists were inclined to believe him. Venter vowed that he would work in collaboration with the NIH genome project, and that the results would be made public, but ethicists were understandably nervous about the prospect of leaving the completion of the project to a private venture.

Near the end of the century in which eugenics rose, flourished, and then all but vanished in the United States, the field of genetics was in a tremendous resurgence. It was rapidly providing practitioners with the tools to identify individuals with a wide range of qualities and susceptibilities as defined by their genetic profiles. What would come of the emerging information? Who would want it, who would be allowed to use it, and for what?

CHAPTER 13

ELSI, the Gentle Watchdog

*—We've made living biological attractions so astounding that they'll
capture the imagination of the entire planet.
—Yeah, but your scientists were so preoccupied with whether
or not they could, they didn't stop to think if they should.*

— Ian Malcolm responding to John Hammond in the film *Jurassic Park*, 1993

THE HUMAN GENOME ORGANIZATION (HUGO), A GROUP
formed to foster worldwide collaborations in genome research, held its
first congress in Frankfurt, Germany, in 1990. The meeting took place
only blocks from the spot where Otmar von Verschuer had dedicated
his racial hygiene institute fifty-five years earlier. Perhaps the only person present who recognized that fact was Dr. Richard Benson, an American Roman Catholic priest and a bioethicist, who had been invited to
address the moral status of the genome effort.

Benson alluded to Verschuer in his remarks and mentioned Verschuer's postwar apologia that he had not been responsible for abuses
because he was "not politically minded." Benson also noted that
J. Robert Oppenheimer had made the same disclaimer about his work
on the atom bomb, and he referred to a "deep philosophical and ethical parallel" between the Manhattan Project and the genome project.

Should a moratorium be imposed on genome research? Benson gave
his own answer to the question. Because humankind has already altered
the gene pool by using medical technology to preserve the sick and
weak, he said, we have "no other ethically right choice than to go forward" and learn how to cope with the consequences: "Human genome
projects offer us hope for dealing with a deleterious situation we ourselves have brought about."

At this point in our history, Benson concluded, we have "only one right
choice regarding our genetic future: We must do what we can, both to
improve our gene pool and to prevent deleterious events." Human

genome projects, he added, "are something we have to do *now*, because *now* we can do them."

His audience of geneticists may have been heartened by Benson's conclusion. But Benson himself later recognized with some chagrin a resonance between his own words and those of early eugenicists, even of Oppenheimer. He had given that speech early in his thinking on the subject, he remarked privately four years later. He had since reordered his thoughts.

During those four years, Benson (now a bioethics professor at a seminary in California) had focused on the risks of overestimating how much we really understand about how to correct problems involving genes. As clinical applications of genetics offer ever more opportunities to predict and prevent human suffering, he went on, "we must be vigilant, lest in our thinking we know more than we do, we attempt more than we should."

Relatively few organizations took the trouble to ask at the outset whether the Human Genome Project was ethical at all, but Benson was not the only person then who pondered its ethical implications. Quite the contrary: people were watching it like hawks.

In fact, the Human Genome Project was the first major effort undertaken by the U.S. government that had its own independent watchdog from its inception. That watchdog was no pit bull, however. It was more of a golden retriever: quite beautiful, good company, not known to be fierce, barks but doesn't bite.

Its nickname — ELSI — brings to mind a different species altogether. The acronym stands for Ethical, Legal, and Social Implications, and *ELSI* has become a term of art in some circles of government policy. These days people in health policy know what it means: big issues.

Since ELSI's inception a large number of similar but unrelated bodies have sprung into being to examine ethical issues surrounding genetics. SmithKline Beecham gave Stanford University a million dollars to start an ethics program in genetics. The Biotechnology Industry Organization spawned another, headed by the chief of diagnostic testing at Genzyme Corporation. In the same year the Institute for Genetic Research (TIGR), the nonprofit organization headed by Craig Venter (who had patented all those genetic tags), established a department of research policy and ethics. (The worst thing for science and society, Venter said, would be to leave the ethical issues up to the "professional bioethicist.") But ELSI was the original, and — despite its tribulations — it still marks the trail.

ELSI came into being at the insistence of James Watson. At the press conference in 1990 announcing his appointment as head of the genome project, Watson came out with the unexpected declaration that the NIH should fund a specific effort to monitor the ethical and social implications of genome research. He evidently made the proposal without consulting anyone at the NIH, but it took root.

"I want to proceed with the [genome] program," he explained at the time, "but I think we also have to be careful that we're not also going to harm people. That shouldn't be on our conscience."

Some bureaucrats at the NIH were skeptical, to say the least. ELSI's first director, Eric Juengst, relates a conversation between one senior NIH official and Watson that same year, just after ELSI had been created. "I still don't understand why you want to spend all this *money* subsidizing the *vacuous pronunciamentos* of self-styled *ethicists!*" the unnamed bureaucrat said. Watson responded that, like it or not, the cat was out of the bag about ethical problems arising from the genome project. "But why *inflate* the cat?" the official shot back. "Why put the cat *on TV?*"

But Congress too knew about the cat and liked Watson's idea. In the authorizing language that created the National Center for Human Genome Research, it specified that the project should include a dedicated effort to scrutinize its own ethics. Initially 3 percent of the center's budget, and after a few years 5 percent, was devoted to the ELSI program.

On the organization chart, the ELSI program got its start as one of four working groups set up by the NIH in 1989 to support a newly created National Advisory Council for Human Genome Research that would help refine the genome project's agenda. It was composed of experts in bioethics, law, social sciences, and genetics, as well as members of the public. ELSI represented a noteworthy innovation in bioethics: Its actions were not driven by a particular crisis such as the controversy over the Tuskegee study or the birth of the first test-tube baby. It was deliberative and proactive, rather than *reactive*.

"No one knew where it was going to go," said Elizabeth Thomson, ELSI's acting chief, in 1995. "It was an idea. Its goals at first were very broad—to anticipate and address all the issues that the Human Genome Project would present." She went on to point out a conundrum that had puzzled the working group from the outset: "These are not measurable objectives. How does one know one has achieved them?"

ELSI's first set of stated goals included anticipating and *addressing* the genome project's implications for society and for individuals, stimulating public discussion of the issues, and developing policy options to "assure" that the information was used for the benefit of individuals and society. These would be daunting tasks for an entire government, let alone for the seven-member working group.

Besides, as genome project director Francis Collins has pointed out, the core assignments to ELSI's members were confusing and perhaps even conflicting. "Were they supposed to be advising the genome [project] about its research portfolio? Were they supposed to be making policy recommendations? Were they supposed to be coordinating research between ELSI and the rest of the [research] world?"

ELSI made impressive strides in some respects, but it was the only one of the four working groups set up in 1989 that had not completed its assigned tasks eight years later. Perhaps by definition this was impossible. As the genome project mushroomed, so would its implications.

The first head of the working group was Nancy Wexler, perhaps the most charismatic figure in the entire history of genome research. The president of the Hereditary Diseases Foundation, Wexler is a most compelling individual, a flaxen-haired woman who personally embodies many of the ethical dilemmas that surround gene research.

Wexler's mother suffered and died of Huntington's disease, so she herself is therefore at risk. She spearheaded the studies, in a remote Venezuelan village where the disease is unusually prevalent, that led directly to discovery of the gene aberration responsible for HD. At that time her picture appeared again and again in newspapers and magazines, often embracing some diminutive person—nearly always a child—outside a lakeside hut in Venezuela. The photos alone make you fond of Nancy Wexler, quite apart from the facts.

"She pours on them a warm contagious care," said Venezuelan physician Americo Negrette, who discovered the cluster of people with Huntington's disease in that village. In the early years of the project, before the genetic mutation behind the disease was found, Wexler traveled tirelessly between Venezuela and the United States, alternately furthering the research in the south and hammering home the uncertainties it raised in the north: Who should take the new test for Huntington's disease when it became available? Who should offer it? What counseling should be required?

Wexler spoke often about genetic testing in powerful images, of Pandora's boxes, of oracles and crystal balls. (The first administrative head of ELSI, Eric Juengst, prefers to compare gene testing to weather forecasting, which is a less romantic but perhaps more accurate parallel.)

Initially, Wexler and the other scientists and ethicists on the first working group set four broad issues for ELSI:

(1) safety and efficacy of testing;
(2) privacy;
(3) matters of discrimination;
(4) improving "genetics literacy" among the public and professionals.

In the following year, ELSI awarded several dozen five- and six-figure grants, allocated among these categories. By the end of its first five years, ELSI had funded $26 million in studies.

One of its first grants was to the Institute of Medicine, to fund a broad overview under the first of those four areas: the risks inherent in genetic testing. The result was its 1994 report entitled *Assessing Genetic Risks* (see page 218). As noted, the report made numerous recommendations about the policy changes that ought to be made to forestall the risks of testing. But much of its wisdom, at least initially, seemed to fall on deaf ears.

Another large-scale effort was more targeted, and in the early 1990s the time was ripe for it. When the genetic test for cystic fibrosis was developed, ELSI provided the ideal avenue for ensuring that the unfortunate history of sickle cell testing in the 1970s would not be repeated, that CF testing would not lead to stigma and resentment.

ELSI therefore created a consortium of clinical research projects to address the personal and social consequences of cystic fibrosis testing. Over the next few years, the results revealed a great deal about the conflicts that CF testing presented to parents and siblings of affected children, as mentioned in Chapter 6. They also gave an early and sobering glimpse of the public's lack of interest in genetic testing, outside the context of pregnancy.

In creating the CF consortium, as Eric Juengst has pointed out, ELSI set a precedent for initiating social and psychological studies at the point when new genetic tests are introduced. Advocacy groups for breast cancer patients quickly seized on this precedent when tests for the breast cancer genes were introduced. Not long afterward the National Cancer Institute set up a network of centers dedicated to studying the implications of the new breast cancer genes—not just the medical outcomes of testing but the psychosocial ones as well.

As to the second broad issue, genetic privacy, ELSI sponsored a cohort of studies designed to review the current status of collection and storage of genetic information. It also funded work to create a model "genetic privacy act," which was widely distributed afterward. Drafted by ethicist George Annas and his colleagues at Boston University's School of Public Health in 1994, the model act has had a strong influence on many of the one hundred pieces of legislation introduced in thirty-three states (and enacted in fifteen) during the years that followed.

According to working group member Robert Cook-Deegan, a physician and one-time analyst of genome research for the government's Office of Technology Assessment, much of the early discussion focused on how far the ELSI program should go in analyzing government policy. There was one intractable problem: While ELSI clearly had a mandate to *speak to* policy issues, it had no power whatever to *influence* policy—and not even any clear and formal mechanism by which its deliberations might inform policymakers.

In congressional hearings in 1992, then–NIH director Bernardine Healy stated as much. She testified that ELSI was "an independent group ... quite removed and quite independent." Congress saw another side to that much-touted independence, noting in a committee report that year that "there is no existing policy process that will use the results of ELSI research to make recommendations."

On the organizational chart, ELSI's powerlessness in regard to policy was clear: it was a subcommittee to an advisory group that reported to two government agencies, the National Institutes of Health and the Department of Energy, which were running the biomedical and technological parts of the genome project respectively. ELSI's advice might be heeded with regard to NIH research procedures, but it was difficult to see any path whatsoever beyond this by which it might affect government policy about genetic research.

The NIH itself all but admitted to this limitation in a strategic planning document about ELSI, issued in 1992. "The aim of confronting these social, legal and ethical problems in research is not to promulgate new regulations or create another layer of research review," it said. "Rather, the aim is to provide the research community with relevant guidance for the conduct of research and to assure the public's understanding of the social benefits and consequences of science."

By that standard, ELSI's job was to guide research and to educate the

BIOMEDICAL ETHICS

Medicine, says one ethicist, saved the life of philosophy. At midcentury it came along with vital issues such as brain death and artificial insemination—and real abuses such as Nazi "experiments" and the Tuskegee study—to rescue a dusty profession from its ivory tower.

The result has been a flowering of advisory bodies and ethics institutes, from the institutional review boards (IRBs) that govern medical research at hospitals, to a series of high-level medical ethics bodies mandated by Congress or the president, to a dozen or so postgraduate programs offering degrees in biomedical ethics. There are even several special centers for biomedical ethics "rescarch" in the United States. In 1996 more than 3,400 citations on bioethics appeared in the medical journal database Medline, up from three hundred only thirty years earlier.

They make strange partners, doctors and philosophers. One profession argues that the other is too theoretical and divorced from real life; the other contends that the first is too focused on finding tidy answers that can't be had. Too often, lamented an Institute of Medicine committee formed to look at biomedical ethics itself, the results of deliberations between them have been either toothless, head-in-the-clouds compromises, or a co-optation of the analytical process by one interest group for its own ends.

Still, the IOM committee set standards for future bioethics panels. Their work should be logical, scholarly, and based on sound judgment, the committee said, representing diverse views with due respect, holding open meetings, and publishing the results. It would also help, the committee said, if the ethics body carried considerable weight with policymakers and the public.

Perhaps the best we can expect from bioethics committees is that they air all the relevant issues from all relevant perspectives and provide a logical framework for thinking about complex problems. It's a common misperception that philosophers and ethicists can find the answers. What they know, at best, is how to argue well.

public, not to affect broader developments in the introduction of genetics to the wider world. "There are dangers here," said working group
member Thomas H. Murray, a biomedical ethicist from Case Western
Reserve University, in 1992. "The public, including public officials,
must not be misled about what ELSI can do, lest it let down its guard."
Whatever its virtues, ELSI lacked the authority, he added, "to decide
what ought to be done." But if not ELSI, then who?

The problem with policy-setting came to the fore with regard to the
third of ELSI's stated issues: discrimination. In 1991, as one of its first
acts, the working group studied the newly proposed regulations from
the Equal Employment Opportunity Commission (EEOC) that had
been created in response to the Americans with Disabilities Act (ADA).
The working group hastily drew up an advisory statement pointing out
that genetic risks should be protected as disabilities, because employees
might be fired (or never even hired) if someone found they were at risk
of a major hereditary illness—whether or not that risk was relevant to
job performance or public safety. In a feverish, last-minute effort, they
faxed these opinions to the EEOC moments before the official period
for comments closed.

At first the EEOC replied negatively to the advice, arguing that because genetic tests indicated only risks, not existing conditions, they
could not fall under the protection of the ADA. ELSI working group
members and grantees pitched into a three-year backstage operation to
amass support for the proposition that employers should not be allowed
to discriminate on the basis of genes.

In the end, they won: In 1995 the EEOC quietly issued some clari-
fications about the definition of *disabled*: ". . . the definition of 'disability' applies to individuals who are subjected to discrimination on the
basis of genetic information relating to illness, disease, or other disorders." The document adds an example, drawn directly from ELSI's
stated concerns, in which an employer declines to hire someone found
to have an increased susceptibility to colon cancer. This would be discrimination under the ADA and therefore illegal.

The statement did not, however, reflect a major concern that ELSI
had also raised in its advisory statement: the fear that genetics might
nonetheless be used to discriminate against unaffected *carriers*, as had
happened in the case of sickle cell anemia in the 1970s. The act did not
prevent employers from obtaining genetic information about job candidates but left it to employees to prove that they had not been hired or
promoted because of some adverse genetic information.

"The ADA experience was important because it indicated limitations in the ELSI working group's ability to analyze and formulate policy," writes Robert Cook-Deegan. The statement was "prepared in haste, and lacked the coherence born of sustained deliberation and systematic data-gathering." Also, it was an *advisory*, not a law.

On the matter of discrimination in health insurance, ELSI took a different tack: it formed an independent task force to study the issues. This took place in 1993, at the inception of the Clintons' health care reform process, and there was every reason to believe that the new Task Force on Genetic Information and Insurance could issue a robust set of policies that would have an important impact on the future.

On paper, the statement it issued was a powerful one. Among other things, the task force recommended that genetic information should not be used to deny health care or health insurance coverage to anyone; that the cost of health care to individuals should not be affected by genetic information; that the health care system should guarantee everyone access to basic health services; and that health insurers should "consider a moratorium on the use of genetic tests in underwriting." (With a national health care system peeking over the horizon, this list of recommendations may have seemed to state only the obvious. In the cold light of hindsight, it makes a remarkably concise list of the bedrock-deep problems that genetic testing still poses to individuals and society.)

The task force members included physicians, biologists, geneticists and genetic counselors, lawyers, ethicists, a spokesperson from a disabilities group, and representatives from state government and from the insurance industry. The cochairmen were bioethicist Thomas Murray of Case Western Reserve University and microbiologist Jonathan Beckwith of Harvard Medical School.

Murray is well known in his discipline, likable and well-schooled in the complexities of the social issues surrounding genetics. He came to the task force with a fine reputation but not the special cachet of a James Watson or a Francis Collins. Beckwith, on the other hand, arrived with well-defined stances preceding him. He is known as a Cassandra about the perils of genetics. He has long been identified with the demise of a proposed genetic study of newborns by some Harvard scientists in the 1970s, on the charge that it would label its subjects for life. (The defect in question, an extra Y chromosome, had been linked to aggression.)

According to some people who observed the task force meetings, neither of the two chairmen was able to forge a consensus, wrestling as they were with a strong ideological divide between some rather strident consumer representatives on one side, and participants from the insurance industry on the other.

Sometime near the end of the procedures, one member of the panel announced that negotiations in the Clinton health care reform process were going so well that universal health insurance would surely be enacted within three months. It was a foregone conclusion that the committee's recommendations would take effect.

It may have seemed so at the time. Nonetheless, the committee's recommendations were opposed by the member who represented the American Council on Life Insurance, on the grounds that it "directly conflicts with ACLI policy in its overall thrust and specific recommendations." The Health Insurance Association of America refused either to endorse or reject the report. (To this day, both organizations continue to insist on their right to collect medical information, including the results of genetic testing, for risk assessment and rate setting, although there is no evidence that in actual practice they do so on a widespread scale.)

Notwithstanding these protests, the recommendations were submitted to the White House Task Force on Health Care Reform and were eventually incorporated into the administration's health reform bill in 1993. The rest, as everyone knows, is history. The ELSI insurance task force disbanded after issuing its report; its conclusions are interesting reading, nothing more.

For all that its stated objectives were ambitious, the ELSI program missed a few issues when it set its own initial goals. Most obviously, it neglected to consider the possible effects of commercial interests on the research agenda of the genome project—an issue that was soon to cause considerable turmoil, when the NIH began applying for patents on gene fragments.

By late 1994 more than two hundred publications had resulted from ELSI research, spread across a wide range of academic, peer-reviewed journals of social science and ethics. In such dispersed venues, buried on university library shelves, policymakers and members of the public are not likely to run across them. Neither, in fact, are journalists.

It's not that ELSI didn't try to be visible. After all, education was the fourth of the four issues it charged itself with addressing. A major focus of the ELSI program in the first few years was to sponsor conferences and workshops, aimed either at defining the issues for further study or at informing the general public about genome research. By September 1991 ELSI had sponsored ten national conferences on topics including prenatal and presymptomatic genetic testing and the ethical issues inherent in doing research on families affected by hereditary disorders. Several other early ELSI grants provided partial funding for books or public television documentaries.

On one hand, this public education was laudable and part of ELSI's mandate. But some critics pointed out that it could also be seen as a public relations exercise for the Human Genome Project. Among others, the ELSI program's first director, Eric Juengst, has been quoted as calling the diversion of genetic research funds to the study of ethical and social issues an "unavoidable political tax" necessary to get the genome project off the ground. In any case, enlightened scientists had a clear interest in informing the public in detail about the real risks of genetic testing, in order to minimize any backlash.

MIT science historian Charles Weiner gave a sharply critical portrait of ELSI in a 1994 book called *Are Genes Us?* He described three strategies that proponents of the genome project used to deflect ethical threats to its existence: selling its efforts to the public through the equivalent of advertising; trivializing ethical problems by focusing only on those that do not weaken the foundations of genetic research; and shunting ethical issues to a branch of the project with no real authority, so that scientists could get on with their work unhindered.

"The decision to map, sequence and interpret the entire human genome is treated as a 'done deal,'" he wrote, "separated from the uses or abuses of the information it generates." Along with the big pot of money behind the genome project that went to the molecular biologists, a smaller pot became a windfall for biomedical ethicists, who had the effect of using it to ensure that the former were seen as respectable.

"Where cash went," writes Robert Cook-Deegan, "ethics followed." In the project's later years, some ethicists (like many biologists) would complain that they couldn't get funded for a project or a study that didn't involve the impact of genetics on a problem.

"ELSI seemed to be looking at safe harbors, not controversial issues," asserts one former ELSI grantee, attorney Ralph Trottier of Atlanta's Morehouse School of Medicine, who failed three times to get refunded for his study of trends in the spread of state-run genetic testing services.

His particular concern was the fact that in some states the same case-workers who oversaw early-intervention services for families with developmentally disabled children (which are part of public health services in about half of the states) were the same people who provided counseling for clients of state-run genetic testing services.

Trottier pointed out the clear potential for conflict of interest: States could gain financially if they could limit the need to provide early intervention services by promoting prenatal screening. He also argued for specific procedures to protect minority groups, because genetic tests might affect them particularly quickly, while they might be slower than others to receive new forms of treatment for genetic services.

Trottier says he was told that efforts to expand or publish his study were moot because his fears were unlikely to become reality. With the subsequent advent of managed care, however, issues of access to genetic services and conflict of interest have become even more critical. (Trottier has since moved on to other interests.)

In April 1993, as the Clinton health reform program was being hammered out in closed sessions, Francis Collins took over as head of the Human Genome Project and therefore of ELSI. (James Watson had stepped down, largely as a result of disputes about the NIH proposal to patent gene sequences.) A practicing physician, Collins had the potential to be an even more effective champion for ELSI than the molecular biologist Watson had been.

Collins had won respect in the gene research community not only for masterminding the discovery of the cystic fibrosis gene but for the way in which he had gone about it. He had chosen to shun the cutthroat competition that was snarling the search for the cause of CF at the time and, for the sake of the families, had proposed to share reagents with his competitors in order to get the job done. His competitors agreed, and the job *was* done.

At the University of Michigan, before taking over as head of the genome project, Collins had been involved in the search for the genes behind breast cancer. As part of the effort, he sponsored psychological studies on the women in the study. "Possessing information about women that had profound implications for their future sensitized me to just how complicated this is," he says, "and to how this information can, besides sometimes being beneficial, be toxic."

A kindly man, an avowed born-again Christian, and the sort of person who would as soon pull up a chair at a table crowded with reporters eating sandwiches as call a press conference, Collins speaks easily and personally about ethical concerns. He has faced them in his own practice. Because geneticists seldom before had much useful information to impart, he feels, they became sensitized to "how we convey that information and what impact it has." In nearly every address he repeats his favorite quotation, from Sophocles: "It is but sorrow to be wise, when wisdom profits not." (The play is *Oedipus*, the speaker Tiresias, who was doomed by the gods to foresee the future but to be unable to reveal it.)

As head of the genome project, Collins saw it as one of his responsibilities to make certain that wisdom does profit. Under his tenure ELSI focused its gaze more closely on the nature and extent of genetic counseling. Collins worried that there would never be enough genetic counselors to inform people about genetic testing, and that doctors and nurses were not up to the task, with everything else they had to do.

"I think we have to move with alacrity in the next year or two," Collins testified before the House in 1995, "because the pressures, particularly from the private sector, in terms of providing these services, will grow. We need to be prepared with a full range of guidelines, and we need to have physicians educated about the appropriateness of these tests. I'm confident that we are on target, but we need to move swiftly."

ELSI was moving swiftly in a number of directions, but its impact, if any, on how genetic advances were to be used was difficult to detect. Certainly during Collins's tenure the program began to show some signs of losing its way.

"What we find *will* be used to establish policy," insisted ELSI's acting director, Elizabeth Thomson, in 1995. "I don't want to call us public relations, because we're not. But we're doing important work. We really are contributing to the body of knowledge necessary to develop sound policies related to genetic services."

Some legislators were not so confident that this contribution would be made in time to protect the public. During the 1995 appropriations hearings, Representative David Obey of Wisconsin had a revealing interchange with Collins about the underlying threats posed by genetic information:

"I think that ninety-nine times out of one hundred, employers and insurance companies will always win out in the political arena," Obey said. "And so I'm very concerned about developing knowledge before we have agreed how we're going to handle it."

Obey's own grandmother used to tell him that just because you can do something doesn't mean you have to. Why, Obey asked (as he had asked, repeatedly, since the beginning of the genome project), should not Congress require the National Institutes of Health to reject applications for research grants from any state that does not have laws to protect people from abuse of genetic information? (At the time only about a dozen states had any protections of this sort.)

"I would be very troubled by that mechanism," Collins replied. "Who would be penalized? Investigators who happen to live in those states, and who have no particular control over the situation. . . . In the process we would in some way be taking away hope from people who are living with those diseases right now. Are we to hold them hostage, on the basis of these concerns about the future ethical, legal, and social consequences?"

Perhaps screening tests should be forbidden until privacy issues are resolved, Obey suggested. Collins countered that the FDA already demands evidence of efficacy before genetic test kits are marketed, neatly steering past the reality that genetic tests are usually offered not as kits but as services, and thus escape regulation, and bypassing the privacy issue.

"I mean the broader protections that I'm talking about," Obey persisted. Collins started to reply but Obey broke in.

"I honestly don't believe that the ethics is ever going to catch up with the science unless we find some way to leverage people into moving forward on this issue," he said. "I mean, you have a hell of a lot more faith in the ability of this society to resist people with economic power than I do."

"We still have a period of a couple of years to get these issues resolved," argued Collins. "And I think there is a reasonable chance we will be able to do that. If we do not have the protections in a couple of years, then I think we may have the potential for trouble."

Obey kept at it. Would Collins then be willing to settle for a halt in funding on the genome project if protections at the state and federal level were not in place within two years, by 1997?

"No, sir," Collins replied. "I would be very uncomfortable with that. . . . To slow down the basic science in order for that step to be achieved will delay the entire Human Genome Project. Suppose you then get those protections in place the next year. You've lost that year. Such a linkage bothers me."

Exactly two and a half years later to the day, on September 23, 1997, when I interviewed Francis Collins, such protections were not completely in place. Legislation did exist to prevent employers from discriminating against people with known genetic risks both in hiring and in providing health insurance, but there were loopholes, and Collins acknowledged them. In hiring, it would be nearly impossible for someone to prove that genetic risk was the reason an employer had turned him down for a job. As for the health insurance protections, they lasted only as long as a job lasted, and they required an employer only to offer the insurance, not to provide it at a reasonable cost. Beyond that, no legislation existed to buffer people who were not part of a large group health insurance plan from the consequences of genetic risk. Anyone who had to buy individual insurance remained in a tenuous position.

"Are we completely where I told Mr. Obey we needed to be?" Collins said. "No, but considering how tough these issues are to move on, I would say we have come dramatically far." He felt there was a good chance that legislation would soon be passed to fill those loopholes. "I hope it will," he went on. "I would be disappointed if it's not."

In the interim Collins himself had become proactive in trying to move the course of policy, not just to talk about it. He hired a policy expert, Kathy Hudson, to work within the genome institute. The result was a symposium cosponsored with the National Action Plan on Breast Cancer, which resulted in a report in *Science* listing six areas of genetic testing that required urgent legislative attention. That night, after the workshop, Collins himself sat up until 11:15 personally drafting the definition of *genetic information* that would recur in most subsequent legislation on the topic.

Like Collins, Eric Juengst also worried that the marketplace would get ahead of policymakers. "One can see it happening already in the marketing of genetic risk assessments using the BRCA1 mutations," he said, "and in the proliferation of commercial firms right out of the genome project . . . which are based on the proposition that a demand can be created for DNA-sequencing-based testing technology."

However, Juengst adds, policy proposals are more easily abandoned than adopted. Perhaps the best defense, he has argued, is to perpetuate ELSI as the prototype "uncommission," a fluid body able to wield influence on a number of levels, gather facts, and recruit advocates as it sees fit. In his dreams Juengst envisions a group of "vocational advocates" for genetic ethics, much like the civil rights volunteers of the 1960s.

Officials of the genome project were not oblivious to the criticisms of ELSI, and in March 1996 they were prodded into making a reassessment of ELSI's role. Some members of the working group, including its head, Lori Andrews, a legal scholar at Chicago–Kent School of Law (who had replaced Nancy Wexler), had been complaining for a long time about constraints on ELSI — especially about threats to ELSI's autonomy from within the genome research center at the NIH.

A particular bone of contention was the working group's plan to spend $20,000 developing an anthology of papers on genetics and behavior. ELSI's parent, the National Center for Human Genome Research, said the cost was too high; but some working group members charged that the scientists were uncomfortable about what they saw as potential threats to the public image of genetic research. Suddenly in March 1996 Andrews resigned.

A year later Andrews discussed her reasons for her resignation with a *Los Angeles Times* reporter. "There is a hostility to scrutiny or to suggestions that there may be impacts that are not considered," she explained. "There really was conflict of interest to have the people who want the research to go forward creating the agenda for what social issues got discussed."

In June of 1996, ELSI's two masters — the NIH and DOE programs for gene research — formed an evaluation committee of independent experts to reassess ELSI's functions and "to recommend an appropriate structure for effectively carrying these out." Although the charge to the committee spoke only of the evolving ethical issues as genetic research began to move from the laboratory to clinical applications, Andrews's protest must have hit home as well.

"Serious concerns have been raised about the Working Group's lack of resources and independence, as well as conflicts with the intramural policy-making activities . . . and the inadequate sharing of essential information by staff at NCHGR," said the committee in a report issued in January 1997. "Strong differences of opinion" exist, it added, about whether the NCHGR staff had been sufficiently forthcoming with the working group about exactly what the funding and research priorities of the genome project were, and how it was carrying them out — matters which were, after all, part of ELSI's original mandate.

A more pivotal concern to the evaluation committee was the most frequent criticism that had been levied against ELSI all along: that its position on the government's organizational chart rendered it almost impotent. "The Working Group is not positioned within the governmental scientific structure so as to fulfill the breadth of its charge," said the committee, which was cochaired by Mark Rothstein, a University of Houston law professor long interested in issues of genetics and discrimination, and M. Anne Spence, a University of California pediatric geneticist. Within the centers at the NIH and the DOE, it said, where the mission is gene mapping and sequencing, policy development is "not logically achieved."

ELSI should not be one body but three, the report advised: (1) a new committee with responsibility for overseeing genetics research grants emanating from the NIH genome center and the Department of Energy; (2) another committee to coordinate the ethical, legal, and social oversight of *all* genetic research at the National Institutes of Health, not just that specifically within the genome project; and (3) a federally chartered Advisory Committee on Genetics and Public Policy. This last should reside at the top of the government's health hierarchy, within the Office of the Secretary of Health and Human Services, to formulate public policy relating to developments in genetics. "The importance to public accountability of providing an independent evaluation and review of ELSI issues cannot be overstated," it said.

Meanwhile, the newly expanded ELSI should continue to charter new task forces. In urging this, the report threw a bouquet at a current task force that had been laboring intensively through all the turmoil. The Task Force on Genetic Testing, created by ELSI in 1995, was working "effectively," even though (like the working group) it was in a cumbersome situation, technically a subcommittee of a subcommittee (ELSI) reporting to both the NIH and the DOE.

Like its predecessor on insurance, this task force faced formidable and urgent problems. It had come into being at a time when federal regulatory agencies were disputing over whether and how to regulate genetic tests. Federal laws governing the quality of medical testing expressly excluded most DNA tests, and many such tests were "home brews" created in university science labs and not marketed commercially. They were provided informally — not as a business, strictly speaking, but as a service within academic networks — and therefore they operate without regulation. Surveys that the task force commissioned showed that some labs that were required to register with federal authorities failed to do so.

Headed by pediatrician Neil Holtzman of Johns Hopkins University, author of an early and influential survey of the use and potential of genetic testing among insurers and health care institutions, the fifteen-member genetic testing task force included representatives of insurance companies and testing services as well as academics, physicians, and members of patient advocacy groups. Officials of three government agencies most closely involved with genetic testing—the Food and Drug Administration, the Health Care Financing Administration (which governs Medicare and Medicaid), and the Centers for Disease Control and Prevention—also attended its meetings, as nonvoting members.

One of the task force's first acts was to commission a survey of laboratories that were engaged in genetic testing, followed by in-depth interviews with twenty-nine of them. Although FDA regulations require organizations developing new medical devices to have their research protocols formally approved by the agency or another outside review board, one-fourth of the 140 nonprofit organizations in the task force survey had not done so; nor had 41 percent of the fifty-four biotechnology companies. In many cases tests were developed and released without any oversight whatever.

And there were many other issues to tackle. At their first meeting the task force members disagreed about whether informed consent should be required and documented whenever anyone underwent genetic testing. (Some people felt that a simple conversation with a doctor was sufficient and that formally signing a document was not necessary.) Another contentious issue was credentialing. Should the task force recommend placing limits on who could order a genetic test? Should patients be allowed to order gene tests on their own behalf, or even family doctors who might not understand the results? If not, who should credential the people who ordered gene tests—and who should monitor the results?

Differences of opinion were inevitable during the task force's eighteen-month tenure, but a change, an evolution, perhaps, had taken place since the histories of the pre-embryo research committee, which had been overruled by the president and Congress, and of ELSI's own insurance task force. The change might have resulted from the increased urgency of the issue, or it might have been that Holtzman himself was able to win respect from committee members of all persuasions. Discussions, though heated, were rarely hostile. According to the insurance industry representative, J. Alexander Lowden, M.D., of Canada's Crown Life Insurance Company, the committee tried to work together toward a consensus—rather than everyone straining toward their own agenda, as Dr. David Lanier, the representative from the government's Agency for Health Care Policy and Research agreed.

The most outspoken consumer advocate on the task force, attorney Patricia Barr from Bennington, Vermont, was firm without being strident. Representing the National Breast Cancer Coalition, she pressed the same point over and over: the introduction of new genetic tests should *always* be accompanied by rigorous research to gain evidence about their effectiveness.

There was never much dispute about her contention. It matched a growing consensus in the entire American health care system that policies in medical practice should be backed by sound evidence of their effectiveness. The problem in this case was how to recommend obtaining such evidence.

In its interim report, issued in January 1997, the Task Force on Genetic Testing proposed establishing a National Genetics Board (NGB) to "assure the protection of human subjects in the development of genetic tests with the potential to predict future disease." The task force provided three separate scenarios for how the NGB might function, but it agreed that in any scenario, one of its chief roles would be to advise other committees, especially the local-level network of institutional review boards (IRBs) that exist to protect human subjects of federally funded medical research at the hospitals and medical centers where studies are carried out.

The task force's interim report appeared on the Internet, soliciting comments within two and a half months. Fifty-six responses were received by the deadline, most of them from professional associations, the gene-testing industry, and university-based medical geneticists. The task force might have reached a consensus, but the world outside did not concur—not at all.

"I am disappointed and alarmed at the apparent goals of this task force," wrote a medical oncologist at Cedars-Sinai Medical Center in Los Angeles. "An active debate has [already] been taking place within the medical/genetic/oncology community regarding the appropriate uses of genetic predisposition testing. I feel certain we will reach the correct conclusion." Systems already in existence can be improved to deal with genetic technology, said a concurring letter from the president of the American College of Medical Genetics. (Who needed more oversight committees, after all?)

The president of the parent organization for gene testers, the Council of Regional Networks for Genetic Services, complained that "the tone of the document remains negative toward genetic testing" and that "genetic testing is unfairly stigmatized as uniquely capable of producing harm if confidentiality is breached."

Some critics argued that gene-based testing was not fundamentally different from any other kind of medical testing. "The performance of gene-based testing need not be regulated in a manner that is fundamentally different from the way other medical testing is regulated," argued the president of the American Board of Medical Genetics.

But the neurologist-researcher who was behind the newest of emerging genetic tests for a predisposition to Alzheimer's disease, Dr. Allen Roses of Duke University Medical Center, was not so sanguine about his profession's ability to settle such issues unilaterally. "It is important that the ethical, social, and legal implications of genetic risk factors . . . become part of public inquiry and discussion," he wrote. A second gene would soon be linked with Alzheimer's, he predicted, and the "reality" of predictions for an incurable and unavoidable disease "is a frightening near-term possibility."

But a possibility that was equally frightening to many of the respondents was the prospect of all those layers of bureaucracy that the task force was proposing to install between the new genetic tests and the market. The proposed National Genetics Board came in for particular scorn, as did the idea of giving the FDA explicit authority over gene tests.

At its final meeting, which was open to the public, the Task Force on Genetic Testing had to confront and resolve these issues. During the first few hours, most of the discussion focused on the fundamental question: What is different about genetic tests that distinguishes them from, say, cholesterol tests, or the PSA test used to target developing prostate cancer?

"The definition [of genetic testing] is everything, and we can't agree on a definition," task force member Stephen Goodman, M.D., of the American Society of Human Genetics, lamented. If the task force were to exclude tests that measure metabolites like cholesterol (which are by-products of normal body chemistry, not genes per se or their direct products) from its final recommendations, he noted, it would be excluding tests for a large number of rare genetic diseases, because metabolites are sometimes the simplest or even as yet the only way to measure a heritable trait.

The definition of genetic testing is not just a problem in semantics, as a member of the audience pointed out. State legislatures trying to regulate gene testing would rely on the task force's report to help them pinpoint the subject of their deliberations. Still, it was a struggle to come up with a useful definition in a field that was growing so rapidly that it would sooner or later encompass nearly all of medicine.

In the end, however, the task force did come up with a way to define and thereby limit what it was talking about. Its final report defines *genetic test* as "the analysis of human DNA, RNA, chromosomes, proteins and certain metabolites *in order to detect heritable disease-related genotypes, phenotypes or karyotypes for clinical purposes* (emphasis mine). The definition was technical but specific, and it went on to describe the purposes of such testing: predicting disease, identifying carriers, establishing prenatal or clinical diagnosis, monitoring, and screening.

The task force report went on to emphasize that it was not limiting itself to predictive tests used in healthy people, nor to tests that screen only DNA. It later defined types of genetic tests that merit special scrutiny from regulators: those that can predict future hereditary disease in people who now appear healthy, and whose results cannot be confirmed by a different kind of test, are likely to be used for that purpose.

Holtzman took very seriously the opposition to the idea of a National Genetics Board. "Virtually everyone who commented objected to the regulatory functions of the National Genetics Board," he said at the final meeting. "There was a lot of discussion on the listserv, but by the time the document was in the Federal Register, I knew it was not even a viable option."

The discourse at the final meeting ranged over the entire vast array of dilemmas that genetic tests present: Should only certain professionals be allowed to order them or give counsel about their results? Should certain uses of genetic testing—to detect criminality, for instance—be explicitly placed beyond the bounds of ethical medical practice? What mechanism should be set up to ensure that the labs that perform genetic tests have adequate quality standards?

Many task force members were concerned that genetic testing was being introduced and rapidly embraced based on nothing more than promotional materials. The issue raised by consumer representative Patricia Barr arose again and again: the need to link the introduction of genetic tests with methods of gathering data and evaluating the use of the tests.

"I'd like to turn a test loose if you want to, but coordinate it with some entity that would test it," she said, and make the practice "not accidental . . . not [merely] something some researchers want to do." That would be a lot of trouble, argued Eliot Hillback, president of Integrated Genetics, and it would cost a lot of money. Some people are in effect working out of their garages to create new tests, another panel member agreed. They wouldn't have the resources to assess them at the same time.

No process in the medical or regulatory system exists to demand such front-end testing at the moment, Barr acknowledged. But, she added, "If the system exists, they'll do it."

"I think you've hit the heart of the matter here," agreed Jessica Davis, a pediatric geneticist at New York Hospital. "All the questions have come back to us because we have no data. . . . For example, look at IVF. What's the end point of that? Did anybody build in a ten-year follow-up? Do we know what all these hormones are doing to people over ten years?" We don't seem to "organize ourselves" to gather that kind of data, she concluded.

Perhaps now was the time to start. Holtzman spoke of using gene tests to train medical science in a "new habit": collecting data as new technologies are introduced. Considerable discussion followed about who should coordinate such data-gathering and who should pay for it. Several panel members suggested the government's Centers for Disease Control and Prevention (CDC), because it is already a well-established focus for medical data-gathering. Muin Khoury, the representative from the CDC, supported the idea. In fact, he was so much in favor of it that he even crafted a paragraph to that effect, which he proposed adding to the final report.

Khoury's exact wording was not included in the final report, but the general idea was, along with numerous concrete recommendations. The final report is clearly worded, succinct, and in the end quite forceful—ultimately a far more powerful document than the interim recommendations that had appeared in the Federal Register and on the Internet. It urges the creation of not four committees but one. It contains many echoes of its forerunner, the Institute of Medicine's *Assessing Genetic Risks*. But the task force's report is more mature, comes from somewhere closer to the center of government, and strikes much closer to home.

Its recommendations are also, unmistakably, ones that policymakers and gene testers could understand and implement—*if* they have the intention, the resolve, and the political power. The task force has no implementation bite, but its bark, at least, is clear and bold:

- The existing federal oversight body for quality in medical labs, created under the Clinical Laboratory Improvement Amendments of 1988 (CLIA), should establish a special internal sub-committee for gene tests and should automatically reserve for special scrutiny any test that "can be used for purposes of predicting future disease."

- Laboratories performing predictive genetic tests should seek accreditation and proficiency testing under an existing program run by the College of American Pathologists (CAP) and CAP should continue to publish lists of those labs that pass.
- Not only should labs obtain informed consent before doing genetic testing, they should document that consent in writing.
- A toll-free hot line should be set up to provide immediate answers to questions about specific gene tests. Hospitals and managed care plans should "require evidence of competence" before allowing doctors to order the kinds of tests defined as requiring special scrutiny under CLIA—as well as implement systematic medical record review to assure that doctors are prescribing such tests appropriately.
- Test developers "must" submit their data about the validity and clinical usefulness of a test to independent review by professional societies and federal agencies before such tests become available for general use. The assessment of these data should be coordinated by an Advisory Committee to the Secretary of Health and Human Services (an entity almost indistinguishable from the one favored by the panel assigned to remodel ELSI).

The task force unanimously approved these recommendations and sent them on to ELSI, which approved them in turn and passed them up to the secretary of health and human services in May 1997.

The following month, the president's National Bioethics Advisory Commission released its hundred-page document on human cloning, accompanied by nationwide press fanfare and laudatory remarks from the president in a Rose Garden reception. Neither the gene testing report nor the advice about restructuring ELSI got any attention whatsoever from the press or the general public—even though both documents are far more likely than issues such as human cloning to have a real impact on us and on our families. If their recommendations are implemented, that is. If there is follow-through.

The rest of us need to keep an eye on the watchdog. At least fifteen genes associated with human disease can now be detected by commercially available tests, and a total of some 450 genetic tests now exist that can help to identify the risks of various diseases. The number will grow.

The head of the IOM committee that drafted *Assessing Genetic Risks*, medical geneticist Arno Motulsky, says that part of the problem with regulating gene tests lies in our multicultural, multisystem society. No single group has the clout to make unilateral rules on this sort of issue. We have to reach a consensus, he says, and enforce it.

"You never know the answer to the question, Will anybody listen?" admitted the head of the new National Bioethics Advisory Commission, Princeton University president Harold Shapiro. "You have to take that on faith."

CHAPTER 14

Identity Crisis

Genetic counseling is preventive medicine and should be so regarded.

— Pediatrician Barton Childs and coauthors in the
New England Journal of Medicine, 1972

JODI RUCQUOI SOMETIMES HANGS A SIGN ON THE door of her little office at Yale Children's Hospital. "Hunks welcome," it reads. "Everyone else stay the hell out."

It's hanging there when she's counseling clients. When it's not, people of all descriptions crack the door with questions, all day long. "We get everything in here—sudden infant death syndrome, neurofibromatosis, PKU, kids with developmental delays, everything," said Rucquoi rather ruefully. "We're what's new in medicine. We are the forefront of technology. The new stuff coming out in medicine—it's all a gene."

Rucquoi is a genetic counselor—the alpha and the omega (as she puts it) in this new world of molecular genetics, the triage station, the traffic manager. "It doesn't stay with me," she adds, "but I'm the one who decides which direction the patient will take." Her office is stacked with papers and files. She needs all that information; it's critical.

Usually, doctors refer patients with genetic questions to counselors, who are trained to give them information about their condition. When the Polish immigrant Anna W. (Chapter 2) had a question about whether her medication could cause birth defects, for instance, it was a genetic counselor who provided the answer. Genetic counselors also see it as their role to offer support, and as a result they often function in part as therapists.

There are roughly 2,000 genetic counselors in the United States. They bear the brunt of the whirlwind, responsible for sharing the good news, the bad news, the news of indeterminate meaning, for explaining it clearly in a few words, and for mopping up the tears besides. Members of this profession have an unmistakable sense of their own value— and of how little others value them. They're in a curious situation: overwhelmed and conflicted about information that others need badly but don't realize they need at all.

A 1995 survey of pediatricians, family doctors, and obstetrician/gynecologists in four states showed that one in three had seen no reason in the previous three years to refer a patient to a genetic counselor. Sixty-two percent of general practitioners felt patients got "not much benefit" from genetic counseling. Among obstetricians and pediatricians, one in ten felt they provide no benefit at all.

Meanwhile genetic tests proliferate, and many experts in the field predict that, by the time the Human Genome Project comes to a close, the bulk of genetic tests will be ordered and interpreted by primary care doctors. Three-fourths of doctors in one survey said they had "heard a lot about" genetic testing. That's the good news. On the other hand, nearly half of them said that they had heard about it mostly in the media, not in professional circles. Perhaps they actually knew no more about it than their patients did.

In that same survey, nearly half of doctors—46 percent—strongly disagreed with the proposal that physicians should obtain informed consent in writing before giving a patient a genetic test. In light of the rest of the survey, how they could inform patients suitably before asking their consent, is an interesting question. Clearly, if the ELSI project intends to shift its focus to professional education, it has plenty to do.

In the interim the bulk of patient education will continue to fall— to the extent that it falls anywhere—on the shoulders of counselors like Jodi Rucquoi. Genetic counselors sense the size of the gap between what they know and what they probably ought to know. What frightens them more, if anything, is the magnitude of the same gap when it comes to those family doctors who don't see the need for genetic counseling services.

"Just trying to keep up with [advances in] the genetic diseases we see most frequently is a challenge," says Rucquoi. We can't do a fishing expedition, she has just told a client awaiting a prenatal test. If we did all the tests that are available now, your baby would probably be entering grade school before you had all the results.

There are so many rare defects, so many labs, so many options for people at potential risk of some defect or other. The way to keep up with new developments is through computer databases, phone calls to help-ful and equally overworked contacts, and a huge box of files that can't ever be entirely up to date.

What can be accomplished in an ordinary half-hour counseling ses-sion for a couple who are testing their fetus just because their doctor said they should—because of the mother's age, for example—is defi-nitely limited. If an actual diagnosis of a genetic defect turns up, it in-tensifies by an order of magnitude the mandate for a counselor to be empathic, caring, and listening. "You can be there a long time," says Rucquoi.

Like many of the clients they serve, the bulk of genetic counselors are fairly young, Caucasian, and women. In one sense Rucquoi does not fit the mold: she is about to become a grandmother.

She has another distinction too: Unlike the vast majority of her peers, Rucquoi spends most of her time on the telephone. In 1995 she and the geneticists at Yale Children's Hospital decided that the bread-and-butter work, the routine prenatal counseling, could be done as well by telephone as in person. And *routine* is the right word for it.

Like many counselors, Rucquoi begins a session by asking the (usu-ally female) client an open-ended, stage-setting question: "Do you know why I need to talk to you today?" She has a few simple goals for the con-versation: to take the client's health and family history, to convey sig-nificant information about the risks of birth defects and the risks and benefits of the relevant testing, and to communicate with her well enough to elicit any special questions or concerns she may have.

The message gets across fine on the phone, she believes, and women probably listen more carefully and comfortably from their own kitchen stools or office desks, in discreet isolation. Certainly it spares them the sterile, forbidding atmosphere of the hospital, and the charts and visual aids many counselors fall back on to explain the intricacies of genetics.

If a client wants a face-to-face interview, of course Rucquoi will meet her. (Couples seldom do.) She is welcome to call back anytime. The counselors are also there when the client has ultrasound or amniocen-tesis, and her chart is reviewed by a medical geneticist. If and when a test comes back positive, Rucquoi is waiting to meet the client in the lobby.

Rucquoi says she would never dream of advising her daughter-in-law to have amniocentesis, to scan for possible genetic trouble in her future grandchild. She knows the couple would not put the pregnancy at any risk, let alone terminate it for any reason.

"That's the first on the list of golden rules in my training," she says. "It's the first thing in the back of my mind. People often ask, 'What would you do in my situation?' I can't answer that question, because I'm in a different place. I'm not in their moccasins."

On the books, the genetic counseling profession in the United States is barely a quarter of a century old, dating to the establishment of a master's degree program at Sarah Lawrence College in Bronxville, New York, in 1969. In fact, the practice of such counseling is much older, dating from the 1940s in the United States when heredity clinics were first established, when it was provided by doctors and geneticists.

Clearly, with the frank eugenics of the early twentieth century, many people provided, however misguided, a form of genetic counseling.

That history of eugenics haunts this profession and confers on it both a rather unique self-importance and a specific professional creed. The earlier "counseling" was directive in the extreme, telling people what they *ought* to do for the sake of society and their family's future. It purported to know more than it actually did know, both about the nature of genetics and about what would be best for everyone involved.

Today's genetic counselors seem to have a deep-seated fear that they will never escape the legacy of those young clerks whom Charles Davenport and his peers sent out from the Eugenics Record Office to track down hereditary "feeblemindedness" and other human flaws and further the campaign to eradicate them. Anyone who spends time with groups of genetic counselors or observes some of their training sessions soon senses this concern. Ethicist Arthur Caplan of the University of Pennsylvania dwelled on the phenomenon at some length during a talk at the National Academy of Sciences in January 1997.

"One of the problems that genetic counseling faces in this country— and has for many, many years now—is that it has been so terrified because of what happened in the Nazi Holocaust of saying anything about what individuals [should] do when they come for genetic counseling or advice or information about genetics or [are] thinking about a breast cancer marker today, or something as simple as an ultrasound test," he said. "We have a counseling profession that adamantly insists that it will be value-neutral. There is no one in all of medicine that talks more about value neutrality than genetic counselors.

"Imagine going to your doctor," he went on. "Your blood pressure is 200 /110, and your doctor says, 'Look, I'm going to give you this information: You have ridiculously high blood pressure. It causes stroke. It could cause an immediate heart attack. You have about a year to live with blood pressure like that. But you do what you want. It's information. Deal with it.' No one talks that way.

"When you get to the genetic counselor, you are told: 'Your child has this trisomy, there are these terrible effects. We don't think this child is viable, but you can do what you want. We will respect your values.' Genetics abhors the thought that it would tempt, push, urge anyone in any direction."

Genetic counseling began to flower in the early 1970s, when amniocentesis was becoming popular. People who could convey the risks and results of the test were vitally needed. Early on, in 1971, at a conference in Virginia on ethical issues in genetic counseling, the profession had "neither certainty nor uniformity of opinion" about what stance counselors should take with their clients: educator, adviser, confidant, or friend.

The consequence today, at the end of the century, is that a moral white-gloves principle suffuses education for genetic counselors, the same philosophy Rucquoi applies to her dealings with her daughter-in-law and with everyone she counsels: nondirectiveness. The ethic runs so deep that when a doctor proposed at a genetics meeting that it would be a good idea to counsel pregnant women not to drink alcohol and to take folic acid supplements, many counselors argued back heatedly that this would be directive and therefore unethical.

Nondirectiveness dovetails perfectly with current ideals such as autonomy and reproductive choice. Nonetheless, it also gives counselors some problems.

What to do, for instance, for the couple who openly avow that they want to know the gender of a fetus so they can terminate it if it is the "wrong" sex? The vast majority of genetic counselors are women, and many of them express discomfort about genetic testing for the sole purpose of gender selection. Still, as a group, their willingness to test for gender in the absence of a risk of gender-related hereditary disease has shifted considerably in the last quarter-century.

In 1972 only one percent of genetic counselors in the United States said they would provide prenatal testing in such a circumstance. By 1985 the figure had risen to 62 percent. In 1991, 85 percent of counselors said they would either provide the test themselves or refer a couple to someone who would. As tests become available to detect more qualitative features—obesity and personality traits, for example— it may become ever more difficult for them to proceed with a moral code that prevents them from expressing an opinion they must undeniably hold, regardless of what it is.

"However much the value of neutrality on the part of the counselor may be espoused," wrote Daniel Callahan of the Hastings Center, reporting on that 1971 Virginia meeting, "counselors do in fact often make decisions for their patients, or at least heavily influence the decisions by the way they present data."

Viewed from one perspective, it is a peculiar restraint for a health professional. As Caplan noted, no one diagnosed with cancer or heart disease expects a doctor to refrain from giving a personal judgment about the patient's best course. That's one thing a doctor is paid to do. The medical profession increasingly expresses an intent to take the patient's wishes *into account*, but no other health profession muzzles itself the same way genetic counselors do.

"We do not expect doctors to express 'value neutrality' about their options simply because the outcome is frightening," write philosopher Robert Wachbroit and attorney David Wasserman of the University of Maryland.

Another level of conflict arises with regard to the language used in counseling sessions. The counselor meets the clients in a medical setting, is perceived as part of the medical profession, and tries to convey a message in medical terms. Other important aspects of the situation, such as the developmental consequences of a disorder, may not even enter the conversation.

Counselors tend to focus on learning and conveying degrees of risk, yet risk may not be what a client cares most about. "Uncertainty is not related to interpretations of risk, to the seriousness or treatability of risked disorder, or to the client's learning of medical information," write Dorothy Wertz and John Fletcher, in a report of a survey about communication between genetic counselors and families. "It is related to questions about desired family size and to concern about how an affected child would affect the quality of life. . . . It is not the level of risk that determines decisions, so much as *what* is risked."

Yet counselors are trained to focus on the former, while they may be more or less unprepared to convey the latter. For instance, counselors are unlikely to be able to answer a couple's questions about the developmental pitfalls a child may experience as an adult, or about his future potential for employment or independence. A genetic counselor may or may not refer a couple to a support group of parents in a similar situation who could impart a deeper understanding of the rewards as well as the challenges of raising a child with a hereditary condition.

(Rucquoi *is* relatively prepared: she worked in an adult mental retardation center for several years and keeps videotapes of families with Down syndrome children to show clients who want more information.)

"A lot of people look at genetics as purely diagnostic," says medical geneticist Golder Wilson of Children's Medical Center in Dallas. "Once you've given the diagnosis, your role is over." Until a decade ago, Wilson saw his role as "helping parents through the adjustment, explaining what Down syndrome is, and sending them on their way."

Then a group of four hundred Dallas-area parents of children with Down syndrome petitioned the hospital to open a special clinic for the care of their children, and Wilson was chosen to oversee it. He began attending national conferences on the syndrome, where he heard young people with Down syndrome give speeches that he says would be "enviable" for any normal person. Gradually he found himself involved in the larger field of special schooling and early intervention for children affected with the syndrome.

Could most counselors conceivably give their counseling the kind of depth Wilson can now provide, whatever the condition? "That's the question I've been dealing with — trying to provide checklists for common genetic syndromes," he says. "I do think once you get involved with that sort of depth, if you allow the genetic counselors to involve those other issues, they can be more effective."

After the Down syndrome clinic opened, Wilson gained a measure of personal perspective that may make his own counseling yet more sensitive: his own three-year-old son was diagnosed as mentally disabled. He found it "most interesting" to watch himself and his wife react to labels like "pervasive developmental disorder" and "retardation."

"It makes you more aware," he says, "of how people can react to callous language."

At the 1996 meeting of the National Society of Genetic Counselors, several speakers urged that the profession rethink its philosophy of nondirectiveness. Sonia Suter, a professor of law at the University of Michigan, likened nondirective counseling to a travel agent providing pictures of foreign destinations but no guidebooks or descriptions. She urged counselors to pursue nonmedical concerns actively when clients suggest they would like to talk about them.

Psychologist Seymour Kessler of Berkeley, California, who trains genetic counselors, said nondirectiveness is "not important" and can even constitute bad counseling. For a counselor to tell a client she would support whatever decision she makes is actually paternalistic and highly directive, he maintained, because the counselor is co-opting the high moral ground and not allowing the client to engage in dialogue or disagree with her—thereby actually robbing the client of autonomy.

Often counselors present too much information in a session, Kessler said, and focus too little on who the client is and what her agenda is. What clients really care about is respect for their autonomy, Kessler said, and above all, empathy.

A survey funded by the New England Regional Genetics Group in the same year tends to support Kessler's contentions. Focus groups of consumers listed as their own top priorities for genetic counselors: respect for persons, professional knowledge and skills (in science, medicine, social and community resources, and personal interactions), knowing when and how to refer, and understanding and admitting to their own limitations. "Making no assumptions about consumers' choices or values" ranked seventh on the fourteen-item priority list. Nondirectiveness did not even appear.

Those who have undergone genetic counseling before prenatal testing generally seem to have positive feelings about their counselors—and indeed most members of the profession appear to be genuine, earnest, and concerned. Wertz and Fletcher's report, however, showed some interesting outcomes: the 44 percent of clients who said they had been influenced by genetic counseling left the sessions with reproductive plans similar to those of the 56 percent who said they had not. More than half who said they were influenced did not change their plans as a result of counseling.

What must be invisible to clients but can scarcely escape the attention of counselors—especially those working in the service of companies that market genetic tests—is the conflict of interest inherent in their role. The counselor is required both to educate the client, as an informed expert working in the service of the provider who has offered the test, and also to befriend the client dispassionately and help her explore her options—one of which should be not going through with the testing.

"The implicit assumption is that the condition should be eliminated—which, given the limitations of present technology, almost always means termination of the pregnancy," write Wachbroit and Wasserman. "The genetic counselor may not share this view; but as the person who mediates the patient's encounter with the technology, she cannot stand apart from it."

Beyond all that, the counselor helps the medical profession fulfill its legal obligation to document informed consent in order to avoid litigation that might follow the birth of a child with a defect that might have been prevented. In the midst of the turmoil of the information revolution, the counselor acts as a legal buffer between the medical profession and the patient.

Sociologist Troy Duster recounts an example of this dilemma from some genetic counseling sessions he witnessed as part of a study:

Male: The odds of having a Down's child [are] 100-to-1 and the odds of miscarrying 200-to-1?
Counselor: Yes.
Female: It sounds like a very small chance to me, 1 in 100.
Counselor: When you were in your twenties, it was 1 in 1,200.
Female: Yes, it's much more likely than I would care to risk.
Counselor: Okay, then, that's why you have chosen to have the test.
Female: Yes, that's why I did it.

The counselor has not only provided the clients with figures about their risk, she has provided perspective that makes it appear considerable, then directed the woman to decide she will have the test.

The quandary is especially clear with regard to prenatal testing, but it may surface in the context of other kinds of testing too, if the interests of doctors and health plans, insurers and employers, continue to blur. Suppose a health plan's case manager refers an employee to the plan's genetic counselor to "consider" testing for a gene related to heart disease, or cancer — or drug addiction. Does the employee dare to refuse? In some cases genetic counselors never speak directly to the patients at all. They merely consult with the primary care doctor. It's anyone's guess what the subsequent conversation with the patient is like.

Counselors themselves are exquisitely sensitive to the conflicts within their roles, as medical anthropologist Rayna Rapp found when she interviewed and observed thirty-five of them in New York City. "The counselors I interviewed were very much aware of the anxiety as well as the relief that their services invoke," she wrote. "Most had thought deeply about why someone might reject as well as accept amniocentesis and possibly abortion."

The National Center for Human Genome Research itself has undertaken a major program to educate genetic counselors. In the light of history, it's difficult to view the outcome of this program with complete confidence. Steeped in the heady world of researchers making genetic discoveries at breakneck speed, genetic counselors trained there would be unlikely to view the enterprise and the culture that surrounds it with any attitude but approval. If the ELSI working group felt considerable pressure from the scientists, wouldn't the genetic counselors feel it too?

On the other hand, in the unforeseeable future of the American health care system (or nonsystem, as it is at the moment), we may all wish for someone who feels herself to be acting as our advocate and educator as we face genetic testing. Yet despite all the money and interest devoted to ethics, social issues, and indeed the training of genetic counselors, the field has been surprisingly slow to sponsor studies of its own methods.

Barbara Biesecker, who heads the NCHGR genetic counseling program, calls genetic counseling an "embryonic field" that has flourished without clarifying or resolving many aspects of its own identity. "We've been asked to evolve into something new before we even know what we do is effective," she adds. "There's a lot of controversy about what genetic counseling is. Some people think what matters is that the client retains information. Others want to set up a relationship, to explore what the issues are, to help people cope—to move forward in their lives, to figure out what they want."

Asking what genetic counseling *is* begins with asking what its goals are, which is an issue the profession in this country began to address a quarter-century ago but has never resolved since. The question came to a head recently in Great Britain, where a modern but nationalized health service has been facing for some years the same problems of cost control and equity that now have the American health system in turmoil. These issues are not yet fully decided, but the terms of the debate are instructive.

"What counts as success in genetic counseling?" asked University of Wales philosopher Ruth Chadwick in the *Journal of Medical Ethics* in 1993. She was responding to a suggestion by medical geneticist Angus Clarke, of the same institution, that in order to avoid such ethically sensitive outcomes as "defective births prevented," the indicator of productivity for genetic counselors should be the number of counseling sessions completed.

Angus Clarke is something of a gadfly in this area. In 1991, in a hotly debated article in the *Lancet*, he argued with the lucidity typical of good British discourse that nondirective counseling was unattainable in pre-natal genetics, and that for geneticists to deny the fact was to cower in the face of abhorrent ethical questions. Being sincerely nondirective about a disorder while aiming to prevent it is impossible, he stated, and is "insider dealing."

"It is immediately apparent that to leave all decisions to the discretion of the parents indicates the low value that our society places upon those with genetic disorders and handicaps," he wrote. "We draw some moral lines for social [motivations for abortion] but none for genetic termina-tion of pregnancy. . . . We must start to discuss whether any disorders, other than female sex, are compatible with a sufficiently good quality of life that abortion for that condition is generally desirable." Otherwise, Clarke feared, geneticists would be responsible (through omission) for the development of prenatal testing for "cosmetic criteria."

Pregnancies terminated would be a handy measure of productivity, Chadwick admitted, one easily translatable into money saved. "There are reasons for wanting to reduce the incidence of genetic disease and these are connected with the consequences of genetic diseases for their sufferers," she went on. "In fact, if medical geneticists do not hold a view of this nature, it is difficult to see how they can justify their service, un-less they *do* fall into the trap of arguing in terms of money-saving."

A fairer indicator of success in counseling, Chadwick maintained, would be whether the interview had truly helped patients to make the decisions they needed to make. But to measure such productivity, it would be necessary to learn whether the counselor had really made the patient aware of all factors relevant to the decision.

"The decisions that people will have to make involve questions about the worthwhileness of lives that future people will live and whether or not it can be said to be better that someone should not be born," she concluded. "These are philosophical questions. How can individuals be provided with the necessary information to make such choices? Should they be acquainted with the latest moves in the philosophical debate about the value of life?"

Chadwick's bottom line is that what people really need in these tumultuous times is not, strictly speaking, just *genetic* counseling. Yet that is what is being offered us, at best—a brief glimpse into the rationales and priorities of the medical profession, while we keep our own counsel.

In the current climate, unfortunately, the advantage of even this limited kind of counseling is anything but a foregone conclusion. Genetic counselors are not only specialists but subspecialists, and managed care controls access to specialists with particular care. Why not leave the explanations to the primary care doctor — or indeed, to the pleasant voice at the end of the customer service line?

At the moment, the former may be scarcely more useful than the latter. Recent studies have shown that more than half of internists and gynecologists miss family histories that clearly point to hereditary breast cancer, and that four out of five patients tested for a pre-colon cancer gene had either received no genetic counseling or had not provided written informed consent. Meanwhile, genetic counselors are in a very tenuous position, because in general their services are not reimbursed directly by health insurance. They rely absolutely on referrals from doctors.

There is hope for the future: The American Medical Association and the National Human Genome Research Institute, together with more than a hundred other organizations of health professionals, recently joined in launching a new education program on genetics for primary care doctors, backed by an Internet site. They are actively promoting new medical curricula on genetics.

All of this takes time. In the near term we may be left truly on our own. We may be offered testing we don't want, or denied testing we do want. We may have helpful counseling, unhelpful counseling, or no counseling whatsoever. As things stand, it's anybody's guess.

CHAPTER 15

Genes and Managed Care: The Bottom Line

Information resulting from the Human Genome Project will change ...
the focus of medicine from treatment of symptoms to prevention—a shift
that will lower the cost and increase the effectiveness of health care.

— Undated backgrounder for journalists,
SmithKline Beecham Clinical Laboratories

DURING THE DARK DAYS OF 1995, WHEN THE CONGRES-
sional budget debate had ground to a halt and nonessential government
workers were put on furlough without pay, a cartoon in the Cincinnati
Enquirer showed House Speaker Newt Gingrich in front of an endless
sea of human beings. At his side stood a lackey, reading from a statement. "On account of the budget," says the caption, "we've had to separate you into essential and nonessential Americans."

Not ha-ha funny but funny sad, especially to anyone who knew the
real agenda behind the budget debate. It was not simply "the economy,
stupid," as President Clinton had proclaimed during the previous elec-
tion. It was the cost of health care.

Essential and nonessential Americans, indeed. Who was essential
enough to deserve the cost of good health, despite the need to balance
the federal budget? Who was expendable? The elderly? Single mothers? The poor?

In a different version of history, that cartoon might not have appeared
(nor this book) because the president would have succeeded in creating a national health system that guaranteed health care for everyone.
Learning about a gene-based condition would not mean risking the loss
of one's health insurance, and therefore losing health care for the very
problem that the test had unearthed.

But that national health care program crashed in flames, shot down
by everyone who would have been involved: doctors who didn't want to

be caught up in a centralized system, employers who didn't want to pay for it, insurance companies that didn't want to go out of business.

But the underlying problem—the high cost of health care—did not vanish with the end of the Clintons' health care reform plan. With 15 percent of the American public already unable to get health insurance, and some 41 million Americans reporting difficulty in getting the medical care they need (57 percent of whom were not poor but middle class, according to a survey by Project Hope), a cartoon with a caption about "nonessential Americans" was no joke at all.

Where does genetics fit in this picture? Just as genetics comes into its fullest flower, the health system into which it must fit is in turmoil. Until the tempest is over, it's difficult to see an obvious place for genetic testing and expensive gene therapy.

This difficulty has not escaped the notice of genetic specialists, and it strikes fear into them. Their future may depend entirely on whether and how they can prove that what they do is cost-effective.

"Geneticists are going to have to form a team, pick the condition, and advertise themselves," declared geneticist Peter Rowley of Rochester, New York, at a session on managed care that he organized for the 1995 annual conference of the American Society of Human Genetics. From the outset, of necessity, the discussion focused on cost—and quickly got to the bottom line.

"The question is how we can demonstrate that genetic services are worth the cost," Rowley told his audience. "A surgeon fixes a hernia, the patient gets back to work, that's obvious. The tests we do are expensive. . . . The subjects of counseling do not go back to work as a result. They may not even be conceived. The fruits of our work—relief of anxiety—are not recognized as cost-effective."

Some of the nation's top experts on the subject rose to the podium to lay out for geneticists the nature of cost-effectiveness analysis and the ways in which genetics provides special challenges. "Certainly any new test has to demonstrate it is cost-effective," said Eugene Washington of the University of California – San Francisco's Center for Reproductive Health Policy Research. Implicit in the question of cost-effectiveness were some others: "From whose perspective? The patient? The provider? The payer? Society? Quite often, as you can imagine, these are in conflict."

Rowley pointed out that according to some studies, averting an unwanted pregnancy with a fetus affected by cystic fibrosis could save about $1.4 billion overall. "Is that a good value?" he asked.

Trying to put a dollar value on matters that are basically ethical, Washington remarked later, is "a way to get guaranteed success if you want hate mail. It's a reasonable way to think about what's likely to generate value. It isn't the way you want to make decisions."

The costly promise of genetic testing and cure might have slipped nicely into the old fee-for-service medical system, when doctors did whatever they thought best and passed the bill on to the insurance company. But that system is no more. During the storm over the cost of health care, it vanished.

What came to take its place was managed care: the principles of big business and competition — cost cutting through efficiency and quality control — applied to the doctors and hospitals. With astonishing speed the large employers who pay for health insurance shifted their employees from fee-for-service policies into less costly managed care plans, and those health plans merged and consolidated. Hospitals and groups of doctors consolidated in response.

Over the last few years Congress — representing the nation's largest purchaser of health care, the federal government — has been taking giant steps toward steering Medicare patients into managed care. For several years it has been encouraging states to steer indigent patients into managed care as well.

Wall Street pundits predict that, when the winds have calmed, the nation will be dominated by only six or seven huge managed health care plans. In 1996, for instance, Aetna Life and Casualty Company purchased U.S. Healthcare Corporation, one of the nation's largest managed care plans. U.S. Healthcare had been a strong proponent of tough cost controls, of penalizing doctors who spend too much, and of per-patient capitation — setting a dollar figure for the price it will pay to provide health care for every covered member. That merger put a price on some 23 million Americans. These days there is a bottom to the pot. Virtually all the major national health care organizations today are for-profit entities.

Selling the promise of genetic *research* to the federal government was one thing; it will be another matter entirely, in the current climate, to sell the existing results of that research — halfway technologies and services that diagnose but do not (yet) cure — to the stockholders of a for-profit health system. As yet, the new genetics offers us no truly satisfying solutions. What it offers so far is only information.

Until genome research generates some undisputed cures, proving its financial worth to the medical system will require placing a value on this information — either by finding some way to justify such intangibles as reassurance, or else by showing a savings from detecting and reducing the extent of disease. Some of the scenarios for the near term, however, are either discouraging or frightening.

In one scenario genetic testing and screening prove too expensive, after all this effort, to be worthwhile, and only the rich or the lucky can

COST-EFFECTIVENESS AND GENETICS

Health policymakers use cost-effectiveness studies all the time, to judge the value of laser surgery, of magnetic imaging, of bone marrow transplants. Some of the cost-effectiveness studies that focus on genetics have had critical flaws. They tend to leave out what matters to the patients, in instances where this may be what matters most.

In such studies, "nonmonetary costs and benefits are frequently overlooked," notes the New England Regional Genetics Group in a policy statement. "Genetics, which occasions individual/family decision-making about reproduction and deals with the analysis of risk, or of variable outcomes, is particularly recalcitrant to accurate and value-neutral cost-benefit analysis."

Many cost-effectiveness studies argue that nonmonetary benefits such as reassurance are "intangibles" and can't be measured — and therefore ignore them. They often set prevention and treatment against each other and inevitably prove that prevention is cheaper. To take this analysis to its absurd conclusion, it is cheapest of all never to have children, which will save us all the cost of schooling.

Obviously, it is also cheapest simply to ignore anyone who cannot ever get well. A pure cost-effectiveness analysis might take this view (as some managed care plans do) because it does not incorporate matters of equity or fairness into the equation. While cost-effectiveness analyses set out to determine value for money, they cannot make judgments about *values*.

A recent study compared two health-screening scenarios; one offered

use them. In another, the behemoth managed care organizations begin to use genetic testing in earnest, for their own ends. A third scenario is that the health care system makes wise collective choices about genetic testing. Setting this scenario in place would require careful planning and vigilance on the part of everyone involved.

To put it bluntly, the most cost-effective service that genetic testing

a cancer-screening test to everyone and saved 1,000 lives, and the other offered it only to high-risk individuals and saved 1,100 lives. In the survey more than half of the members of the public favored the first—and less cost-effective—option, because, as one of them put it, "Equity is more important than efficiency." It's only fair: everyone should get a chance, in other words, even if that way more people will die.

"Cost-effectiveness analysis operates on the assumption that the primary goal of health care spending should be to maximize health care benefits across a population rather than to distribute those benefits equally," wrote the authors. "Many of the respondents who rejected the more effective test did not accept this assumption." Although our health care system seems to operate more and more according to the bottom line, when the proposition is put to the test, many of us reject it.

One critic has argued that nearly all cost-effectiveness studies of prenatal testing are flawed according to simple logic and mathematics, because they leave out of the equation both the cost of potential fetuses allowed to be born and the potential value of those aborted. From that perspective, the only potential of the aborted fetus is cost, and the entire future of the yet-unborn healthy child represents positive value. But what if the healthy child becomes a drug addict or an embezzler? The analysis doesn't work that way.

In the real world, notes Theodore Ganiats in the journal *Medical Decision Making,* neither side frames the debate this way. Pro-choice advocates place value on individual freedoms. Pro-life advocates argue that killing the fetus is wrong. Neither side, Ganiats points out, is arguing on the basis of the potential value to society—the expected utility—of the unborn child. Cost-effectiveness arguments about prenatal testing, whatever their usefulness to policymakers in public health, ignore the elements that are most important to the public debate.

could offer to managed care at the moment would be a way to avoid the cost of keeping people at risk of hereditary illness alive and well — either by making them disappear before birth or by keeping them out of the health plan afterward. The industry has a term for the latter approach: cherry-picking. Should they choose to, health plans could use genetic testing to assure that they do not undertake to provide health care for anyone at hereditary risk of getting sick. In most states, there is now nothing to prevent them from doing this.

"In ten years we have to have universal coverage," said medical geneticist Susan Pauker, of Boston's Harvard Pilgrim Health Plan, after a symposium on cost-effectiveness and genetics. "Do you mean," I asked her, "it's inevitable?"

"No," she replied. "It has to be. It just has to be." Some congressman will discover he was at risk for some illness, she added, and health reform will push through.

"Eventually I think that's where we will have to go," agreed Francis Collins in an interview. "But I think we can find a partial solution that will be pretty good until such time as we finally recognize that our current system of health care is inherently unfair and heartless."

Maybe we will reach that solution; maybe not. People who want to blow away debate over cherry-picking point out that we all carry genes that predispose us to some hereditary illness. But that fact alone won't stop managed care plans from picking and choosing their risks if they want to. On the other hand, if people can withhold from insurance companies the knowledge that they are *not* at risk of major disease — and therefore don't need to pay to insure themselves against it — they may well drop out of group insurance plans, skewing the odds for high-cost medical care within the group and ultimately causing health insurance costs to skyrocket for those who remain in the group.

At some level insurance works only if the cost of care is spread across a large population of healthy people, who collectively pay for the care of the ill. Once we have complete information about everyone's genetic risk, it may be still be possible to create large and diverse enough groups to spread the risk of illness equitably. In the interim, however, with only some adverse genes identified, the situation remains tenuous for those with known risks.

When a working group of the National Association of Insurance Commissioners looked at gene testing in 1996, it reported that in general insurers were not asking insurance applicants to undergo genetic testing as a prerequisite to gaining coverage, but that if the information existed in a person's medical record, they would use it. "The viability of a voluntary insurance system is dependent upon insurers' capacity to avoid or limit the impacts of adverse selection," said their report. ". . . To do this, insurers must have access to the same material knowledge as the insurance applicant." The working group engaged in "substantial discussion" about developing a model act or regulation that would resolve this thorny issue, which resulted in "substantial disagreement." Thus, even the advisory body for regulators of insurance plans could not come to terms with how to reconcile gene testing with fairness in health insurance policies.

"The decision has got to be made that [genetics] is part of basic medical care," said John Mann, chief of genetics at Kaiser Permanente–San Jose, part of one of the nation's largest and oldest nonprofit health plans and one of very few to have its own staff geneticists and clinical lab. "That's what we geneticists have to convince the world to pay for." A laudable opinion, but it comes from an authority within a well-regarded nonprofit plan. How many of his counterparts in other managed care firms share it?

In *badly* managed care, genetics brings other potential perils. Cost cutting may prompt managed care firms to order genetic tests from labs that have poor records for reliability, leaving members falsely frightened or falsely reassured. Doctors may order tests without providing counseling, if the former is covered but the latter is not. Standard approval procedures could lead to delays in prenatal testing beyond the point where couples can act on the test result and have a pregnancy terminated if they wish, or to delays in counseling during which a depressed patient ends the waiting with suicide.

On the other hand, a managed care plan that is privy to gene test results might try to force a couple to abort an affected fetus by refusing to pay for its care after birth, or pressure them in more subtle ways. One such case is already on record, involving a fetus affected by cystic fibrosis. (The couple threatened to sue, and the plan backed down.) Because of clauses in their contracts with managed care plans, physicians may not be at liberty to discuss all the alternatives with their patients, and may steer them in directions they would not choose if they were given full information.

The editors of *The New England Journal of Medicine* declared in 1996 that managed care plans involve an "inherent conflict of interest." The United States has "embraced a financing and delivery method that rewards doctors, sometimes quite directly, for doing less for their patients," Marcia Angell and Jerome Kassirer warned in an editorial. "Most doctors are now double-agents—working for their patients, but also for their companies."

Legislators have been slow to reach the same understanding. In a comprehensive 1995 report on state laws regulating health maintenance organizations, the Los Angeles–based Center for Health Care Rights noted the states' "almost total failure to address the problem that financial considerations by the decision-maker might directly affect medical decisions." At that time only two states had laws that even contemplated the possibility that financial factors might influence a health provider's medical conduct.

But the states are swiftly catching up. In 1995 state legislatures began to adopt a wide range of measures to constrain the activities of managed care plans, including prohibitions on "gag clauses" that would limit what doctors can tell patients about their options (adopted in nineteen states during 1995 and 1996), limits on financial incentives to restrict costly kinds of care, and other measures to expand the independence of health care professionals.

Like children who consider their dysfunctional family to be normal, we and our legislators have grown up accustomed to a peculiar situation. The health care system most of us have always taken for granted—in which almost everyone who works, and his or her family, gets health insurance through the employer—is a peculiarity of American history that dates back only to the years after World War II. At that time strong labor unions were demanding higher wages, and employers offered them health insurance instead, as a benefit.

The employers could not have known what they had bargained for. As medical science progressed, it offered ever more ways to make or keep people healthy—at a price. As experts in health policy like to say, the incentives were misaligned. Doctors and hospitals provided the care, the employees got the benefit, and the insurers passed the cost along to the employers, who, until fairly recently, paid up without giving the situation much attention.

But in the 1980s the cost of medical care became a noticeable item on the corporate ledger. (It also became noticeable to Congress, which had to pay the bills for Medicaid and Medicare, the federally funded medical insurance programs for the indigent and the elderly.) Between 1965 and 1990, the annual per-capita cost for health care in the United States rose from $1,200 to $3,000. Gradually, the concept of prepaid health care—insurance plans that guaranteed to provide medical care for a population of defined size at a set fee—looked very attractive indeed.

In 1988 (two years before the Human Genome Project moved from concept to reality) about 30 percent of Americans were enrolled in some form of managed health care. By 1995, when gene research was in overdrive, the statistics had flipped: only about three in ten Americans still had traditional fee-for-service health insurance.

Meanwhile, because of corporate downsizing, fewer and fewer Americans had employers who paid their health care costs. From 1987 to 1995 the proportion of the nonelderly population receiving health care coverage through their employers fell from 69 percent to just under 64 percent. Many people who lost their jobs and hence their insurance were unable to replace it. There was a term for them, too: the "medical homeless."

All but heedless of this turmoil in the health care system, genetic researchers began their big campaign to map human genes, beginning with the ones involved in diseases. At some point the two juggernauts— health insurance and genetics—are bound either to merge or to collide, because they deal with opposite ends of the same phenomenon: risk.

Health insurance takes on the risk of catastrophic medical problems and tries to make money while spreading the risk around. Efforts to understand the human genome will inevitably clarify who is at risk of what. Unless our society finds some way to reconcile these opposing goals—probably by guaranteeing health care for people whatever their risk of hereditary illness—we will unquestionably violate one of our deepest and oldest moral principles: equity.

"Above all," says medical geneticist Susan Pauker, "it's an issue of justice. There's nothing *just* in the medical system about our genes. We don't choose our parents."

So far, there is little direct evidence that employers and insurers are using genetic testing in discriminatory ways. All that exists are isolated anecdotes, stories of people who have been denied jobs or insurance because of something that turned up in their records. In fact, a 1996 article in *Business and Health*, a magazine intended for employers, advised that "general population screening rarely pays" and that "there is still no conclusive evidence linking [genetic] testing to lower costs or improved outcomes."

Still, some evidence does indicate that employers and insurers are attentive to the possibilities of genetic testing. A 1989 survey released by

THE OREGON PLAN

In 1989, hoping to provide medical care for its 120,000 uninsured people under the Medicaid program, Oregon health officials drew up a list of more than seven hundred medical treatments and asked an expert committee to rate their effectiveness. To assess the cost side of the equation, it surveyed the public: Which priorities in health care did citizens value the most? Prevention, pain relief, and maternity care topped the list.

Then state health authorities sorted all the treatments into a master list, which was 744 items long. They determined how much money they had for providing care, analyzed what each treatment would cost, and, somewhere near the bottom of the list, drew a line. Above the line are treatments the state Medicaid program will pay for, for those who have no insurance. Items below the line are those that the state cannot afford.

The line moves according to the state's annual budget. Funding stopped at line 606 in 1993, but in 1995 it went only as far as line 581. Today health interest groups who believe that a certain treatment should be covered no longer lobby the legislature. They have to find a logical way to convince the authorities that the treatment's position on the list is in error—and that's harder.

The Oregon plan has aroused tremendous controversy. Many critics revile such rationing, and the U.S. Department of Health and Human

the Office of Technology Assessment (just after the genome project began) found that only twelve of 330 Fortune 500 companies were using genetic tests for any reason. But more than half of the companies said they found the idea acceptable, and four of ten said that an individual's insurance costs might affect his or her chance of getting a job.

"Even if employers do not use genetic testing," wrote a joint committee of the ELSI program and the National Action Plan on Breast Cancer in 1997, "they still may have access to the medical records of their employees and prospective employees, and thus will be able to find out if these individuals have certain predispositions to disease."

Services, overseeing Medicaid-funded health care, rejected an early version of the Oregon plan as discriminating against the disabled. But its supporters say that the plan buys medical care for more than 100,000 people who would lack it otherwise, and the items above the line seem generous indeed. For instance, coverage for Gaucher disease treatment is safely high at line 51, and treatment for problems in eating, swallowing, and bowel and bladder function fall on line 213.

Treatments on the margin include repair of dental appliances, at line 581. Treatments for impulse disorders, sexual dysfunction, and thrush—candidiasis of the mouth—fell below the line in 1995.

The system's defenders argue that it is a rational and laudable way to apply public values to the problem of health care costs. "We can't buy everything, and we won't buy everything," says Michael Garland of the Oregon Health Sciences University. "But we should buy those things that are most important to us." Ordinary folks have a "richer" set of values than academics, he adds, and the Oregon process has found a way to include them in the debate.

The plan is not perfect, however, and it may face a stormy future if health care costs rise again. People with no income will be covered, but those who are at or just below the federal poverty level may have difficulty affording the sliding-scale premiums. A provision that would have forced employers to provide benefits for treatments on the list was repealed in early 1996. Even with the Oregon plan, many Oregonians are unprotected by health insurance, yet according to one analyst's 1997 report, the plan is "on a budgetary tightrope."

At least thirty states have now adopted laws to regulate use of genetic test results or to prevent discrimination by employers, according to the National Conference of State Legislators. The protections provided by these laws vary from state to state, however, and their definitions of *genetic testing* and *genetic discrimination* are often too vague to be workable.

Add to this situation the chilling statement of Francis Collins that "the notion of collecting all the information about a patient's DNA within the next decade or so is not science fiction," and it's easy to see why there is widespread concern about the potential for abuse of this information.

"You didn't get to pick your DNA," Collins said at the introductory gathering of the new National Bioethics Advisory Commission. "I didn't get to pick mine. Genetic information about you should not be allowed to deny you insurance or a job. It's a civil rights issue." He went on to cite a 1996 Harris poll in which 60 percent of respondents said they were "very concerned" that genetic information might be used against them by an employer or insurer.

Congress and the administration are well aware of these issues and have been working steadily to resolve them. Proposed legislation relevant to genetic testing was introduced in both 1996 and 1997, although with the exception of HIPAA (the Health Insurance Portability and Accountability Act)—which applies only to people who have health insurance from their employers—no legislation has passed.

Both President Clinton and Vice President Gore have been active in promoting federal legislation against genetic discrimination. In January 1998 Gore released a new administration report urging legislation that would protect against genetic discrimination on the job and ensure that genetic information is not released without an individual's explicit permission.

Clinton was embroiled in a sex scandal at the time, however, and Congress was busy with oversight responsibilities relating to health legislation passed in the previous two years. At this writing it seems unlikely that any broadbased new protections will be in place soon, and as always with Congress, it is very difficult to predict when federal legislation will be put in place to fill the major loopholes in protection against genetic discrimination.

Even if outright discrimination is outlawed, the health care industry still may be able to use genetic information to its advantage in subtler ways. The latest proposed solution to the problem of rising health care costs, for example, is a phenomenon called "disease management." Although it's something doctors were intended to do all along, private companies now offer it as a business.

Disease management means many things to many people, but here it means an integrated effort to track all aspects of care for a patient with a major disease, according to a comprehensive plan aimed at delivering the most effective care in the most economic fashion possible. Disease management programs usually coordinate health care strategies for people with expensive chronic health problems such as diabetes, chronic lung disease, heart problems, or mental illness.

Pharmaceutical companies like disease management, because it offers them the chance to steer doctors and patients to a particular medication. The programs include some counseling and education, coordination of referrals to specialists, close monitoring of patients' progress, and active efforts to ensure that patients are taking their medicine as needed.

In a document prepared for prospective customers, Integrated Disease Management, a subsidiary of the pharmaceutical firm Eli Lilly and Company, described its operating philosophy as follows: "At the heart of our approach is an orientation toward prevention as well as treatment, the adoption of tactics that empower patients to take on more responsibility for their own health as well as foster greater rapport with providers, and the pursuit of cost efficiencies achievable through elimination of over- and underutilization of care modalities." The firm added that it puts its money where its mouth is, setting contracts by which it makes a profit only when it is able to reduce the total costs of caring for patients with a specific disease.

As a marketing strategy for pharmaceuticals that treat life-threatening conditions such as diabetes, this approach seems not only shrewd but actually laudable. But what exactly would it mean if a genetics diagnosis laboratory marketed its services by offering to "manage disease"? Helping people to remember to track their blood sugar is one thing. When the management extends to other family members, the issues may not be so simple.

The first organization to tumble to the marketing potential of genetics in disease management was a Scottsdale, Arizona, firm named Genetrix, which introduced its genetic disease management program in 1995. Originally a cytogenetics lab offering results for amniocentesis procedures, the company prudently spurned the word *disease* in labeling its services. Instead it called its product "The Genetic Health Network," and billed it as a program to provide comprehensive care for prenatal management of genetic disorders. Genetrix offered to provide everything in one coordinated package: testing, counseling, and backup referrals to specialists.

"This is all about cost containment in health care," said product manager Sheila Shuster, speaking at her company's booth in the exhibit hall of a genetics conference. "Right now, we are providing case managers. We are contacted by the plan when someone is pregnant. Immediately we send a letter urging them to go to the doctor. We give them an embryological brochure [as an incentive] when they go."

Genetrix coordinated its services according to predetermined clinical pathways, she added. "Our case managers are in contact with the patient. The patient gets a first information packet with a general history form [that they fill out]. They send it back to us, and we decide if they are normal or at increased risk. Then they get into one of two paths. We tell them what the next necessary step is. The high-risk path takes them to a counseling session.

"We want to tie prenatal diagnosis back to outcomes, validating our critical paths," she added. "Plans are very interested in that." Most patients are not offered gene testing, she went on. "We encourage those who feel they need it to get it. It's really a matter of education."

But the education was aimed at increasing genetic screening, as Genetrix's own promotional material showed. The brochure promised to increase triple-marker screening of pregnant women under thirty-five from 50 percent to "access to" 100 percent, as well as reducing by two-thirds the number of undetected chromosome abnormalities—an "efficacy proven in outcomes."

What were these outcomes? Those listed on the firm's reports included the number of "induced losses" of pregnancies as well as the reasons for them, and the incidence of two dozen fetal abnormalities. Clearly, Genetrix offered to manage disease by encouraging the use of genetic tests and enhancing the odds that any unfavorable result of conception would not be born.

Whose disease is being "managed" in such programs—that of the patient, or the entire family? What would an insurer do with information that related to family members other than the patients? What are the implications when "managing" the disease involves detecting a predisposition to it before it has emerged—a predisposition that the patient may not want to know about? When the predisposition is discovered, precisely how is the patient "helped to decide" what to do about it? What if the patient's desires do not, in fact, lead to a cost savings for the health plan or the disease management firm—or in fact (as we have already considered) the public purse in general?

Genetrix may hold the claim to being the first genetics firm in disease management, but it is far from the only genetics laboratory to do so, and there are giants in that league. Molecular genetic testing "will initiate a major change in health-care delivery by shifting emphasis to disease prediction and prevention rather than post-symptomatic treatment," promises a document prepared for reporters by the pharmaceuticals firm SmithKline Beecham.

During the same year that Genetrix entered into managing genetic disease, SmithKline Beecham—which was investing heavily in Craig

Venter's effort to find and sequence genetic fragments—launched a new central DNA testing lab to work in concert with its well-established nationwide network of medical diagnostic centers.

"We've never had a specialty in genetics before," explained molecular geneticist Jean Amos, who had just joined the company after heading the DNA diagnostics lab at Boston University School of Medicine. "We want to regain our position of scientific leadership."

The firm Vysis, which promotes itself as offering "molecular disease management" by marketing DNA tests, put things somewhat differently. "Although the current market for ... 'research-use-only' chromosome detection systems, reagents, and imaging systems is still in its infancy, the mid- to long-term market potential for the company's products is huge," states a background document about the company. "The molecular disease management market is estimated to exceed $10 billion over the next decade. Key segments of this market are expected to include $6 billion for early disease detection, $2 billion for prenatal disease tests and $1 billion for disease predisposition tests. As the link between genetics and cancer grows, analysts estimate this market alone to be upwards of $800 million by the turn of the century."

"Theoretically there is no limit to the number of mutations we can identify," said Tony Shuber, manager of technology development at Integrated Genetics, describing a new technology he had developed which in a single test could pinpoint hundreds of patient DNA samples simultaneously for the presence of more than a hundred mutations. The firm, a subsidiary of Genzyme Corporation (which sells medications, such as growth factors developed using genetic technology), portrayed the new technique as a way to detect any one of scores of mutations that might affect a single gene. (A few years later there were thousands of DNA fragments on single chips, and the technology was being used to look for alterations in different genes that work together to cause complex medical problems such as mental illness.)

Integrated Genetics' first application of the technique would be to develop a program to test for disease predispositions, said its vice president for marketing, Ann Merrifield. In the parent company's annual report for the same year, 1994, however, Genzyme described another major goal: the development of a commercially viable method for separating and analyzing fetal cells in maternal blood. Would the firm be able to resist melding the two technologies?

Parallel to all of these developments, and vital to their ultimate success, is the trend toward integrating medical records into computerized databases. When a patient's record can be tracked from the doctor's office to the hospital and back, it will finally be possible for managed care plans to establish whether a treatment is truly effective.

Although the idea of linking all the medical records in an entire community is seductive from the public health point of view, it has proven very difficult to accomplish. One of the major barriers is that it's very expensive to retool all existing medical records systems so that they all speak the same language; another is simple mistrust. In general, people don't want their medical records officially centralized and available for scrutiny. This issue alone brought down a movement to reform the health care system in the state of Washington.

By the end of 1995, the model privacy legislation sponsored by the ELSI program had served to inspire lawmakers in some of the ten states to pass resolutions protecting the privacy of medical records. (The model was introduced intact into the Maryland legislature but did not pass.) By 1997 more than one hundred genetic privacy bills had been introduced into state legislatures, and at least fifteen states had enacted laws limiting the use of risk information gained from genetic testing of currently healthy individuals.

A number of medical privacy bills have been introduced into Congress, including one sponsored by Senator Robert Bennett, a Utah Republican, that was touted as a privacy bill but actually gave virtual carte blanche to a wide variety of people, including insurers, researchers, and public health officials, to use the information as long as their research proposal had passed a hospital review board. (The controversial bill never reached a vote.)

The privacy of medical records remains a hot issue in Congress, but that hardly guarantees a quick resolution. In late 1997, as she proposed new standards for medical records privacy, Health and Human Services Secretary Donna Shalala predicted that "this is the beginning of a long discussion with Congress."

The Kennedy-Kassebaum Health Insurance Portability and Accountability Act, passed in 1996 and intended primarily to allow employees to maintain their insurance coverage if they change jobs, mandates new genetic privacy legislation by August 1999. But it also has provisions mandating the creation of electronic medical records systems by the government and large corporations based on a "unique identifier"—a code number representing an individual. It has already been estimated that during an average hospital stay nearly eighty different people come in contact with paper medical records. In order to receive reimbursement from insurance companies, most people sign a blanket release allowing unspecified individuals access to information about their medical treatment and history. How much easier will it be for even more strangers to access medical records in electronic form?

While the 1996 law also mandates fines and imprisonment for anyone who violates the confidentiality of medical records, it does not prevent health care plans from increasing their premiums or excluding employees with certain conditions, as long as such an act is not targeted at a particular employee. It is difficult to imagine that such plans, and others with access to large numbers of electronic medical records, will not be able to use the information to their advantage.

An editorial in the Pittsburgh *Tribune-Review* called the provision about electronic medical records "the latest in a long line of chilling privacy invasions," pointing out that employers or insurers could easily examine medical information without a person's consent and reject him or her for "confidential reasons." Will the privacy legislation have teeth? Will businesses find ways to get around it?

Without a doubt, managed care plans *could* use genetic information in databases to the disadvantage of people with genetic predispositions to disease; the pertinent question is whether they *would*. But others could use the information too, and are very eager to gain access to it, implying a certain willingness to use it. Unable to gain access to patient databases from hospitals and insurers, for example, the pharmaceutical firms that want to market disease management programs have been buying up companies that own the databases themselves. The future is not in lab tests, one director of a national diagnostics firm confided privately. It's in information.

In 1995, for instance, SmithKline Beecham acquired a minority stake in a small company called Buckstel and HalfPenny, which specializes in creating networks of health information. The company had contracts to build a score of health information networks in the Atlantic states, and one of its patient-record systems was in use by four thousand physicians. SmithKline Beecham promoted the software to every physician who used its nationwide laboratory services. The following year the pharmaceutical giant Glaxo-Wellcome formed a $50 million joint venture with another informatics company, the Physician Computer Network.

Bearing all this in mind, it doesn't take much imagination to come up with a whole new spin on the push toward prevention. "Preventable illness accounts for about 70 percent of the burden of illness and the associated costs, according to some reports," said Carson Beadle, managing director of the benefits consultant William Mercer, in a special supplement to *Business and Health* in 1995. "Focusing on the needs of the 20 percent of us who use 80 percent of the services obviously will reduce the cost of health care."

GENETIC PROTECTION LAWS

Depending on how one defines *protection*, some thirty states have now enacted legislation to protect the public against discrimination based on information about their genes. These laws have come in two waves. The first, in the early 1970s, responded to the introduction (and frequent misinterpretation) of screening for sickle cell disease and Tay-Sachs carrier status. Many of the early laws made specific and limited references to these diseases.

The second wave, beginning in the early 1990s, reflected concern about the increase in genetic testing heralded by the Human Genome Project. The extent of the laws' coverage, and the rigor of their language, was patchy. Although they referred broadly to "genetic" conditions, many limited the information that insurers or employers could use to that gained from "genetic tests," thus allowing them to discriminate on the basis of biochemical tests that are not genetic, family history, and other kinds of information. Life and disability insurance were often omitted from the protections.

Attention to these issues is growing. In the first half of 1997 alone, nine states enacted new legislation against gene-based discrimination (Alabama, Arizona, Connecticut, Florida, Illinois, Indiana, Oklahoma, Tennessee, and Texas). A law passed in New Jersey in 1996 was hailed as a model, because it extended "genetic testing" to "genetic information" as the focus of protection and extended some of the limits it imposed to employers and life insurance.

The clamor for genetic protection at the federal level as well is ever louder. The Health Insurance Portability and Accountability Act of

Prevention programs like Weight Watchers, stop-smoking campaigns, and "wellness programs" within large corporations are laudable
efforts. But prevention programs that involve genetic testing, especially
in a health plan trying to optimize costs by minimizing the need for
care, have another meaning.

"If you think about the future of nanotechnology and information

1996 (P.L. 104 – 191) was the first nationwide stab at the problem. It forbids employers to exclude people from group health plans, including
those self-funded by the employers, based on genetic information. But
health plans are allowed to limit the benefits or charge higher fees for
genetic conditions—as long as everyone with the same genetic type has
the same type of coverage.

No sooner did the legislation pass, however, than state insurance
commissioners discovered that individual companies were setting policies to get around it. A common evasion was to set much higher rates for
new policies written under the law—a blanket 35 percent surcharge was
common—especially for people deemed to have preexisting conditions.
For some individuals, said California Democratic representative Pete
Stark, the new federal law was "a hoax."

Moreover, the provisions of this law do not apply at all to the 40 million Americans who have no group health coverage. In early 1997 President Clinton weighed in with his own legislation, broadly based on two
bills sponsored by Republican senator Olympia Snowe of Maine and
Democratic representative Louise Slaughter of New York. Both would
extend similar protections, including nondisclosure of genetic information, to health insurance of all kinds.

The genetic privacy issue, oddly, rears its head within the Kennedy-
Kassebaum act, which encourages the creation of uniform nationwide
databases of genetic information. It also includes provisions meant to
create the corresponding privacy protections around those databases,
protections that must be in place by the end of the century. At the moment (according to an unscientific survey of attendees at a 1996 conference on electronic medical records), only 37 percent of health care
organizations have taken steps to preserve the confidentiality of electronic medical data, and another 42 percent are starting to work on it.

technology, and trying to use it to [achieve certain] ends, the kinds of issues that are only now beginning to percolate down to employers — we're going to see some very interesting wrinkles about how far employers can go, how much information they can have, what they can test for, and what they can demand from employees," says ethicist Philip Boyle of the Hastings Center, who has completed a survey of ethical issues facing executives in managed care. "We're going to have a set of choices we didn't have before."

The nightmarish image of managed care plans amassing detailed genetic information on thousands of people and using it to fine-tune medical and economic decisions may be about as likely as cloned Hitlers and Frankenstein monsters. In general, when managed care plans have played tricks to try to improve their economic situation, they have engaged in fraud on a relatively unsophisticated level, such as falsifying patient records to get larger fees from Medicare or having enrollment meetings on the top floors of buildings without elevators to discourage the infirm from joining up. How long will plans wait to discover and adopt the financial advantages they could gain from genetic testing? Are they already doing so? Who knows?

It's difficult to see who will advocate for health care consumers if they do. There is as yet no effective nationwide consumer movement that represents health-insurance beneficiaries the way, for example, Ralph Nader and Consumers Union keep the automobile industry on its toes. Medical consumer advocacy is most effective with regard to specific conditions, such as a physical disability or breast cancer, notes Indiana University attorney and health policy analyst Marc Rodwin, the author of *Medicine, Money and Morals: Physicians' Conflicts of Interest*. "Our system lacks strong institutions or groups that advocate more generally for medical consumers or that can serve subscribers within their own managed care organizations," he wrote in the journal *Health Affairs*. "The near absence of proposals to foster organized advocacy for consumers of managed care is striking."

Our traditional advocates, the doctors, are caught in a vise between their desire to help sick people and the pressure to contain costs that managed care imposes upon them. "What you're seeing over and over again," says Vincent Riccardi, a medical geneticist who has worked as a consultant for several companies in managed care, "is that doctors are couching medical decisions in terms of benefit decisions: 'I'd really like to give you this, but the plan won't cover it, so I won't.'

"What I see happening is the genetics people essentially caving in to what the managed care issues are," Riccardi adds. He points to a recent article in a journal for geneticists that urges them to respond to the crisis that managed care poses to their professional identity simply by learning all they can about the new system, in order to improve their own odds of success within it—and by hiring a new person specifically to handle the confusing jumble of claims from all of those different health plans. Not a word of the article advises them how to deal with the new conflicts of interest they may confront by having to weigh their own interests, the insurer's, and the patient's.

Riccardi now runs a for-profit company called American Medical Consumers, which represents and advises people involved in disputes with their health plans. Doctors need to challenge insurance companies, he continues, and perhaps genetics is the place to start. "We need to stand up to insurance companies and say, 'Hey, you can't do that!'"

Genetic discrimination is the kind of compelling issue that energizes people, says Francis Collins. "They say, 'What? This can happen in this country? People can have this information used against them? That's not right!" Because the argument has "such a strong moral underpinning," he adds, "virtually everybody except the insurance industry agrees: We have to fix this."

Meanwhile, physicians on the front line providing genetic services report that managed care has not embraced genetic services with particular enthusiasm, especially when it comes to providing care for those situations in which affected children have already been born. "The characteristically unique quality of the team approach to comprehensive genetic services is seriously threatened by managed care," says human geneticist Maimon Cohen of the University of Maryland, since health plans may see integrating laboratories, doctors, genetic counselors, and social services as inordinately expensive, involving as they do a variety of subspecialists.

At the very least, managed care plans have a tendency to parcel out different types of care to the least expensive providers, regardless of location. This tendency is especially notable for laboratory services and can lead to considerable inconvenience for patients as well as disruptions in care. Thus, for families with children who have birth defects, managed care may actually represent a de facto barrier to effective disease management, because managed care plans often fail to link or even to provide the necessary care.

What could happen to genetics under managed care may be foreshadowed by the experience of the state of Tennessee, which gave over health care for its medically indigent population to eighteen managed care organizations when it established its state-run TennCare program in 1994. The program had a notoriously disorganized birth, because the state established it after only eight months of planning, deciding to iron out problems as they arose. Obviously genetics programs were not the only medical services affected by the tumult, but the particular tribulations of genetics patients and their providers are instructive.

Genetics services (and the attendant care for the handicapped that had always been provided under the state-run genetics clinics) had previously been offered to any Tennessee citizen who had or was at risk of having a genetic disorder, regardless of ability to pay. Under TennCare these services suffered serious disruption. The greatest casualty in the state-run genetics units was time: time for phone calls between clients and health care personnel, time for counseling, the time required to make (and obtain) approval for referrals (which had never been necessary before).

Many of the state's earlier guidelines about genetics services, which clinic personnel were required to uphold, were in direct conflict with the policies of the managed care organizations. Furthermore, friction arose between the primary care doctors, who were now required to act as "gatekeepers" controlling access to the genetics specialists, and the specialists themselves. Often the result was a disruption in continued care for children with chronic hereditary conditions such as sickle cell disease.

States that are considering the adoption of managed care for their Medicaid patients need to "pay very close attention to the continued and adequate care for not only genetic patients but also for the children and clients who require chronic, specialized care," says Jewell Ward, M.D., professor of pediatrics at the University of Tennessee Center for Developmental Disabilities. Such advice might seem of interest only to welfare recipients, except that people who are found to be at risk of genetic disease are also at risk of being denied insurance coverage and becoming medically indigent. Will states interested in cutting costs heed Ward's concerns?

"When motives are mixed, financial considerations tend over time to displace other values," writes historian Diane Paul in her book, *Controlling Human Heredity*. "One clear lesson from the history of eugenics is this: What may be unthinkable when times are flush may come to seem only good common sense when they are not."

There are major differences between geneticists in 1990s America and the eugenicists of the past, especially the Nazi era. Ours is not a totalitarian regime. Today's geneticists have a much clearer idea of what they are doing and how to accomplish it. Most importantly, we are not proposing to actively do away with "nonessential" Americans. But thus far we are doing little in any organized fashion to provide them with decent medical care.

Diane Paul tries to discourage people from using the word *eugenics* in debates about modern medical care. She finds that it's a conversation-stopper: It defines geneticists as immoral by association, they reject the accusation irately, and the dialogue deteriorates.

"It's more productive, in my view," she says, "to ask, What are the failings or the problems with this policy? What's inappropriate about this kind of analysis? Should we stop using it, or should we modify it?"

What *are* the failings or problems with our policy? Taking a broad view, we have plenty to ponder.

On the environment side of the ledger, we deny poor women federal funds for abortion, yet we set strong limits on publicly funded child support—while neglecting to offer such women reasonable options for child care so that they can find jobs for which, in any case, we have not given them an adequate education or training. We fail to provide adequate public services for the legions of children who, for whatever reason, do not receive sufficient care from good parents, although we do provide them with increasing opportunities to attend prison. We still fail even to guarantee a substantial proportion of our nation's children—regardless of their genetic heritage—basic health care.

Meanwhile, we enthusiastically grant federal funds for research into the genetic precursors of mental retardation, mental illness, attention deficit disorder, and substance abuse. We continue to encourage the development of genetic tests for a wide variety of troublesome conditions, yet we often leave it to the medical profession, to business interests, or to sheer chance to determine the use of prenatal and predictive testing for such conditions. When today's infants are teenagers, will we have sophisticated molecular ways to predict which of them are more susceptible to "social problems"? And how do we intend to use that information?

We continue to dodge the haunting question of who should pay the high costs of health care for people who have hereditary problems or (by extrapolation) for those at genetic risk. As it stands, the people most in need of expensive care for a disease that has been dealt them by the genetic lottery may be the very ones who risk either catastrophic financial losses or poor medical care because of it.

Year after year we have been leaving such matters to the free market system. That is, after all, our national philosophy — much as the optimum health of the *Volk* was the national philosophy in another place at another time. Perhaps we will not leave it to the system much longer. It is heartening to see the president and legislators continue to press the issue of individual rights in the context of genetic testing — yet frustrating to see how slowly we gain progress in their interest.

As at the turn of the previous century, our society today is feeling overwhelmed by the cost of caring for those who cannot afford to care for themselves. High health care costs are only a part of this problem, albeit a large part. This time around, however, a mean-spirited attitude of laissez-faire has marked our thinking about the problem. We no longer bother to clothe self-interest or cost-cutting motives in grandiose language purporting high-minded motives such as trying to improve the human breeding stock.

That has always been the dark face of American opportunism, the attitude that those who do not succeed did not deserve to in the first place. Fin-de-siècle genetics merely provides us with a way to confirm it.

CHAPTER 16

Pandora's Box

Momma related times without end, and without any show of emotion,
how Uncle Willie had been dropped when he was three years old
by a woman who was minding him . . . She felt it necessary to
explain over and over again to those who knew the story by heart
that he wasn't "born that way."

— Maya Angelou
I Know Why the Caged Bird Sings, 1970

FROM THE OUTSET OF THE GENOME PROJECT, SOME
people have been claiming that it could offer solutions to major social
problems. In 1989 Daniel Koshland, the editor of *Science,* wrote an editorial strongly backing the project; among his major arguments in its
favor was the implication that mental illness and even homelessness
might have genetic roots, which gene research could help to resolve.

"The costs of illness, the difficult civil liberties problems they cause,
the pain to the individual," Koshland wrote, "all cry out for an early solution that involves prevention, not caretaking. To continue the current
warehousing or neglect of these people, many of whom are in the ranks
of the homeless, is the equivalent of providing iron lungs to polio victims at the expense of working on a vaccine."

Who could argue against improving on warehousing and neglect of
the indigent or mentally ill? If we found the genes that cause problems
such as mental illness, Koshland implied, then we could do something.
What that something might be, he did not specify. Nonetheless, for almost every kind of social distress, genetic researchers are now working
to find information that actually could be meaningful.

Name the social issue—someone is looking hard for its genetic un-
derpinnings. Not only alcoholism and drug addiction but also mental
illnesses (predominantly manic depression and schizophrenia), homosexuality, aggression and impulsivity, aspects of intelligence, and ethnicity—all have been the subject of research efforts in genetics in recent
years.

GENES AND SEXUALITY

Sexual preference: is it inborn or ingrained? In the early 1990s two studies seemed to point to an answer.

In 1993 Dean Hamer, a cancer biologist who had grown weary of studies in yeast and mice, published a startling report about genes involved in homosexual behavior. He had recruited forty pairs of openly homosexual brothers, took DNA samples, studied their family histories of sexual preference, and looked for patterns among the relatives. Noting that homosexuality seemed to pass most often along the mother's side of the family, Hamer focused on the X chromosome (which men get only from their mothers), and soon he found a linkage. Homosexual brothers tended to share the same genetic pattern from the same region at the tip of the X—although unrelated homosexuals did not all share the same pattern that the homosexuals showed, and heterosexuals did not have these patterns at all.

The study seemed to bolster an autopsy study published two years earlier, which had reported similarities in the brains of a small number of homosexual men that differed from such structures in brains of heterosexuals. Together, the two studies generated tremendous controversy. Were their methods valid or flawed? Would they create tolerance for homosexuality as an inborn trait, or instead lead to discrimination?

Hamer and the author of the autopsy study, Simon LeVay, wrote a joint report of their research in *Scientific American* in 1994. Hamer hired a writer to help him create an autobiography depicting his trials and triumphs in the search for a "gay gene."

Hamer has since switched his attention to the subject of genetics and impulsivity. Two researchers from the University of Western Ontario, trying to confirm Hamer's results, said they had found "not even a trend" in Hamer's support. They have yet to publish their study in the medical literature.

So is homosexuality nature or nurture? We're back at the beginning. Even the question—let alone the issues it raises—is unresolved.

A review of *The Reader's Guide to Periodical Literature* from 1976 to 1982, notes sociologist Troy Duster, shows a 231 percent increase in articles that attempted to explain the genetic bases for crime, mental illness, intelligence, and alcoholism. Between 1983 and 1988 articles that imputed a genetic basis to crime appeared more than four times as often as during the previous decade. This increase was an outgrowth of what researchers were finding, of course, but it was also a reflection of what they were choosing to look for — which is in turn a reflection of what our society was willing to pay them to do.

Take the enigmatic figure of David Wasserman, an attorney who works at the University of Maryland's School of Public Affairs. A slight and soft-spoken man with the demeanor of a philosopher, Wasserman has become personally identified with the most controversial aspect of the entire field of behavior genetics: proposed links between genes and crime.

On the eve of a hotly disputed conference that he had proposed and organized on that subject, Wasserman admitted that he was "still somewhat skeptical about research in this area" and went so far as to add: "I dread the idea of being identified as being in genetic research." Still, as he explained later, genetics "seemed one of the most promising areas to get funded."

One day in 1995 psychologist Irving Gottesman, a pioneer in the field of behavioral genetics, rose to open the controversial conference about genes and crime. After three years of delay and debate, it was finally going to take place. Wasserman had taken great care with the title he chose for the meeting: "The Meaning and Significance of Research on Genetics and Criminal Behavior."

The title was decidedly *not* "Genetic Factors in Crime: Findings, Uses, and Implications." That title had sent up red flags three years earlier, because it implied that there *were* known genetic factors in crime.

Back in 1992, goaded by outraged objections from critics in behavioral research and from black political leaders, the National Institutes of Health had summarily withdrawn a $78,000 grant to support the conference. Some people construed its name and the description of the conference in the brochure as implying that efforts to prove and address environmental causes for crime had failed, and that a link between genes and crime was now accepted.

The proposed conference was also doomed by association with activities going on in the federal government in 1992. The Bush administration had begun a million-dollar anticrime program called the

Violence Initiative, which was intended to identify and seek treatment for predispositions to crime. The initiative itself was controversial as social policy; the prospect of a conference addressing the genetic tools that an anticrime program might employ was too provocative for some people to ignore.

At a press conference announcing the government anticrime initiative, psychiatrist Frederic Goodwin, then director of the federal Alcohol, Drug Abuse and Mental Health Administration (an arm of the National Institutes of Health), stoked the flames with an incendiary remark. Goodwin quoted studies showing that roughly half of male monkeys in the wild die by violence. Male monkeys that are hyperaggressive tend also to be hypersexual, he observed, adding that there were interesting evolutionary implications. He went on to draw an analogy with "high impact inner city areas," adding "maybe it isn't just careless use of the word when people call certain areas of cities 'jungles.'"

This remark cost Goodwin his high-level job (he was demoted, interestingly, to the post of director of the National Institute of Mental Health, one of three institutes within the administration that he had previously headed). It also cast a further shadow over Wasserman's proposed conference. Whether or not they were related, press reports about the cancellation of the conference almost invariably alluded to Goodwin's remark as well.

"It's another way for a violent, racist society to say people's problems are their own fault, because they carry 'bad genes,'" charged psychiatrist Peter Breggin, a hotly outspoken critic of the use of medication to treat behavioral problems of all kinds and one of the chief opponents of the conference. Although Wasserman heatedly denied that anything about the conference linked genes and crime *to race* (in fact, several members of the review board that initially approved its funding were African-Americans), he later acknowledged that this was what people assumed.

"On a radio talk show," Wasserman pointed out, "the callers were about equally divided between whites who endorsed the conference because they always knew that 'those people' were predisposed to crime, and blacks who opposed the conference because they objected to being so destructively stereotyped."

If he wasn't already aware of them by that time, Wasserman quickly learned of the dangers inherent in linking genes to crime. "There will be considerable pressure to use those genes or markers for detecting criminal tendencies in young children and assessing dangerousness in convicted offenders," he acknowledged in early 1995.

By then, numerous sobering studies had hinted at a genetic basis for traits implicated in crime, such as aggression. One of the most controversial (the molecular geneticist involved was no longer talking to the press about it) had begun in 1978, when a woman stopped by the office of Dutch geneticist Han Brunner at University Hospital in Nijmegen, asking for his help. She said several men in her family were mentally retarded. Before having children, she told Brunner, she wanted a genetic test to see if she could avoid passing the problem on.

Looking closer, Brunner found that the men's basic problem wasn't actually mental retardation at all. What was common to some of them was a tendency so distressing that a male forebear had compiled family records about it decades earlier. One man in the family had raped his sister and then, confined in a mental institution, gone after a warden with a pitchfork. Another forced his sisters to undress at knifepoint, and still another angrily tried to run his boss down with a car. Altogether, Brunner reported later, fourteen men in the family exhibited some form of "aggressive" behavior such as arson or rape.

The fact that the family's behavior problems were confined only to some of its men strongly implied that, if genetics were involved, the explanation might lie within the X chromosome. Because women inherit two X chromosomes (one from each parent), but men get only one (their fathers contribute a Y instead, whereby they become boys rather than girls), men are uniquely at risk for genetic peculiarities that can be passed along on the X. (In the absence of a second X chromosome, an unmatched recessive gene can exert its effects to cause a disease. Color-blindness and hemophilia are well-known X-linked disorders.) Did some of the men in the Dutch family suffer from an unknown X-linked disease?

Brunner began run-of-the-mill genetic studies on the family, using some newfound markers on the X chromosome, and fairly quickly located a pattern that seemed to implicate a particular region of the chromosome, in the vicinity of the genes that underlie a system of enzymes known as monoamine oxidases, or MAOs. It was a tantalizing discovery.

In the brain the MAO enzymes act to break down neurotransmitters such as serotonin and dopamine. Acting together, these chemical messengers are signals for the "fight or flight" responses to stress. Studies of skin and urine samples from members of the Dutch family showed that affected males (and some of the women, presumed to have one of the putative genes because their sons were affected) showed biochemical abnormalities that hinted at a malfunction of one of the MAO enzymes. The consequence, presumably, would be a buildup of fight-or-flight signals in the brain. It was possible to conjure up all sorts of theories about the behavioral result.

Across the ocean in Boston, Xandra Breakefield of Harvard University, who had isolated two different MAO genes in 1988, was waiting to find a family with a pattern that suggested a mutation in that region of the genome, in order to provide some confirmation that her purely biochemical finding had a logical role in a known human brain function. After Brunner contacted her about the Dutch family, Breakefield ran tests on their cells and found what she had been waiting for: a single-point mutation—an exchange of one genetic molecular subunit, from cytosine to tyrosine—at the same location on the X chromosomes of all males in the family known to show the untoward behavior pattern.

Bracing themselves for the reaction, Brunner and Breakefield reported the finding at a genetics meeting and in a journal later that year. "These people have a metabolic defect," Breakefield told *Science*. "They also have difficulty handling stress and regulating their blood pressure. But it would be a mistake to assume a cause-and-effect relationship even in this kindred. We have shown an association, but not necessarily cause and effect."

The distinction was too subtle for the general press, which quickly reported on the discovery of an "aggression gene." Just as quickly, critics began to minimize the importance of the finding.

"I'm not sure what they've found means much of anything," remarked Robert T. M. Phillips, deputy medical director of the American Psychiatric Association, at the time of the Breakefield report. "I'm not sure we can make a quantum leap from what we know in one family. One has to understand the context of those behaviors and what they mean in that society."

In addition, microbiologist Jonathan Beckwith of MIT raised the specter of a massive screening program for MAO mutations aimed at finding babies destined to become aggressors. Beckwith himself was remembered as a key figure in a protest during the 1970s, which led to the demise of a Harvard study that had proposed to screen boy babies for an extra Y chromosome, XYY, rather than the normal XY.

The XYY genetic type had been linked to criminality because a high proportion of prison inmates appeared to possess it, but it was never clear whether the physical qualities that went with the genetic type—an odd, lanky appearance and sometimes mental retardation—might have caused environmental problems that contributed to the risk of crime. The Dutch study had never specified rigorously what it meant by *aggressive*, Beckwith pointed out, and a number of family members who had the mutation appeared to behave quite normally.

After several months on the firing line, Breakefield feared that the political ramifications of her finding might ultimately prevent her from pursuing it further. "This is something that could be a positive thing for society," she said wearily, pointing out that there might be relatively simple ways to address a MAO defect of the type she had helped to identify. "If it gets seen in the wrong way, people won't even be allowed to do research on this. . . . If people jump to conclusions before we get the data, we may never get the data."

Controversy may put an unpopular observation in the shadows for a while, but if there's something to be seen, someone will eventually perceive it. Although nothing further was heard of the unfortunate Dutch family, barely two years later, in June 1995, researchers in France stumbled on another piece of the same puzzle.

The researchers, at the Institut Curie in Orsay, were involved in something unrelated to aggression. They were testing a new gene therapy for AIDS treatment, which would involve inserting a gene for the antiviral substance interferon into the cells of AIDS patients. There was a possible hazard: if the gene kept churning interferon out forever, uninterrupted, it might cause harm—perhaps something just as bad as AIDS. The French team looked for the answer by inserting the gene for interferon into mice and waiting to see what happened.

What happened was that they inadvertently created what are known as "knockout mice": the inserted gene knocked out something else when it arrived in the cells. Completely by accident, in some of the mice the gene for interferon wedged its way into the middle of a MAO gene, causing abnormalities in the same enzyme that was implicated in the study of the Dutch family.

"The males had bite wounds all over their bodies," said Edward De-Maeyer, director of research at the institute, "whereas normal mice don't have such wounds and don't fight."

The French team added that their serendipitous discovery bolstered the idea that, whatever was causing "the particularly aggressive behavior of the few known human males" with a similar defect in their MAO gene, it was not social problems but "a more direct consequence" of the underlying biochemical deficiency. At this point, commented a researcher at the Marion Merrell Dow Research Institute in Cincinnati, using such MAO mutations for possible diagnosis of aggressive human behavior "is a reasonable expectation."

No one wanted to pursue the implications of that statement too openly. But some years earlier, before these revelations about MAO and aggression, German geneticist Benno Müller-Hill had foreseen the darker implications of such a finding. The author of an exhaustive book about abuses committed by German doctors in the Nazi era, he could easily see what social consequences might flow from the ability to detect a gene or genes that predisposed people to unacceptable behaviors.

"I have little faith in the notion that treatment of mental diseases will truly benefit from knowledge of the culprit genes and gene products," he wrote in the journal *Nature*. "But I have no doubt that diagnoses will flourish. Cheap tests will be developed which will allow everyone to be tested for the variants of genes determining psychiatric ailments or psychic qualities outside the doctor's office."

Will governments follow by endorsing the view that carriers of such genes are bad and inferior? Will they stress privacy and "cleverly" leave the selection to market forces, he asked, or will they "resort to legal measures to speed up the process of the 'physical disappearance of the unwanted'? And what will the geneticists themselves say? Perhaps they will simply be relieved to find that their own mental genotypes are 'healthy.' But will some of them propose ways to eliminate the 'bad' genes from others?"

That some ideas are so dangerous that we dare not entertain them was the implication behind the scuttling of the 1992 conference. Wasserman and the University of Maryland strenuously objected to this. Rejecting the "air of Greek tragedy—that he who touches the subject is doomed," Wasserman rewrote his grant application and changed the conference title, somewhat reworked the program and the list of scholars who would participate (by invitation only), and reapplied for funding. In the end he won a considerably larger grant—$133,000, this time from the Human Genome Project's ELSI program—and relocated the event to a remote retreat center in the woods an hour's drive from Washington and Baltimore, on an estuary east of Chesapeake Bay.

It's a lovely area, flat and spare, a place where sharecroppers' cabins still survive from the old plantation days. Beyond the lobby door stood groves of trees and then the distant bay. The only sounds were birds. It was remote from intrusion, certainly, but considering the subject at hand, the setting also conferred a certain sense of unreality. In such surroundings crime seemed hypothetical.

As Gottesman began his opening remarks, the atmosphere was quiet, even tranquil. Whatever Wasserman had said beforehand about Greek tragedy, the event certainly had its elements of theater.

In the first moments of the conference, Gottesman invoked the book of Genesis: "Of the tree of the knowledge of good and evil you shall not eat."

A pioneer in his discipline of behavioral genetics, Gottesman proceeded intrepidly, noting that numerous recent studies supported an association between various behaviors and hereditary factors. These included comparisons of behavior patterns or criminal records between identical twins, who can be presumed to have an identical set of genes, and fraternal twins, who share no more genes than other siblings. Gottesman showed tables from studies assessing whether people who were adopted as infants are more similar in their behavioral traits to their biological or their adoptive parents.

Always courtly and jovial, he peppered his remarks with caveats, starting with an appeal for consensus "that a resurgence of draconian efforts at social engineering and misequation of genetic influences as opposed to genetic cause are things we can deplore in unison." Keeping a smile fixed on his face throughout, he noted that there is no firm agreement as to what constitutes "crime," which can in diverse times and places include rape, murder, jaywalking, spitting on the sidewalk, and bringing 1.5 liters of Scotch into Dulles Airport from Heathrow.

Gottesman recited study after study supporting estimates that various antisocial behaviors—whatever the definition—are roughly 50 percent heritable. "Pooled studies from four countries support the heritability of adult criminality," he concluded.

After each presentation, Wasserman had scheduled time for dissenting remarks from individuals likely to have a contrasting point of view. The first to react to Gottesman was a neuroscientist from San Diego, Evan Balaban. Many events in the home environment or even the womb, he pointed out, could equally well explain the results Gottesman had just presented, without invoking genetics.

Internist Paul Billings followed, with comments more heated. A prominent activist against discrimination based on genetic testing, Billings retorted to Gottesman's stated assumption that everyone present would deplore such discrimination. "There is absolutely no consensus within the scientific or medical community about the properness of genetic discrimination," he asserted. "I can assure you

HERITABILITY

Press reports about genetics and behavior often refer to the claim that a trait is *heritable*. Popular reports sometimes use the term interchangeably with *inherited* and *hereditary*, and readers may infer that the word actually means "immutable" and "inescapable."

But that's not at all what scientists mean when they use the term, which has a precise scientific definition and a most indefinite implication. The controversy around the 1994 book *The Bell Curve*, and in fact most arguments about intelligence and race, arise around heritability. It's a dangerous word, easily misused and misunderstood.

Heritability is a fraction, a ratio. It is the proportion of the variance between the occurrence of a trait in a particular group in a particular environment that can be explained by genetic factors, set against the total variance between individuals in the group. A scientific study might conclude that, say, a preference for the color blue is 60 percent heritable among urban Americans. That would mean that 60 percent of this preference could be explained by genes, and the remainder by other causes.

However, even if a trait is 100 percent heritable, that hardly means it is unchangeable. Environmental factors can have a tremendous influence on completely hereditary traits. For instance, height is the most heritable of all human traits. Whether among Caucasian American males or starving North Korean males, it is 95 percent heritable. But environment still plays a part. Average height in the former group has increased noticeably in recent decades. Improve nutrition among North Koreans, and their average height might eventually surpass that of white American men.

By the same token, whatever the degree to which intelligence is heritable, environment may play a much more immediate role than genetics. Whatever differences in average IQ exist between American blacks and whites today, they might vanish quickly if differences in the educational environment disappeared.

that the insurance industry does not agree with Irv, and there is no consensus in society at large."

Billings observed that the conference was proceeding in the midst of a "public health campaign" directed against violence. The government's Centers for Disease Control, he noted, had recently declared violence to be within the realm of those health problems worthy of medical attention. In America's past, he pointed out, eugenic information had been used for public policy "which hurt people. How do we know that modern studies are not going to lead to that kind of outcome?"

The conference proceeded in the same vein through Friday evening and into Saturday morning: scholars in the genetics of behavior and experts in brain research quickly summarized the best evidence from their fields linking something familial to something antisocial, and others followed—some calmly and some not—with reasoned rebuttals.

"Because of the regularity of data on twins and adoptees, we infer that something is going on in the DNA," said University of Colorado geneticist Gregory Carey, "much like Gregor Mendel ended up deciding there was something in sweet peas in terms of what he called hereditary factors. This is simply a first step, as Mendel's was. Mendel never saw a gene."

Psychologist Andrew Futterman, taking his turn, asserted that researchers looking into the genetics of crime were trying to track a "moving target." Definitions of antisocial personality change time and again, he observed, not only from study to study but even in succeeding versions of the official diagnostic manuals created to define them. What is antisocial depends on what society is. Nobody today, Futterman said by way of example, would ever think of inquiring into the genetic roots of heresy. We don't consider it a behavior problem.

Later, geneticist David Comings of Duarte, California, recounted his exhaustive studies of attention deficit disorder in children, which is often accompanied by disruptive behaviors. If you compare the ADD scores of the most severely affected first, second, and third graders with those less affected, he said, you will find much later that there is a significant difference in the number who finish high school, get arrested, or wind up working as laborers. Any parent might look to educational or family problems as the link between crime and ADD. Comings turns to genes.

Comings has studied genetic markers tirelessly, most notably those involving the neurotransmitter dopamine, in families affected by ADD and other "antisocial" behaviors, including alcoholism. Twenty or thirty genes affect dopamine activity, he told the conference, and "people who have a certain number of these genes—maybe five, ten, or fifteen—form the pool from which children with ADD and conduct disorders are drawn."

Psychologist Adrian Raine of the University of Southern California recounted his search for biological factors common to boys who have run-ins with the law. Among other subjects, Raine had studied heart rates, electroencephalograms, and skin conductance measures (essentially lie-detector test results) among fifteen-year-old schoolboys in Britain, then followed up nine years later to see who had been convicted of a crime.

"Criminals-to-be have significantly lower resting heart rates and skin conductance," Raine said—adding the caveats that the tests were imperfect and that the same factors held true for some very respectable risk-takers such as bomb-disposal experts. "We cannot use any single measure to predict who's going to become a criminal," he added.

Whatever its troubled past, the secluded conference had all the hallmarks of an ordinary scientific meeting: Ladies and (mostly) gentlemen met in a quiet chamber where they discoursed politely. Dialogue was well ordered and mannerly. Points were made and counter points raised, slides flashed onto screens.

In some ways, granted, it was less insular than many other conferences. The participants approached the topic from widely different perspectives, using the tools of a range of academic disciplines. But as with most scholarly gatherings, they made a tacit agreement that they had come to discuss politely and to learn.

There were some gentle and even poignant moments. Adrian Raine acknowledged that he felt extremely hurt when people accused him of being a racist. "All our knowledge to date is based on whites," he declared. "We can make no substantive statements at all" about a possible biological basis for racial aspects of crime, "simply because there has been no such study to my knowledge."

A few minutes later, Andrew Futterman stood up and addressed Raine. "I haven't talked to you yet," he said kindly, "but I—I'd like to talk to you." People chuckled genially. "I don't think this issue of racism is meant as a personal thing. It's about policies being racist, and I think we should address that in this conference. It's not directed at you personally at all, or anybody. The direction is really with respect to policy,

RACE AND CRIME

One harsh truth, above all others, bedevils efforts to study race and crime in America: The justice system is tougher on blacks than on whites. Over and over the studies show that blacks are more likely to be arrested, convicted, imprisoned, and executed than whites suspected of the same crimes.

The statistics, which are mind-boggling, defy explanation by mere genetics. Almost four of ten black male Californians in their twenties are either in prison or on probation or parole. Blacks account for a mere 7 percent of the population of California.

Nationwide, a third of black men in their twenties are under the control of the justice system—up from a fourth five years ago. That's certainly too fast an increase to be explained by genetic factors. One recent survey in California found that under the new "three strikes" sentencing law, blacks were seventeen times as likely to be convicted as whites. Roughly half of all U.S. murder victims are black, yet 85 percent of executed murderers have killed a white person.

Social critics can use these raw statistics to argue that the entire social system is guilty of criminal behavior toward young black men. So if you're a researcher using arrests, convictions, or imprisonments to define *crime* in your genetic study (and how else should you define it?), you have no way to adjust for the possible effects of racism in the social system. It's no wonder the search for "criminal genes" is controversial.

because that's what history's about in some sense—how it gets used—and that's the fear."

There was an immediate rumble of applause. For all their disagreements, people were bonding.

Outside in the reception area, though, tempers were beginning to fray. "I'm sorry, I just can't tell you anything more," a staff member was saying on the telephone—and as she rang off, she overheard on the other end of the line: "The nerve!" Someone else was talking to a television cameraman: "Whatever you're going to do, you have to clear it with the police."

On the podium psychologist Martin Daly of McMaster University in Ontario was taking issue with a point someone had made about evolution, when he was interrupted mid-sentence. "You've really got to puzzle why creatures ever take life-threatening risks at all—" Daly was saying, at which point a door at the back swung open; fresh spring air burst in. So did a line of strangers. They were chanting: "Maryland conference, you can't hide! We know you're pushing *genocide*!" Some of them were waving red flags.

It soon emerged that these were members of the Progressive Labor Party, accompanied by representatives of Support Coalition International, a group of self-described "psychiatric survivors" who protest the use of psychiatric medications. Someone lifted the microphone off the podium.

"We're having our own conference!" she shouted. The intruders began to berate the conference participants about the use of medications for hyperactivity, about the devaluation of the Mexican peso, about unemployment and the poor quality of inner-city schools.

"Why don't you leave?" shouted someone from the audience. "Jobs yes! Racism no!" they chanted back. "Genetic conference has got to go!" If they meant that literally, though, they made no physical move to evict the participants.

By and large, the audience sat impassively. It was not clear what would happen. There was some nervous laughter. One conference participant did stand up and take a swing at a protester; but except for that, the protest remained as choreographed as the conference it was interrupting.

Occasionally a conference participant would try to argue back: Adrienne Asch, for instance, an ethicist at Wellesley College and an outspoken advocate for the disabled.

Asch stood up and lifted her head skyward, as she often does when speaking in public, as if to address the ceiling. Asch is blind.

"You don't know what the purpose of this conference is," she shouted, "and you're standing here trying to tell us not to have it!" For that moment, surely taken off guard by the very sight of her, the protesters were quiet. "There are a lot of people here who have many reservations about biological or genetic determinism," she went on.

"Then why hasn't it been an open forum?" someone retorted. "Why do you have to hide it in the backwoods?" And the chanting began anew.

As they doubtless intended, the protesters had swept into the calm oasis bringing with them all of the world outside. Outside, the president and Congress were engaged in an ongoing battle over how deeply to cut welfare benefits and Medicare insurance while trying to pass a tax cut. Outside, one in every three young black men was involved in some way with the criminal justice system, for reasons fair or foul. Outside—and far away from that room—were guns and drugs. Immediately outside also, by that time, were the police.

At length David Wasserman rose from his seat in the middle of the audience, red-faced and visibly shaking. It was difficult for him to make himself heard over the shouting—he is normally a soft-spoken man—but he managed. "Look!" he began. "There's a hell of a lot of people attending this conference who think the dangers of genetic research are as great in the long term as the dangers of atomic energy. Let the scientists confront their critics!"

Ironically, the demonstration had interrupted the conference just moments before it was scheduled to turn to the very issues the protesters were shouting about—including an unusual item still on the agenda: whether the agenda should exist at all. The demonstration had truncated an esoteric discourse near the end of a late-morning session. The most controversial dialogue was scheduled for that afternoon. If the protest had been orchestrated, it could have chosen no better moment for the interruption.

Wasserman—older and presumably wiser than three years earlier—was ready with a plan, and he put it into action. "You don't want to talk to us!" called out his University of Maryland colleague, Robert Wachbroit. "We're small potatoes. You want to talk to the media. Let us make a gift to you: a press conference."

Within minutes, the intruders and the interested were clustered in small groups on a lawn at the back. News helicopters hovered overhead. Most of the conference members strolled calmly to another building for lunch.

It was an opportune moment for six of the scheduled participants to launch a quiet protest of their own. They presented a manifesto they had prepared arguing that the conference they were attending should not have been held in the first place. There is no credible way to identify genetic determinants for subjective qualities such as "violent" and "aggressive," contended the signers, who included Futterman and Billings. Such a conference "can play upon and feed into racist stereotypes," they went on, and scientists must not provide academic respectability for "racist pseudoscience." Just because phenomena are biological, the statement added, does not mean they are caused by genes.

Furthermore, "at a time when many people face large cutbacks in pay, social services, health-care benefits, and educational opportunity, the emphasis on a genetic basis for crime scapegoats those who are most hard-hit by current economic conditions." Intellectual debates about the implications of biomedical research on people with so-called aggressive tendencies, they commented, seemed to resemble much earlier discussions about whether there were scientific grounds for slavery or the innate inferiority of some ethnic groups.

The manifesto presented, everyone had lunch and then went back to the conference room. The protesters had vanished, the skies were silent, and they went on to the next order of business. With the science (or "pseudoscience") behind them, the participants turned to the issues.

They heard some history of eugenics. They pondered long and hard whether there was even any point discussing the "heritability" of some human trait or other, since the term was designed for animal breeding and not for studies of free-living human populations. They noted that genetics may seem attractive to policymakers because it seems to hold out the promise of a "quick fix," and they generally concurred that they ought to be cautious—without deciding what that meant.

At the end of the day, what was most striking of all was how often the disputants actually had agreed with each other. Above all, they agreed—as most authorities in the field had long since acknowledged—that there is no point in arguing about whether genes or environment cause behavior, just as there is no point in arguing about whether a cake is really eggs or flour.

"For the last twenty years, I'd say most individuals in this area have cleaned up their act," declared Gottesman, "and we're well aware of correlations between genes and the environment, and various other components of variance. What we're dealing with here are shorthand descriptions that don't do justice to what's happened." No one stood up to argue with him.

No one argued either when behavioral geneticist Gregory Carey said researchers had "moved beyond" trying to decide what percentage of a trait is heritable—"and we are wasting valuable time talking about it." Historian Diane Paul came up with a telling illustration of why heritability is irrelevant: because it may reveal nothing at all about genetics. A generation ago, she pointed out, wearing an earring was a gender-linked trait in American culture. Today it's not. The heritability has changed dramatically, but all the explanations worth talking about are environmental.

Curiously, the meeting that began as a Pandora's box closed the next day, by putting everything back where it started. The criminologist among them, Diana Fishbein of the U.S. Justice Department, opened her remarks by observing that the reason people don't pay much attention to successful programs like Head Start is because they don't seem "very sexy." People "find genetics much easier to write about," she said. In the end, she barely alluded to genes at all.

"I do have a very idealistic part of me that wants to help people improve their quality of life," she went on. "I think this research highlights the importance of environment. I think what we can do is attempt to create an environment that is sensitive to the human condition and to our basic human needs, and I hope that is where this research will lead us."

Although she set as her top priority "establishing the incidence of biological disorders in offenders," Fishbein stressed that "measures of biological function may or may not be expressions of gene function" and that much more research was needed to identify what these factors are. (You can cause serious brain damage, as someone had noted earlier, by shaking a small child.)

Researchers had yet to prove that behavior could be manipulated by "biological controls," she added. "The research we have now shows that a combination of [environmental approaches] works best. At this point in time, only the privileged have access to this kind of treatment. The underclass do not and unfortunately are relegated to the criminal justice system." The woman whom most listeners had expected to be touting genetic tests for markers of crime ended her remarks by calling for better prenatal clinics and social services.

After all the shouting was over, and the well-mannered discourse as well, Adrian Raine sat in the next building eating a leisurely lunch. What had he, one of the most prolific authors of studies trying to predict criminal behavior (and the frequent target of antiracist sentiment), gained from the conference?

"I'll be more careful in the terminology I use," he said. "I'll be more careful in dealing with the press. And I really gained a lot from hearing the history of eugenics. I always used to think the science was shoddy back then, and that we've moved so far now we don't need to worry about it. But the speakers yesterday showed that was not true. They [the early eugenicists] were not as naive as I thought. We do have to pay attention to the concern about the uses of our research in society."

It had also helped, he added, to learn that many of the people who had concerns about his research were rational and earnest—not just ideologues, as Raine put it, but "sensible people."

Would the man who had tested children's hearts and brain waves and then watched to see whether they fell into crime as they got older change his line of research? No, he said. "I still feel very strongly that it can be beneficial. We need to beware, and take responsibility for our research—but we also need to take responsibility for the interests of the victims of crime." Just suppose, he said, that gene research leads to some treatment that *does* prevent aggression?

Clearly in two days the parties had come no closer to resolving their fundamental disagreement: Is research that seems to link crime to genes moral or immoral? Reflecting on the conference much later, Wasserman himself decided that the participants' differences were too "profound" to be reconciled.

Critics of research into genes and crime see an insurmountable problem in the fact that *crime* is poorly defined and dependent on social factors, he observed. But researchers merely see this as a challenge. Critics expect genetic effects to be slight; researchers see them as complex and interesting. Critics find the term *heritability* misleading and meaningless; researchers are willing to downplay the heritability of behavioral factors because it has served its purpose in defining the problem at hand. Thus, although they could converse politely, the two sides were talking past each other.

Nonetheless, the research continues. It is likely, as Wasserman notes, that we will "discover markers and genes that are loosely associated with [antisocial] behavior. That discovery will be highly susceptible to abuse by agencies of social control, from school to parole boards, because those markers and genes will be easy to detect and tempting to employ in programs of screening and preemptive intervention."

His conclusion reveals the obvious reason why the conference participants could not resolve the real issues behind the Wasserman conference. These are not really matters for scientists to address. They are ours.

CHAPTER 17

Traces

Cultural influences have set up the assumptions about the mind, the
body, and the universe with which we begin; pose the questions we ask;
influence the facts we seek; determine the interpretations we give these
facts; and direct our reaction to these interpretations and conclusions.

— Swedish sociologist Gunnar Myrdal, 1944

WHAT SHOULD WE MAKE OF THIS PHOTOGRAPH, REPRO-
duced in *Scientific American* in 1991? A white man sits at a table, smiling broadly. Lying across the table in front of him are the instruments
for bloodletting and also an arm, with a tourniquet above the elbow.

Sitting to his left is the woman who has extended that arm. She is
barechested and wears ornamental bands across her forehead and rib
cage. She stares toward space off camera, away from her arm.

Is she passive? Pensive? Resigned? Is her expression any different
from what mine or yours would be—a glance away when someone is
drawing blood?

Because of who she is, and because of what people can read into the
photograph, this question is not trivial. "Genetic sample is taken from
a member of the Aka tribe of African Pygmies by the author," reads the
caption.

The impact of genetic progress on our own culture, clearly, is complex and often troubling. When we propose to take genetic samples
from people in other cultures, the questions deepen. Michael Kaback
and Josef Ekstein faced them, to a degree, when they became involved
in offering Tay-Sachs testing to the Jewish community—seeking information that would sometimes prove unpleasant for the donor. Both succeeded by finding a way to introduce it from within.

This approach may not be possible, however, when the other culture
is so remote from ours that terms like *gene* and *molecule* can have no
meaning to its members. The population geneticists who seek genetic

samples from native or indigenous populations are after information
that is basically neutral to the donor himself or herself—the frequencies of blood types, for instance—but issues of autonomy and discrimination can still arise. If anything, they can be even more spiny.

Genetic research is "not a priority for indigenous peoples," said Debra
Harry, one of the native American Paiutes, speaking before the United
Nations Educational Scientific and Cultural Organization, UNESCO.
Not *their* priority, but *ours*. What then?

The man in the photograph, Luigi Luca Cavalli-Sforza, is a world-
renowned population geneticist who has carried out genetic studies on
African Pygmies for more than a decade. He speaks of those people with
obvious affection and admiration. "Many of them are very brave," he
writes in his 1995 book *The Great Human Diasporas*. "Some have made
important discoveries regarding animal behavior, and others have invented new medicines and hunting techniques. They have survived in-
finite dangers, trials, and hardships." At the moment the photographer
snapped the photograph, he says, he was smiling in anticipation that the
woman at his side would soon look at him for reassurance.

Cavalli-Sforza first learned about Pygmies as a child, when his father
took him to see a film about them. Later, when he resolved to try to
learn how they had retained their uniqueness through millennia of evolution, he recalled hearing that Pygmies were very fond of salt. Thus he
would give them salt, as well as soap, tobacco, and medicine, in exchange for samples of their blood.

He says that a far more important factor in gaining their confidence
was that he offered them what many local people did not: respect as individuals. His writings and his conversations on the topic reveal Cavalli-
Sforza as genuinely concerned about the Pygmies' own concerns.

"We are stealing their forest from around them because it suits us,"
he writes, "and we don't care in the slightest that we are destroying their
way of life without being able to offer them an alternative one; and if
we could, it would be infinitely worse than what they are losing."

In the early 1970s, when education professor Arthur Jensen of the
University of California at Berkeley was trying to prove that blacks are
intellectually inferior to whites (and proposed giving a $5,000 incentive
to any black woman who would agree to be sterilized), Cavalli-Sforza
appeared several times in public debates at Stanford, opposite Jensen's
chief ally, physicist William Shockley. The physicist tried to persuade
his audiences with a barrage of charts and statistics, Cavalli-Sforza recalls, but his ideas about the mechanisms of genetics were misguided.

"The idea of race in the human species serves no purpose," Cavalli-Sforza has written bluntly. "Every classification is equally arbitrary."

These hardly sound like the words and actions of a hardened and heartless imperialist. Cavalli-Sforza, however, had to endure being portrayed as a "planner of genocide" and a mercenary man, because he has proposed and promoted a project to survey genes among hundreds of isolated and endangered ethnic groups around the world. At one point fairly early in its troubled history, the proposed Human Genome Diversity Project took on a nickname that Cavalli-Sforza regards as beyond derisive: critics began calling it the "vampire project."

"You have to learn to avoid getting too angry," he remarked recently, "if you want to remain sane."

The original impulse for the proposal was pure scientific inquisitiveness, but there was an urgency to it. Cavalli-Sforza and his colleagues argued that the Human Genome Project was ignoring "a vanishing opportunity." Endangered ethnic groups "cry for immortalization," they wrote in the journal *Genomics*. The scientists wanted to extract blood or other cells from individuals of isolated populations around the world, so that they could preserve genetic information about them and analyze it by the exciting new techniques of molecular genetics or by any other new method that might arise in the future. The basis of the scientific interest was not the individuals themselves, but what the samples could reveal collectively about the evolutionary history and genetic relationships of different subgroups of the human population.

In addition to its failure to document vanishing population groups, the larger Human Genome Project was vulnerable to a serious charge of discrimination. In the effort to create the first reference gene sequence for the human race, almost every single human whose genes were under intense study was a white person of European origins, like most of the geneticists themselves. As a record of the human genome, the Human Genome Project was destined to be woefully incomplete. A human genome *diversity* project would fill in major gaps and (perhaps preeminent in the minds of those who proposed it) "make enormous leaps in our grasp of human origins, evolution, prehistory, and potential."

Five years after it was proposed, however, and as the Human Genome Project was rolling along at full force, the smaller but no less ambitious diversity project had stalled. There was some genetic-diversity work in Europe and a few countries elsewhere, but certainly no organized and centrally funded worldwide network of projects to create genetic profiles of specified indigenous groups. "We will not proceed," said Cavalli-Sforza, "until the ethical situation is completely cleared."

The motives of the diversity projects' founders have been impugned repeatedly. A British television documentary portrayed the project as a "genetic gold rush" and featured critics who used words such as "exploitation" and "colonialism." The critics of the diversity project had also targeted an unrelated biomedical experiment in Papua New Guinea, and were accusing the American scientist in charge of "stealing genes" (see "Who Owns the Hagahai Man?" on page 320).

Certainly in the United States—where the original land holdings of the indigenous population have shrunk dramatically over two centuries but the individual tribes have been deemed "a distinct political society, separate from others" by the Supreme Court and have been given by Congress local authority to set water-quality standards—the native population did not view with great favor the proposal that they donate their genes to scientists who are mostly of European ethnic origin for a study of genetic diversity.

Of all the clashes of values in the late twentieth century, in a world polarized across cultural and ideological lines, the debate over the diversity project was an archetype among political challenges. The geneticists, driven by a characteristic scientific curiosity about human origins that is shared by many nonscientists in the developed world, saw the concept of the project from a viewpoint that was bound to be inscrutable to the prospective subjects, the overwhelming majority of whom had never stepped outside their isolated villages. In retrospect, however distressing and unfortunate the controversy, perhaps it is not surprising that it arose.

At first the organizers promoted the project as a way to learn about human origins. Later, under fire as racists, they defended it as a campaign against racism.

"As a student from Berkeley in the 1960s, I'm actively concerned that if people with the right motives don't get involved [in comparative studies of genomes among different ethnic groups] it could go the same way as before," insisted Mary Claire King, who besides working on BRCA1 had a history of actually using genetics in service of human rights. (She had used genetic studies to help identify remains of the "disappeared" in Argentina.) "The more we learn that our diversity is a diversity of *in-*

dividuals," she insisted, "the better we will be able to use genetics as a weapon against racism."

In the last analysis, examining the motives of the researchers into human diversity is fruitless. What matters is what will be done with what they find. Is it possible to assure that someone who *is* racist will not use newfound knowledge about the genetic differences that do exist between ethnic groups—such as the high incidence of the BRCA1 gene or the gene behind Tay-Sachs disease among Ashkenazi Jews—as means to racist ends? Gene research may be new territory, but crafting the policies to prevent discrimination is the true frontier.

Furthermore, why should desert nomads or the remnants of hunter-gatherer societies care anything at all about how people in distant empires classify them, or have any sympathy for our reasons to want some of their blood, which many of them consider sacred? What's in it for them, really? The studies might help indigenous groups by drawing attention to their various plights. "The number of evils that have been perpetrated on them is incredible, and still continue now," says Cavalli-Sforza. But most of his rationales for the project are to the benefit of science. "Knowing about things is what matters," he says. "That in my view is the major benefit." A few moments later he adds another advantage: "I believe that it will generate an enormous number of questions, and it will also decrease conspicuously the cost of doing this type of work, which will make it much easier."

To judge from news reports about protests against the proposed Human Genetic Diversity Project, those few members of indigenous populations who grasped the nature of the project could see no good reason to make genetics much easier, or to help the rest of us fight racism, or to learn about our origins, or (as promised by the pharmaceutical companies who sometimes sponsor independent expeditions to remote areas) to create new medicines. Many of the medicines that might arise from study of their blood are irrelevant to the lives of people in those cultures. The proponents of the diversity project left themselves open to charges of exploitation because, at least initially, for all their lofty ideals about combating racism, their proposal was not directed at preventing the extinction of isolated populations themselves. It was intended only to document their genes.

"Our land, our culture, our sub-soil, our ideology, and our traditions have all been exploited," said Leonora Zalabata, a spokeswoman for the Arhuaco people of northern Colombia in the British documentary (referring to a study sponsored by a pharmaceutical company). "This could be another form of exploitation, only this time they are using us as raw materials."

Face to face Cavalli-Sforza himself, a gentle-mannered scientist who was born and raised in Italy, comes across as someone heartily opposed to all forms of exploitation, and genuinely fascinated with the origins of diversity (in the politically correct sense of the term). Those same fundamental questions about the human race seem to fascinate us all: Where did we begin? How did we come to be here?

Who isn't intrigued to read about a prehistoric human found mummified in ice, or about the ancient bones that give scientists a glimpse of the species that predated ours? How were they like us, and how were they different? Even a small child will ask: Who would I be if I had been born someone else? All of which leads to that most basic of questions: Who am I?

Which always carries with it another, less innocent inquiry: Who am I not? And there's the rub. As with the study of crime, a fascination with human evolution has kept Cavalli-Sforza on a path along the boundary of a social and moral thicket.

As a university student in Italy in the 1930s, Cavalli-Sforza could hardly have ignored the question of racial distinctions, because students of many origins mingled in the cloistered academic world while, outside, the forces of racism were gaining strength. "I began to wonder whether Europe really does contain all these different races after all," he writes in *The Great Human Diasporas*. "I decided to pinpoint the factors I relied on to identify nationality. Hair and eye color were of immediate help, of course, but other features were much more important: shoe shape, the style and color of clothes, and above all, haircut, all of which are entirely cultural." It was one of those early perceptions that helped shape his future.

At the same time, he was trying to decide which courses of study to pursue at the university. General biology in the 1930s seemed too vague and descriptive to answer the questions about human variation that intrigued him. It provided no hint of a way to understand the origins of variation — merely alternative ways to define it. "There was no detail for understanding what it is that distinguishes one human being from another," he recalls. "If you did a course like that and then you learned about genetics, you realized that there shouldn't be two subjects. There should be just one."

Two events steered the young Italian medical student in the direction of genetics: the discovery of a new book in the early 1940s (the first book ever written about the genetics of microbes) and a visit to an eminent geneticist in Germany in 1942. As a medical student, Cavalli-Sforza was exempt from military service. For a summer research project, he was using mice to try to measure the virulence of bacteria. The study was not proceeding well: it was difficult to obtain enough mice by buying them from local farmers, and he had run into some scientific difficulties.

The only person who could help, according to one of Cavalli-Sforza's professors, was a certain eminent scientist in Frankfurt, Germany, who was knowledgeable in both statistics and bacteriology. Cavalli-Sforza decided to seek a scholarship for a month-long visit to his laboratory. In the interim, another mentor—a professor nine years older who had befriended Cavalli-Sforza—said he would be going to Germany at the same time for a visit to the Russian geneticist Nikolai Timoféeff-Ressovsky, who was working at the Kaiser Wilhelm Institute in Berlin. He suggested that Cavalli-Sforza add a visit to Berlin before his month in Frankfurt, and Cavalli-Sforza did so. The visit to Timoféeff-Ressovsky changed his life.

The Russian scientist with the long name was interested in two subjects: population genetics and radiation biology. His passion was infectious, and with regard to the first of those two subjects, Cavalli-Sforza was stricken. "I really decided to go into genetics because of Timoféeff," he says, "because he was such an overwhelming personality. He was enthusiastic, warm and friendly, talkative."

The Russian scientist is an enigmatic figure, a man who unconcernedly expressed his disdain for the Nazis and whose own son, an avowed anti-Nazi, was captured and killed in prison. He was also an avid proponent of using science to discover what he called "weaknesses" in genes, the clues to origins of human variation.

"In humans in whom natural selection is less intensive (especially in civilized populations)," Timoféeff-Ressovsky wrote in 1933 in Verschuer's journal *Der Erbarzt*, "the conditions for the preservation and spread of strongly pathological qualities are even more favorable" than in animals. He went on to argue for the study of the geographic distribution of mutations, and was intent on studying the genetic effects of radiation and on estimating the spread of mutations through populations.

Cavalli-Sforza says he never worked directly with Timoféeff-Ressovsky; they just talked. But his stay in Germany gave Cavalli-Sforza a glimpse of what scientists could accomplish with sufficient support. His bacterial studies in Frankfurt the following month were a resounding success, in part because the professor there could supply him with hundreds of mice of a specified weight and gender from a central breeding facility. Cavalli-Sforza says he achieved more in a few months in Germany than in all the years previous. The month in Frankfurt produced three published papers about bacteriology in German, but after he finished medical school, Cavalli-Sforza shifted to population genetics.

Both the Russian and the Italian were captivated by the idea of tracing the ebb and flow of various genes in the course of human evolution. Timoféeff-Ressovsky was fascinated by one of the major forces in that current of evolution: mutations. Cavalli-Sforza focused on another: genetic drift, the role that chance plays in expanding or eradicating certain genetic types among isolated populations through inbreeding.

After the war he did postdoctoral research at Cambridge University and then returned to Italy to study human variation in earnest. He started with a set of isolated populations close at hand: the residents of remote villages in the hills above the Parma Valley in northern Italy. With a small grant from the Rockefeller Foundation and the assistance of a student who was a priest, Cavalli-Sforza began what he calls a "brute force" study during the 1950s, transcribing local church records to track marriages, births, and deaths. He also began to track how the frequencies of traits such as blood type varied from village to village.

The same motives took him to Africa in 1966, to study the last remnants of the hunter-gatherer Pygmies. They were of interest for two main reasons: because of their unusually short stature, and also because, in preserving the cultural remnants of an early phase of human history, they were perhaps closer to our genetic origins as well.

"They are hunter-gatherers, and hunting and gathering has been 99 percent of the way of living of humans," says Cavalli-Sforza. "Farming people take a really different way of life. It's necessary to settle down. . . . I thought that might have had some genetic consequences, so why don't we look at what it is that determines population structure, the way people form social units, how much the social units exchange genetically and so on. Ours was one of the first systematic studies of that."

Cavalli-Sforza has focused heavily on the related but distinct influence of culture and genetics on evolution, but he has also thought and written extensively about the contributions of environment to physical characteristics—forces such as those that lead to dark skin and short stature among the Pygmies. At the same time he has been a vociferous critic of attempts to link these obvious physical traits to the inheritance of intelligence.

The earliest attempts to track the inheritance of such traits led to a largely racist body of science in the late nineteenth and early twentieth centuries that purported to link qualities such as intelligence to physical features such as head size. This entire literature has been discredited, as Stephen Jay Gould describes in detail in his book *The Mismeasure of Man*.

Conclusions about evolution based on external characteristics are bound to be misleading, Cavalli-Sforza has argued, because none of the inherited differences that are visible to us, such as skin color and height, correlate with the inheritance of other kinds of variations. "We automatically assume that differences of similar magnitude [to skin color or height] exist below the surface, in the rest of our genetic makeup," he states. "This is simply not so; the remainder of our genetic makeup hardly differs at all."

The first humans were dark-skinned meat-eaters. Light skin developed, Cavalli-Sforza says, as humans spread to Europe and developed agriculture. Their diets began to rely more on grains, which, unlike meats, contain none of the essential vitamin D. They do, however, contain a precursor that is converted to vitamin D if exposed to sunlight through the skin. Only fair-skinned farmers could obtain enough vitamin D from a cereal-based diet. Thus fair skins were an adaptive advantage that evolved far from the equator. The Inuit people of Alaska are an exception that substantiates this theory: meat and fish are mainstays of their traditional diet, and even in northern latitudes their skins are dark.

Climate has molded body shape because of the influence of heat. Large bodies are advantageous in cold climates, because they have proportionally less surface area and lose less heat than leaner bodies. In hot climates it is preferable to be thinner, to have more body surface per unit volume.

Cranium size tends to correlate with body shape and size. Early in this century, when anthropologists tried to equate head size with intelligence and that in turn with various ethnic qualities, they overlooked this fact. Larger northern bodies would be expected to have larger skulls for physiological reasons alone.

When the blood groups were discovered in the late 1920s, scientists for the first time had an objective neutral quality to use in the study of human variation. Blood types are purely biochemical variations in a common blood protein, which did not seem to portend any *meaning-ful* difference in the way people behaved or functioned, lived or died (unless you transfused someone with the wrong type). You couldn't in-fer someone's blood type just by looking at him or her. Here perhaps was a bias-free way to study the flow of genes within populations.

Many studies immediately tried to use blood types as markers for var-ious human weaknesses, including criminality and mental illness. But Cavalli-Sforza was among the first to use variations in the inheritance of such "neutral" factors as clues to the migrations of human subpopu-lations. At one stage during the 1960s he feared that his chosen work would come to a dead end.

The problem was that there were not enough of these blood-protein variants, and not enough variability within each of them, to resolve ma-jor questions about the biohistorical relationships between groups of human beings. For instance, by what routes were the Americas popu-lated? Prehistorically, where did Europeans come from, and when? Ge-netics might have provided the answers, but it didn't—or not then.

In 1970 Cavalli-Sforza relocated to Stanford University, where ge-neticists in the biochemistry department were beginning to discover the molecular scissors that would revolutionize their field. Molecular meth-ods were emerging to analyze DNA. The variation among DNA frag-ments was rich almost beyond imagining. Suddenly it seemed that DNA would provide an almost limitless amount of neutral human vari-ation to be analyzed in the effort to trace the currents of individual pop-ulations within the river of human evolution.

Cavalli-Sforza quickly compared notes with others who were intent on using the new molecular tools to address questions about evolution. Among them was geneticist Kenneth Kidd of Yale University. Eventu-ally Kidd and Cavalli-Sforza collaborated on analyzing genetic diversity among some twenty-five aboriginal populations around the world.

In 1987, a team headed by Cavalli-Sforza and Kidd published their study, analyzing variations in the inheritance patterns of forty-seven DNA fragments among five populations in four continents: North Americans of European genetic origin, people born on mainland China but now living in San Francisco, Melanesians from the Solomon Islands, and two different groups of African Pygmies. The same genetic variations found in the Caucasians "almost always exist at reasonable frequencies in the Pygmy, Melanesian, and Chinese populations," they wrote, adding that "since these populations represent the three primary population groups . . . one could conclude that the usefulness of DNA [variants] found in Caucasoids . . . can be extended to all or most populations." In other words, the new tools being tested among people in the most technologically advanced countries would probably prove useful in studying anyone's genes anywhere.

Ironically, however, the populations of greatest interest to the study of human evolution were rapidly disappearing. The Yanomami of Brazil, for instance, were dying off at a rate of some 13 percent per year, felled by malaria and other diseases of the "outside" world. In addition, "isolated human populations are being rapidly merged with their neighbors," wrote Cavalli-Sforza and the four other geneticists in 1991, when they proposed the Human Genome Diversity Project, "destroying irrevocably the information needed to reconstruct our evolutionary history."

"We must act now to preserve our common heritage," they declared, calling for a concerted international effort to collect blood, hair, or tissue samples from "numerous" indigenous populations. Their appeal in the journal *Genomics* refers to twenty population groups in particular.

"How can we afford to ignore diversity and not study it when we have a chance?" argued molecular biologist Allan Wilson of the University of California at Berkeley. "It's an insult to a lot of people." What he did not appear to realize was that some people would see the proposal itself as an insult.

In a series of workshops beginning in 1992, Cavalli-Sforza, Wilson, Kidd, and others began to set plans for the project, proposing to seek funding from institutions such as the National Institutes of Health, the National Science Foundation, and the United Nations. The final plan was to draw blood from twenty-five individuals at each of at least four hundred sites. Among the chosen populations were the Yanomami of Brazil and Venezuela; the Hazda of Tanzania (who resemble the East Africans but speak a language of Bushmen from the south of Africa); and the Yukaghir reindeer hunters of Siberia, some of whose ancestors may have crossed the Bering Strait to populate the New World.

After the samples were drawn, they would be rushed to centralized labs, where they would be transformed into permanent cell lines at a cost of about five hundred dollars each. The idea was to collect hair and saliva from even more people, using these samples for quick analysis of DNA without immortalizing them in permanent cell lines. The total cost of the entire project was estimated at somewhere between $20 and $30 million over five years—a lot, on the face of it, but less than one percent of the budget for the larger Human Genome Project, of which they saw it as a part.

Just before the third planning workshop, Cavalli-Sforza and two geneticists working in Italy, Paolo Menozzi and Alberto Piazza, published a tantalizing hint of what could be accomplished. In a long article in *Science*, they showed detailed maps of human migrations, based on computer models drawn from existing genetic studies of human variations. The authors called it "genetic geography."

At first glance the maps look just like topographical maps. Rather than indicating elevations, their concentric rings represent genetic distance from an evolutionary source. Beginning with sites where a large difference exists between the frequency of certain gene fragments among separate populations, the concentric rings of genetic variation move apart, much like the ripples caused by a pebble dropped into a pond. Painstakingly comparing and overlapping these gradients, the authors created a genetic map of the world.

These maps are much different from the genome map based on molecular studies of DNA. This atlas results from mathematical modeling based on the gene frequencies compiled from thousands of different studies of untold numbers of family trees. It is not a chart of chromosomes but rather a topography of gene frequencies overlaid on the standard world map—a compendium of information about human genetic variability, based on the geographic distribution of genes around the world.

The work behind the atlas offers some fascinating insights into human cultures. The Lapps of Finland, the maps imply, were originally Siberian Asians, and they still diverge considerably from the Europeans who surround them. It is possible to infer the spread of the nomads who domesticated the horse from the steppes of Eurasia westward toward Europe and southward toward Iran and India.

It also points to the probability that the Basques of northern Spain are, as they themselves argue, unique among Europeans. They appear to be the nearest descendants of the ancient Cro-Magnon people, who left behind the legendary cave art of France and Spain. Genetically they are distinct from other Europeans, who appear to descend from later immigrants to the area.

On one level, revelations like these are intellectually satisfying. Politically, however, this particular one is unsettling, because it has the potential to bolster Basque claims for independence — or someone else's attempt to discriminate against them. It also shows how the study of genes, whatever the motives of the researchers, can be used to support political ends. As Troy Duster inquired at a UNESCO conference about genetic diversity, what could be gained from a genetic map that provides information about early migrations of Palestinians and Jews? The peril lies not so much in the researchers' motives as in the power of their findings.

In retrospect, the organizers of the Human Genome Diversity Project were almost endearingly naive. Although they paid lip service to the importance of culture in evolution, they seemed to ignore completely the divergent evolution of their own culture and those of their prospective subjects. Henry Greely, a Stanford University attorney and chair of the ethics group for the project's North American committee, later spoke of a "misperception among some participants that it would be easy to . . . create a wish list of interesting populations . . . and [the populations] would agree."

The proposed diversity project did not long escape the notice of a thriving and organized worldwide network that represents numerous indigenous ethnic groups. The existence of the network, however, had escaped the notice of the project's founders, who neglected to consult it.

In March 1993, the Rural Advancement Foundation International (RAFI), a Canadian group formed to protest the exploitation of plant species from developing countries, heard press reports about plans for the diversity project and sent out a warning on E-mail. Individual groups quickly fired off protests online.

The South and Meso-American Indian Information Center sent an E-mail message to Greely complaining that no one had consulted them about the diversity project, or even stated a mechanism by which they were to be consulted. The Onondaga nation of New York demanded that the project be halted. At its international meeting in December, the World Council of Indigenous Peoples unanimously denounced the project after a long and emotional debate. The $20 or $30 million, it argued, might be better spent on "healing and community development" for the endangered populations in question.

By that time some anthropologists had also begun to express disquiet. Alan Swedlund, head of anthropology at the University of Massachusetts, told the British magazine *New Scientist* that the project was "21st century technology applied to 19th century biology." Another outspoken critic was Yale University's Jonathan Marks, who addressed the

American Academy of Anthropology in 1994 with a talk that began as a history of eugenics and ended as a critique of the Human Genome Diversity Project. It was an important audience, because the cooperation and direct involvement of anthropologists were essential to the project's success.

Arguing that the project could never establish the genetic basis of anything without a systematic plan for identifying and recording the overt physical characteristics of each individual who donated DNA and linking these characteristics to the DNA, Marks lambasted the project as "lacking . . . a contemporary conception of human population or culture history." The "allocation of megabucks to open the veins of the indigenous peoples of the world," he added, was a "significant political act."

Anthropologists have their own history to atone for, Marks said, because not only did their European predecessors fail to avert eugenics, many of them actually abetted it. He implied that anthropologists now had the opportunity to make amends. The project "needs to reformulate itself at the most basic levels before it has the potential to be much more than an international scientific embarrassment as an anthropology project," he wrote in *Anthropology Newsletter* in April 1995.

The ethical controversy around the diversity project involved two separate issues: informed consent and rights of ownership. As to the first, ethicist George Annas of Boston University pointed out a dilemma that might be insoluble: Unless the individuals whose blood was being drawn understood the real reasons behind the effort—and it would be a daunting task to explain those reasons in any terms that, say, a Kalahari Bushman might comprehend—they would be giving blood without informed consent. But if the subjects really did understand, it was likely that many of them would refuse.

The other question focused on the ever-contentious issue of who owns the DNA in tissue banks and who has the right to profit from it, if it proves possible to learn something commercially useful by studying it. Over and over, from the outset, Cavalli-Sforza and others behind the project repeated that any profits that might be gained as a result of the diversity project would be shared with the ethnic group that donated the blood, and they set about to create legal mechanisms to ensure that it would.

Third world countries would profit in other ways too, Cavalli-Sforza pointed out in an impassioned address to UNESCO in 1994:

"One of the exciting aspects of the . . . project is that it offers all countries a unique opportunity to become involved in, and contribute to, the global human genome initiative by undertaking the collecting and typing of samples from their own region as well as other studies of local interest." The transfer of skills involved in the new genetic technology to third world scientists, he said, along with all the potential they held for medical science, would be "a major benefit" of the project. Above all, Cavalli-Sforza hoped that UNESCO would find a way to funnel work from the project directly to the countries involved, to provide them with involvement and expertise but also to protect the subjects from being exploited in the effort.

Establishing ethical rules was an important priority, Cavalli-Sforza added. He promised that the project would define clear rules for informed consent, give local groups a strong role in designing questions to be studied, and create a body to review ethical issues. He also vowed, yet again, that a "reasonable share" of any profits would return to the groups under study. Then he closed with a long and forceful argument that the project, far from being racist, would lay racial supremacy to rest.

"The truth is that there is no documented biological superiority of any race, however defined," he said, adding later that "humans thrive by remaining individually different from one another. In fact, the concept of race can hardly be given a scientific, careful definition."

A year later UNESCO held a conference to explore issues of genetics and diversity. A UNESCO committee on population genetics criticized the project's planners for failing to anticipate the objections of some indigenous populations to their intentions but noted that the project's planners had responded by producing "ethically sophisticated and detailed procedures for obtaining informed consent." Nonetheless, UNESCO declined to provide funding for the project.

The UNESCO conference participants also drafted a set of principles "on the human genome and human rights." Among other points, they declared that the applications of genetic research must be "regulated" to guard against any eugenic practice that runs counter to human dignity and human rights; that an individual cannot be reduced to genetic characteristics alone; and that everyone must respect whatever these characteristics are; and that the human genome contains "potentialities" that are expressed differently depending on the environment and other factors of an individual's circumstances such as education.

The Human Genome Diversity Project has not died, but it has not

WHO OWNS THE HAGAHAI MAN?

One morning in 1995 Carol Jenkins, a medical anthropologist working with the Papua New Guinea Institute of Medical Research, awoke to the rude news that she was being accused on the Internet of stealing genes from the Hagahai people, with whom she had worked for ten years. RAFI was campaigning online again. RAFI's members learned that researchers had applied for a patent on a cell line derived from a blood sample taken from one Hagahai man. Using words like "vampire," the release charged that "an indigenous man of the Hagahai people . . . ceased to own his own genetic material." While they were at it, the RAFI protesters again took a shot at the diversity project, accusing it of "bio-colonialism."

What the Hagahai man had actually ceased to own was a culture of cells derived from his blood, a viral preparation derived from the cell line, and three different tests to determine whether other blood had been infected by the virus. The research might well benefit these in-

yet come to be. There are pilot projects around the world — in various parts of Europe, in China, and even among native Americans. But these are not coordinated, as Cavalli-Sforza and the other planners had hoped. Nor will worldwide progress be as swift as they intended.

In a sense, to an armchair observer, the history of the Human Genome Diversity Project and all its related issues have echoes of an adventure story: it raises questions about the nature of human origins, the pattern of prehistoric migrations, and about who owns DNA from endangered populations. It has a little of Rudyard Kipling to it. But it also has elements of immediate relevance, because a great many of us (especially Americans) are descendants of indigenous populations of one sort or another. We just don't look at each other that way very often.

The obvious exception, of course, is the issue that divides us still: skin color. But at this moment in American history, who would dare to look closely at the genetic differences between "blacks" and "whites"? Her name is Georgia Dunston. She is a biologist and a professor at a

digenous people, because it might lead to a test for a cancer-causing virus that is common among them but quite rare in the rest of the world. As Stanford attorney Greely pointed out, the man could obviously continue to use his own DNA to operate his own body, or patent anything else he chose to patent from it—except that particular cell line.

The cell line was also interesting, and potentially profitable, because although some Hagahai are infected with a virus known to cause T-cell leukemia, they do not develop the blood cancer. Researchers at the National Institutes of Health who had derived the cell line and the tests had sought a patent, in part in order to clarify the rights of anyone who might want to develop a commercial test from the discovery.

"I think most people would agree that the rights of people in the Third World should be respected when biological discoveries of potential commercial benefit are made from biological samples of any kind," the director of the Papua New Guinea institute, Michael Alpers, told Science.

There will be no royalties in any case: largely because of the protests, the NIH withdrew the patent application in late 1996.

bastion of higher education for African-Americans, Howard University. Dunston is director of the immunogenetics laboratory, where she helps to match organ donors with transplant recipients. What would the racial hygienists of the early twentieth century have made of her?

Without a collection of genetic markers drawn from their own population, Dunston says, blacks will never benefit fully from the genetic revolution. Otherwise, "an aspect of our diversity is not going to be represented in a whole new area of medicine," she says. "It's very important. If we are going to be beneficiaries of what science is going to offer, we have to understand our own genetics." This is not a matter of mere scientific interest, however: for some blacks it can be a matter of life and death.

Like Cavalli-Sforza, when she was young Dunston was preoccupied with the origins of human differences. She focused not on hairstyles and clothing but on skin color. As a schoolchild she wondered why God had decided to make people different in the first place. If everyone were the same, she figured, we would have had a lot fewer problems.

Dunston's curiosity drove her first toward biology and then, like Cavalli-Sforza, toward genetics. Coming to the science a generation later than he did, she focused not on ABO blood types but on the issue that was hot when she was in graduate school in the 1970s: typing tissues for organ transplantation.

As in so many other aspects of medical care, organ transplantation is not as successful among African-Americans as among Caucasians. Rejection rates are much higher. This is discrimination at the cellular level: the panels of immunity reactants used for tissue typing, designed to avoid transplanting an organ that will be rejected, are derived largely from the majority population, Caucasian. Molecules are apolitical; their variability is not in itself discriminatory in any social sense. But it can prove fatal.

Survival rates after transplantation have improved considerably in the last decade, Dunston says, but it's still not uncommon to find tissue samples from a black person whose immune system would reject *every-thing*—meaning that no one has yet discovered a tissue type that matches theirs, so no one can identify a donor organ that their immune system would recognize and accept as "self."

The reason that matches cannot be found is because we don't know nearly enough about the variety of tissue types among African-Americans. The origins of human evolution lie in Africa; African populations have had more time to evolve variations than the rest of humanity; and Americans of African origin embody a rich genetic diversity unmatched among other ethnic groups and more or less unrecognized by current genetic research. Those who see all blacks as a homogeneous group are oblivious to how much they differ from one another genetically.

Moreover, even among the known tissue types, the number of possible combinations is almost astronomical, Dunston says, and it's difficult to find a match for anyone who doesn't have an identical twin. Like panels of reactants for tissue types, reference panels for genetic testing derive largely from whites of European origin. Because of this medical quandary, it is not at all racist in this sense to seek to learn how blacks differ genetically from other American ethnic groups. In fact, it might be racist *not* to inquire into the difference, because the result would be a continuing difference between Caucasians and African-Americans in the mortality rates for organ transplants and hereditary diseases.

"When it comes to genetics," Dunston said, "the reality is that Caucasians just cannot be a reference for African-Americans." As she spoke, she was on sabbatical from her job at Howard University and was working at a lab inside the National Center for Human Genome Research in Bethesda, Maryland. Laboriously, she was typing breast cancer genes in blood samples from black women — fully aware that what she found would not match the pattern among whites. Two genes had been identified that were associated strongly with breast cancer among members of that relatively homogeneous group, the Ashkenazim. How long would it take, she wondered, to find all the genes that contribute to breast cancer among black women?

"Africans are totally diverse in a way we're not aware of, because we haven't looked at all," said Dunston. She had proposed to look.

Even before the Human Genome Diversity Project emerged into public debate, Dunston had begun planning a smaller, more focused version, which she called G-RAP: Genomic Research in African-American Pedigrees. Like the diversity project, Dunston proposed to create a supplement to genomic databases that would include ethnic populations that were under-represented.

Dunston had to grapple with the same questions that the diversity project faced: Whose blood to draw? Where? How many samples? Originally she thought she would try to take a random sampling of American blacks, but bioanthropologist Fatimah Jackson of the University of Maryland, who had been studying the ethnohistory of African-Americans, came up with a far more compelling strategy. Jackson suggested turning the project around, organizing the sampling design around ethnohistory and ethnogeography by defining the populations for study based on their distinct origins in Africa.

Fortunately, information about the arrival of black families in early America is relatively complete, because slavery was an important business and record-keeping was extensive. Jackson and Dunston proposed using shipping records at the sites of importation to define the African origins of various groups of slaves, using courthouse records in eighteen southern and eastern states to trace their movements away from the seaports. The survey they had in mind would make *Roots* look positively trivial. They meant to follow the records search with interviews and profiles of some three hundred African-American families, tracing their ancestors back to distinct regions of Africa.

Dunston also began making contacts in Africa who might be able to provide blood samples to bolster the ethnic history. Through a cancer researcher at the National Institutes of Health, she met with researchers in Nigeria, Cameroon, Zimbabwe, and Benin. They were eager to be involved and went so far as to structure a contract about the arrangement. Researchers at a hospital in the Transkei area of South Africa offered to provide five hundred samples a year.

Dunston proposed to set up a center at Howard University to carry out the genotyping and maintain all the cell lines. A biostatistician offered to undertake the effort to keep all of the genetic information in a database. Administrators at the human genome center in Bethesda, however, declined her application for funds. G-RAP was simply peripheral to the interests of the established genome project, Dunston said she was told; it did not fit neatly into any of their priorities.

Given time, however, an important piece of the project did find a home. In the spring of 1997, Dunston won funding from her own university and from the National Human Genome Research Institute to carry out a collaborative study with scientists at hospitals in Ghana and Nigeria, searching for pairs of siblings who were both affected by adult-onset diabetes. Doctors there had expressed interest in being part of G-RAP and had maintained continuous contact with Dunston about its fate. They had their own compelling reasons to hope for progress. The new project would draw blood from up to four hundred pairs of siblings, and ship it to Howard and the U.S. genome institute for analysis.

The story of diabetes is of particular importance among West Africans and also among African-Americans, for whom the risk of the adult-onset form is far higher than for other American ethnic groups. Genetically, West Africans are far more homogeneous than African-Americans, and they are far less likely to be overweight (a major contributing factor to diabetes in the United States). A study of West African genes should hold important insights to the origins of adult-onset diabetes in both groups and would also hold out the prospect of earlier diagnosis and better treatment. Even white Americans might benefit, but that is not the goal at the moment.

While the ambitious megaexperiment known as the Human Genome Diversity Project was still facing roadblocks in several regions, including the United States where the proposal originated, doctors in West Africa began drawing blood for Georgia Dunston's lab. Here were the details that made the difference: West African teams had been directly involved from the outset. The project had compelling interest and clear promise to help people on both sides of the Atlantic. The originator could be seen as having an identity with the subjects. For once, all the elements are right, and the project may succeed.

This tale has a curiously fitting conclusion. In time, an indigenous need finally prompted the National Institutes of Health to start a broad-based genome diversity project of its own. As with Dunston's collaboration, the proposal arose as a way to meet a regional need. It just so happened that the region was as broad as the United States, the indigenous researchers were Americans, and the need was to address the tremendous variability within the American gene pool.

By the time these words appear in print, if the plan goes according to schedule, a small new genetic database will be in place at the Coriell Institute for Medical Research in Camden, N.J. Funded by the U.S. government, and mirroring the true diversity of the American population, its contents will be available to all researchers.

What ultimately drove this development, oddly, was not scientific curiosity or altruism, but the NIH's long-standing face-off with the biotechnology industry over patent rights to gene sequences. Sometime in late 1997, Francis Collins began to signal his alarm at the fact that many big university laboratories and private companies had been plunging eagerly into the business of amassing genome databases—leading to a knotty tangle of property rights over genome fragments.

Officials in other areas of the NIH who had a growing interest in applying gene research to their own needs shared Collins's concern. The disease-oriented institutes that focus on specific groups of illnesses—heart disease, diabetes, cancer, and so on—required information that reflects the genetic diversity of the entire American population in order to use genetic information in search of cures. But existing public-access genome databases, such as the one created by Merck at Washington University, focused overwhelmingly on genomes derived from European populations. They were no longer suitable for answering questions about the origins of diseases important to the entire American population.

As a result of these concerns, in January 1998 Collins's institute—the genome research arm of the NIH—announced that it would provide grants for scientists to amass cell lines and DNA samples from unrelated individual Americans. Never mind traveling to South America or Asia; the pertinent DNA samples would be found inside the United States. The NIH proposal specified that they should represent Americans of African, Mexican, Asian, and Native American ancestry as well as those of European origin (and it stated the corresponding proportions), in order to maximize the chances of discovering a broad range of variations within particular gene sequences. Although ethnic origin would be noted, links to individual donors would be "irreversibly broken," the proposal said, adding that "the intent of the sampling strategy is to improve the chances of discovering genetic variation, *not* to draw conclusions about relationships among populations."

Genetics provides us with novel ways to be racist, indeed. It also advances important reasons *not* to be racist. To benefit fully from what science has to offer, we have to understand our own genes—and we have to understand all of them.

CHAPTER 18

On Human Evolution

*As natural selection works solely by and for the good of each being,
all corporeal and mental endowments will tend to progress towards
perfection.*

— Charles Darwin, in *Origin of the Species*

WE MAY BE EXCUSED FOR FEELING SOME PRIDE,
Charles Darwin wrote in the final paragraph of his last great work, *The
Descent of Man*. We cannot take credit for natural selection; but
nonetheless, he asserted, we have "risen . . . to the very summit of the
organic scale." That we have risen so far through evolution (rather than
being created through divine power), he added, may give us "hope for
a still higher destiny in the distant future."

Those visionary words appeared in 1871. For two generations afterward, his followers held to that hope. Many of the evolutionists were
idealists, and some of them tried to help evolution along toward the goal
that they imputed to it.

More than a century later — in a world at once growing in population, shrinking through telecommunications, and still riven with brutal
territorial conflicts — it is appropriate to inquire whether we are indeed
"rising." Besides its implications for us as individuals, modern molecular genetics seems to confront us even more urgently with the question
that fascinated the early eugenicists: Where is evolution taking us? Is
there, in fact, anything wrong with helping it along, using information
we have gained from our own genome?

Actually, the initial premise contains several flaws. For a start, we are
not necessarily tending "upward." Darwin, like many religious, political, and social theorists of his time, took it for granted that evolution had
a purpose and direction, that it was biology's mechanism for "progress."

That assumption still underlies popular opinion about evolution, although mainstream biologists have abandoned it.

Several decades ago the eminent Australian immunologist McFarlane Burnet invited Darwin's grandson to dinner at a small dining club of scientists in Melbourne. Sir Charles Darwin (who was a physicist, not a naturalist like his famous ancestor) had published a book called *The Next Million Years,* in which he speculated about the future of the human species, given a long enough timespan for humans to evolve into something else.

The two scientists spent a warm and lively evening, Burnet recalls. As they were parting, Darwin congratulated him on the wine, then suddenly burst out with an unforgettable question. "Burnet," he said, "do you think that anything *good* will ever come out of it all?"

"The processes of evolution, including human evolution," Burnet wrote as he recounted this, "are not to be interpreted in terms of human values." Evolution is inherently neither good nor evil, in other words; it is simply there.

The epitome of today's objective posture toward evolution is the stance of geneticist Richard Dawkins, who argues that human beings and all other species are merely tools by which DNA makes more of itself. "The universe we observe," he writes, "has precisely the properties we should expect if there is, at bottom, no design, no purpose, no evil and no good, nothing but blind, pitiless indifference."

A feminist theologian, Sara Maitland, takes an entirely different view of the same nonplanned state of affairs. What seems like indifference to us, she says, is God's decision not to impose upon us a predetermined universe, but to leave creation open to creativity. "Randomness, like determinism, shapes how the world will be tomorrow," she writes, "but it does it quite differently. . . . Time is not just the unfolding, the reading off, of an already written text, a mere turning of the pages; it is an active, creative force that cannot, of its nature, be predicted.

"God has built risk in," she goes on, "has created things thus, so that, not merely at the moral and individual level but at the cosmic level, the creation can participate in its own creativity." Thus her God leaves us free to make of ourselves, and of our world, what we will.

Whichever philosophy you prefer — atheist or radical Creationist — one observation is inescapable: Evolution does respond to particular environments, and if any force is driving changes in the environment these days, it is we ourselves. We not only define progress, we either create it or confound it by our actions and our interactions with our surroundings. This idea is nothing new. What *is* new is our capacity to create or confound evolution directly, by manipulating human genes.

We used to refer to this as "genetic engineering." Writing on the subject in 1967, Nobel laureate Joshua Lederberg alluded to the imminent developments he foresaw for human genetics. He compared the public's "panicky reactions" to the prospect of genetic manipulation and "tampering" with nature to the uproar that greeted *The Descent of Man*.

"How would an ape-prophet's relatives," Lederberg asked, "have greeted his predictions about the upsets their species would soon experience?" It is worth noting that he referred to the evolution of that ape's species not as "progress," but as "upsets."

Darwin assumed that evolution was moving in a certain direction. The latter-day view is that it has been merely taking place, drifting — and in our own case, perhaps not even that. We do all we can to thwart the efforts of natural selection. As a matter of course, we protect our infants from major causes of death. We shield ourselves from the natural environment with Gore-Tex and Thinsulate, with mosquito repellent and sunscreen. We know how to adapt and survive, and we use our heads to do so. We have been doing this for many generations; indeed, that is one of the qualities that defines us as human.

Whatever improvements genetic research brings to medicine will only extend the reach of health care interventions that have already been common for more than a century. We have always done more than respond to our environment; ever since the advent of agriculture, if not even earlier, we have shaped it to our needs. Gene therapy defies natural selection, but so do air filters, central heating, and refrigeration. Long before we were able to identify specific genes, we were hamstringing natural selection by cleaning up municipal water supplies, improving waste disposal, and training doctors in antisepsis. In the industrialized world, natural selection hasn't had a chance for a long time.

We don't view our situation in terms of natural selection anymore. Certainly Merck, one of the world's most successful pharmaceutical firms, does not agonize overmuch about interfering with natural selection when it uses genome-based information from its open-access database to identify children at risk of diabetes.

Scientists involved in genome research don't tend to mention defeating natural selection as a motivation; they are more keen to talk about unlocking nature's secrets. For Merck, "with the new genetic markers, we should be able to very accurately identify people at risk and have the opportunity to intervene, either with a vaccine or with drug development," says the company's senior vice president for research, Thomas Caskey, M.D. Profits for the firm, health for the children: the state of the gene pool doesn't seem to enter into the equation.

Similarly, the stated goal of the massive Collaborative Study on the Genetics of Alcoholism (COGA) is not to try to eradicate the predisposition itself but to help those who have it. The objective is "learning how the disease develops," says psychiatrist Henri Begleiter of the State University of New York Health Science Center, coordinator of the COGA project. "Knowing the etiology should lead to some treatment," he continues. "That's the plan."

At the time of the two world wars, when geneticists were fretting about the gene pool, some of them contemplated the possibility that modern society was sowing the seeds of its own decline by preserving the lives of people with hereditary diseases, and therefore the genes that caused them. Upon reflection, most scientists who thought about it realized that if this effect did happen, it would happen so slowly as to be meaningless.

The practice of screening pregnant women for recessive diseases, for example, would actually have the effect of preserving the genes that cause the diseases. Without prenatal screening, many couples who have had a child with a severe disease such as Tay-Sachs would resolve never to bear any more children in order to avoid the risk of having another affected one. But few couples would abort a fetus that would be a carrier, simply to avoid transmitting the single recessive gene to a grandchild. Thus prenatal screening would actually select *for* the recessive gene, not against it.

In fact, it has been calculated that ultimately amniocentesis and abortion of fetuses affected with cystic fibrosis might actually *increase* the incidence of carriers of the CF gene by 50 percent, from fifty out of every thousand to seventy-five. But that would take fifty generations — about 1,500 years. What are the odds that in a millenium and a half, the medical problem of cystic fibrosis will be solved, or at least irrelevant? More than likely it will happen within only a matter of decades. It is debatable how long it may take to mold information from the genome into real and practical cures, but almost unquestionably it will happen more quickly than genetic diagnosis will produce any noticeable effects on the evolution of the entire human genome.

One important understanding that will emerge from the Human Genome Project is that everyone possesses a certain, if small, number of potentially lethal mutations. Often—as with diabetes, cancer, and heart disease—the medical profession labors valiantly to compensate for them, and often, with medical interventions, it renders these potentially lethal genes impotent. Plenty of "former lethals" are completely irrelevant these days, such as the genetic changes that took away our fur and those that made some of us nearsighted, or that took away some people's ability to digest milk as they matured to adulthood.

Conversely, genes that seem dreadfully deleterious to us now in their recessive form may have survived because in the past or in other parts of the world, they have conferred advantages as single copies. Thoughtful scientists do not dismiss this possibility, because it may prove significant in the future.

The classic example is the genetic variation that causes sickle cell anemia. Studies have shown that the same deformation of red blood cells that causes painful crises in sickle cell disease also limits the survival of the malaria parasite. Carriers who have one copy of the variant gene, and make some normal and some sickled cells, are far more likely to survive malaria than people who do not possess the variant gene at all.

This advantage may seem arcane to readers in the United States, where carriers of sickle cell genes are rarely at risk of malaria unless they travel to the third world. But it remains highly relevant in sub-Saharan Africa, whose population suffers 90 percent of the world's two million or more malaria deaths today, the vast bulk of them small children.

The Tay-Sachs gene may have persisted for similar reasons: because the carrier state conferred resistance to tuberculosis in the crowded Jewish ghettos of eastern Europe. Cystic fibrosis may be with us here and now because a single copy of the gene defended carriers against cholera in other times and places. We know about these once-unsuspected advantages only because we chanced to inquire.

Overall, "we are quite ignorant about the potential advantages in a rapidly changing environment of single copies of recessive genes," says geneticist Kurt Hirschhorn, arguing that by preserving the lives of people with hereditary diseases long enough for them to reproduce, we may actually gain an advantage.

Anyone with diabetes who survives to adulthood, Hirschhorn points out, has the potential to endow his or her genes to thousands of descendants. Imagine that a massive catastrophe at some point in the future wiped out worldwide supplies of insulin. No doubt all of those descendants who actually had diabetes would die, but the other descendants would live on—and so would their countless other genes, unrelated to diabetes, that have unknown survival benefit.

In diabetes, Hirschhorn chose an interesting example. As James Neel suggested in 1962, diabetes may have survived as a remnant of the time when all humans were hunter-gatherers. The disease is exceptionally common in some aboriginal groups today; perhaps the genetic variants involved are advantageous in times of famine, when it becomes necessary to be able to store starches and sugars in the body, just as a camel or a cactus can store water in the desert.

Thus the genes involved in diabetes are not inherently "good" or "bad." Their value depends on the context. Whether people with diabetes would be more likely to survive a worldwide famine we cannot now know, and we don't want to find out either. The far more urgent question is how to deal with the disorder it represents *now*, in the most effective manner that is feasible.

On the face of it, the long-term eugenic motive seems inconceivable these days. It is probably difficult for anyone today to contemplate *not* trying to save the lives of people with diabetes by medical means or any other, simply to eliminate it from our descendants' genomes. We are too familiar with the disorder, and we know and appreciate too many diabetic people, to contemplate eradicating or even sterilizing someone solely because they are diabetic.

Meanwhile, molecular genetics goes on detecting variations among us. It helps to remember that in many cases it is our environment and often simply our society that defines these variations as "disorders." Diabetes is a serious problem in the United States partly because the American diet contains so much sugar to metabolize. Hypercholesterolemia, an inherited disorder that causes dangerously high levels of blood cholesterol, can also be exacerbated by a typical American diet. But it's not much of a disability in cultures where people survive on a diet of boiled grains and rice, vegetables, and fruits.

Asthma poses one of the greatest public health problems for American children today, especially in inner-city environments that are rife with respiratory irritants—pollution from cars, cigarette smoke, and dust. The leavings of cockroaches present a special hazard. The children of nonsmokers in affluent families in rural Arizona, however, are not particularly at risk for asthma. A variant is "normal" only if it is "functional" (and abnormal only if it is dysfunctional), but in many cases it is the situation that defines the function.

Obviously Huntington's and Alzheimer's truly deserve the appellation *disease*. *Dis-ease*, in fact, seems far too benign for describing them, since these conditions represent inevitable derangements, true dysfunctions that cannot be ameliorated. But in many cases the definition of *dysfunction* is fluid, depending on how far the rest of us are willing to go to accommodate disabilities. Despite the slow deterioration in my eyesight as I age, I can still hold a job; my company's insurance policy will even help pay for eyeglasses.

Other employees, who have certain limitations in the resilience of their wrists that reduce the time they can spend working at a keyboard, are less "functional" than they would have been a decade ago. If a genetic variation underlies repetitive strike injuries, it would have been silent fifty years ago. These same people would be quite functional working on a farm. It is the environment, not the underlying biology, that has changed.

"The reality . . . is enormous genetic heterogeneity, with all of us harboring genes capable of expressing themselves as deleterious diseases and disorders," writes attorney and bioethicist Susan Wolf. ". . . We are all part of 'them.' The category of people whose genetic burdens can be labeled today is simply a function of what genetic mapping has occurred so far. The category will grow tomorrow."

The fact that we do not worry much about the gene pool these days, or that we work deliberately to defeat natural selection, does not, however, protect us from an affiliation with eugenics. Decisions about what constitutes a disorder, and how much we are willing to pay collectively to address the consequences of such decisions, are unavoidably eugenic in nature whenever they address a hereditary condition. To the extent that we attempt to address them using genetic information—and especially if we invoke implications that involve a whole population, or the cost to society of a particular ailment—we are inevitably practicing a form of eugenics. With every passing week and every new genetic discovery, the opportunities for doing this grow in number.

What is fascinating—and perhaps ultimately heartening—is the fact that discussion and deliberation on these issues is becoming as vigorous and visible as the research itself. Constant news attention to genetic discrimination may scare the public and irritate researchers, but it may also prod our representatives to formulate enlightened policy that allows the research to continue without causing harm to individuals—drawing us closer to the vision that has always impelled Francis Collins:

a world in which geneticists can be not just "bookies" but "fixers," as he puts it, using the results of genetic research to offer not merely predictions but cures.

H. J. Muller, perhaps the last prominent American geneticist to campaign actively for eugenics, did not focus on its potential to rid society of costly disease. Above all (like so many others), he hoped to improve humanity by optimizing our genes and thereby our character. Muller was a high-minded positive eugenicist if there ever was one, among the last true believers in the idea of using genetic manipulation wholesale to improve the genome. Not only was he not *amoral*, like most eugenicists he was a staunch moralist.

In the early 1960s Muller proposed the creation of a voluntary sperm bank, where people could choose fathers for their children. (He also hoped for ovum banks, but at the time that seemed impractical.) In his particular vision, people would select sperm donors according to what he felt were the truly important traits: health and intelligence, of course, but also such virtues as warmth of fellow feeling and intellectual and spiritual values.

People could bear a child derived from the union of "reproductive cells, one or both of which may have been derived from persons who exemplified the ideals of the foster parents," Muller suggested. He did not ever seriously ponder how one might measure warmth of fellow feeling and spiritual values — much less ensure that they were present in a particular sperm sample.

Inspired by Muller's ideas, a California millionaire established a sperm bank, the Repository for Germinal Choice, which is still in business today in Escondido, California. A few hundred children alive today were born to mothers who used its services to ensure that their own genes mingled with others that were, as the repository's founder, Robert Graham puts it, "top notch."

One single mother who bore a son through artificial insemination says she chose Graham's Repository because, with most other semen-donor programs, "all you're told is their race, religion, and that they were medical students who were paid twenty dollars per sample. . . . I felt my unborn child should be guaranteed the best genetic material possible."

The son who was born as a result of her efforts had an IQ of 170 at the age of five. In discussing her rationale for seeking out the blue-ribbon sperm bank, the mother does not mention hoping for a donor known to be empathic or good-natured, matters that would have weighed heavily on Muller's mind. In fact he dissociated himself from the facility when it became obvious that Graham wanted to focus on intelligence and not much else. (Its first donors were Nobel Prize-winners.) Muller's own intentions were nobler than that.

"With the shrinkage of the world, and the suicide that is being committed by war, if it does not murder us first," he wrote in *Man's Future Birthright*, "each man must ever more strongly identify himself with humanity in general."

Such idealism, which spans the whole world and all of the future, is rare among geneticists today. Perhaps they feel it's dangerous. A few years ago, when James Neel had their undivided attention en masse while giving a summary address at the annual meeting of the American Society of Human Genetics, he chided them for being "markedly silent" about the future of the gene pool—whether through fear of being labeled as eugenicists, or simply from their intense fascination with the molecular mechanics of the system.

He proceeded to lay out the near-term future of our species in this fashion: The earth's population is 5.7 billion, and we are rapidly using up its minerals, its water, and its other resources. By the year 2020 the population should reach about 8 billion. The kind of worldwide catastrophe Hirschhorn played with in his scenario about diabetics, Neel predicted, is between twenty-five and fifty years away.

"To most economists and politicians this seems comfortably distant. But to a geneticist one or two generations seems frighteningly close." Our children will live to see it. The Malthusian scenario that inspired the idea of natural selection is evidently just over the horizon.

"Some would say, let natural selection do its work," Neel went on. "Unfortunately, in the grossly aberrant environment we now live in, selection is not natural, it's manmade."

What, then, should geneticists do with the genome in the next century, once they have read it and translated it? Unlike their intellectual forebears of a generation or two back, the geneticists in his audience did not believe that evolution is thrusting upward. Should they have the hubris to nudge it in some direction?

"I propose we should leave the gene pool as it is," said Neel. It's "almost Kafkaesque," he went on, "to contemplate genetic therapy directed at genes whose role as part of our evolutionary birthright is still so poorly understood."

It's an old argument and one not often heard from an eminent geneticist: let's not mess with nature until we understand it better. But

Neel was not arguing about hubris in that address. He was arguing that once the genome is an open book, scientists will have far more important ways to devote their exertions. His tone was far more sober than idealistic.

Neel devoted most of his attention to "euphenics"—an old-fashioned term, as dated as eugenics, but with the opposite meaning: efforts to improve the environment.

An hour of exercise a day and avoiding obesity will eliminate 60 percent of diabetes, Neel said, far more effectively than gene therapy. As our romance with the genome loses its ardor, he said, we should turn to cultural—not genetic—engineering. For instance, he suggested, we should take a hard-nosed, scientific look at the matter of violence on television.

As the genome project culminates, "eugenic voices will be heard," Neel concluded. But they would be missing the point.

The philosophy that directed society in Darwin's day was progress. In ours, if anything, it is adjustment—to change, and to rapid and constant upheavals. Furthermore, by our insistence on networking, mingling, and relocating, we continue to frustrate any natural forces that might foster some directed biological human evolution. We have done so since the Stone Age, but the process is working much faster now that we have jet planes and the Internet.

In *Future Shock* Alvin Toffler pointed out that the rate of social change is accelerating. Humankind was now in about its eight hundredth sixty-two-year generation, he calculated, of which 650 have been spent in caves. Within one single generation, early in this century, agriculture lost its place as the dominant activity in human economy. Today it is industrial processes that are losing their dominance in our society, ceding their place to information technology. To adjust to this kind of rapid change, Toffler said, "we must be able to operate at a level of adaptability never before asked of human beings." At that pace of change, the adaptability required is not genetic at all. It is cultural.

A few moments pondering recent history makes the idea of directed efforts to improve the gene pool seem almost laughable. In the mid-1980s, when the seeds of the Human Genome Project were planted, no one could have foreseen the tumultuous political, economic, social, and technological changes that were to turn the world upside down within one brief decade.

At midcentury geneticists devoted a great deal of discussion to the threat of global nuclear war to the genome. Within only a few years, near the end of the century, that peril seems to have vanished from our collective thoughts altogether. Today our chief concerns about the future of our species focus more on global ozone depletion. There is still no worldwide or even national consensus on its origins and implications, let alone effective agreement about whether it is necessary or even feasible to do anything about it. In this context it is difficult, almost ridiculous, to imagine that human beings could mount concerted effort to improve the human genome in order to foster our success as a species. Could we ever reach collective agreement about the specific ways in which it needs to be "improved"?

Such agreement is not likely, because we hardly concur even about the meaning of success. People in European and American societies tend to equate success with economic prosperity, but population geneticist Cavalli-Sforza points out that there are other measures that we could easily use, such as happiness or cooperation. Having created scales to measure genetic distance between neighboring populations, he notes that no such scales exist to define cultural distance. He predicts that if the means existed to make the comparison, we would find that culture is far more complex than genetics.

One thousand years ago, for example, southern Scandinavia was inhabited by a race of exceptional navigators who were also fearsome warriors. The Vikings migrated to Scotland, Ireland, northern France, and Iceland, and they even reached America.

Today Scandinavians as a rule are mild-mannered and calm. As a culture, they are dedicated pacifists, and their political systems are models for communitywide sharing. Could this difference be explained by thirty generations of steady genetic change? "Cultural evolution," writes Cavalli-Sforza, "strikes me as a more convincing explanation."

As one of the world's preeminent evolutionists, Cavalli-Sforza has been trying to find ways to measure the influence of culture. In the early 1980s he and biologist Marcus Feldman carried out a study in which they surveyed college students about all sorts of factors, from their tastes in food and leisure activities to their religion and politics.

Many of these clearly cultural factors are just as "vertically transmissible" from parents to children as genes are, they found. Religion and tastes in food pass on particularly well, without any apparent genetic influence. Other factors, such as fashions in clothing, he says, are transmitted horizontally among unrelated peers. Still other factors, such as someone's birth order within a sibling group, can have definable effects on human nature for reasons that are purely cultural, not in the least genetic, and that arise by accident rather than by any kind of transmission — vertical, horizontal, or otherwise.

This entire line of reasoning makes a mockery of the idea that within our kind of society directed eugenics or even human cloning could go very far to create a specific kind of human being. As any parent knows, too many indefinable factors intervene between birth and maturity for genetic endowment to determine the nature of any individual, let alone a whole population.

The early human geneticists, by and large, did not attempt to separate the effects of culture and biology. In fact, they appeared to regard them as one and the same thing. For instance, when Count Joseph-Arthur de Gobineau (not actually a geneticist but an anthropologist who had a very strong influence on the early German eugenicists) argued in his essay *The Inequality of Human Races* that the Germans were the superior culture, he used their physical appearance to distinguish them from other Europeans but their cultural characteristics to define their success and superiority. The unstated assumption was that the inherited biological characteristics somehow endowed the desirable cultural qualities.

Gobineau's writings inspired Hitler to try to re-create a "pure" race, but it is obvious to geneticists today that the concept of a "pure" race is as corrupt scientifically as it is abhorrent morally. There never was a pure "Aryan" race, nor any other pure human ethnic group for that matter. There aren't even any genetically "pure" families. The only genetically pure populations are pairs of identical twins, purebred livestock, and laboratory animals. In general, by comparison with "wild types" or mongrels, purebred populations do not tend to be very robust.

Racists, like the poor, will probably always be with us. But if they want support for their fantasies, they will have to look elsewhere than genetics. If genetics leads us anywhere, it leads us not toward purity but toward a new understanding of variation. In a brief span of time, close scrutiny of the human genome has shown clearly how difficult it is to decide what is "normal" and what is a "mutation," what is relevant and what is meaningless.

Throughout history human beings have classified one another into contexts and categories for cultural reasons. Biology is oblivious to such pigeonholing, as the tissue-typing system makes clear. Many African Americans are much more similar genetically to whites than to other blacks, Georgia Dunston points out, whatever our eyes tell us about their skin tone. As the Human Genome Project proceeds, it will make folly of our cultural divisions and our centuries of obsession with race. It should subtly change our understanding of normal and abnormal, healthy and unhealthy.

The genome project "is going to totally disrupt some concepts we have," Dunston predicts. "Do you want to understand biology, or do you want to hold on to your concepts?"

We will find purpose neither in natural selection nor in the test tube,

LINGUISTIC SELECTION?

Language has had an undeniable impact on the development and adaptation of human societies (defining, in fact, our distinction from other primate species), yet languages themselves evolve and mutate. Cavalli-Sforza has done exhaustive and fascinating studies that show how linguistic evolution actually parallels human genetic evolution.

Linguistic changes over time can be tracked and portrayed as linguistic trees, which appear strikingly similar to evolutionary trees. The similarity is fact, not only appearance: the picture that linguistics provides of human migrations through prehistory and history is almost identical to the image of migrations provided by population genetics.

Cavalli-Sforza's gene map shows that the major clusters of human populations (Africans, Caucasoids, Northeast Asians/Amerindians, Southeast Asians, and New Guinean/Australians) correspond almost identically to linguistic groups. Where there are exceptions, there are good historical explanations. For instance, in genetic terms Tibetans resemble Northeast Asians, but the language they speak resembles the Sinotibetan group of dialects spoken in China. Chinese history holds that the Tibetans originated from pastoral nomads in the steppes north of China, which would explain their distinct genetic origins.

Language must have had a major impact on humans' ability to expand around the world, Cavalli-Sforza maintains, because "more efficient communication can improve foraging and hunting techniques, favor stronger social ties, and facilitate the spread of information useful for migratory movements."

Dunston thinks, but she also thinks purpose could be waiting for us elsewhere in the genome project. She is not referring to the kind of purpose most people expect to find in the genome, however. It's something much more surprising.

"There's something fundamental about the genome project, something about helping us to get beyond a certain point in our evolution," she said. "To get to that point, it's got to be done as a group. It's got to be done as a whole. We have to find a way of reconnecting, a way to get where we want to go." The genome project itself is a case study in cooperation.

Ironically, the field of genetics, since Charles Darwin first introduced us to the concept of evolution, has concerned itself with the opposite, Dunston points out: competition. The theory of evolution itself was inspired by eighteenth-century economist Thomas Malthus's gloomy projection that the growth rate of the human population would soon outpace its resources for survival. This led Darwin to his revolutionary and historic musings about the nature of competition for scarce resources. Over the subsequent century, the theory of evolution in turn led many others to inquire into the precise mechanisms by which reproductive success, and therefore natural selection, is achieved.

The upshot of all this inquiry is the Human Genome Project, an undertaking so vast and intricate that its proponents realized from the beginning that the only way it could succeed—the only way the scientists could make sense of all this information—would be not to compete but to collaborate. Dunston restates the deeper challenge underlying the genome project: "Do you want to see the puzzle? Do you want to get the answers you are being driven to ask?" If so, then scientists studying the genome have to learn to cooperate, to share information—as they have been doing, on the Internet and through other worldwide networks of collaborative research. Patent disputes notwithstanding, the breakneck pace of the genome endeavor has been more the result of worldwide sharing than of global competition.

A science that began as an inquiry into the nature of competition (red in tooth and claw), and later evolved into the brutish and erosive pseudoscience known as eugenics, emerges at the end of the century as an object lesson in cooperation. Cooperation is most important for the scientists involved, but a similar challenge faces the rest of society as it decides how to use the results of genome research. We can use them cooperatively and humanely, or we can use them for competitive advantage against each other, individually and collectively.

An old-school eugenicist might say that allowing the cognoscenti and those with the most resources to take the fullest advantage of genetic testing and gene therapy is simply enhancing the progress of natural selection, another example of the fittest surviving. But such a view presumes that by definition natural selection pits individuals and groups against each other, and that such niceties as working together toward a common goal are irrelevant and superfluous to evolution. That is a popular assumption today, and perhaps it is a logical one. But it is also limited and out of date.

An emerging theory in population biology today holds that cooperation and altruism are themselves forms of adaptation and may operate to influence natural selection at a between-groups (rather than an individual) level. Birds and small mammals, for example, endanger themselves by giving out warning calls in the presence of a predator. There are numerous other examples in nature of such apparently selfless behavior, which helps to preserve the group at the expense of an individual life. A recent line of research also attempts to correlate the characteristics of whole societies with their survival and adaptation, to inquire whether there are measures beyond population statistics that may indicate evolutionary success, and strategies beyond mere survival that may enhance it.

The sweet irony about the genome project is that it *could* represent part of our own evolution in an unanticipated way. In order to gain full advantage of a molecular knowledge of "ourselves," perhaps we must engage exactly those aspects of ourselves and our society that we do not associate with the actions of molecules: collaboration, coordination, a degree of genuine altruism.

For instance, we could begin to look at the potential of genome research in a less self-centered way—as James Neel urged in his address to the genetics conference. A few years earlier, in 1992, the French geneticist Jacques Cohen had begun working to establish an institute for genome research in the third world. It was no esoteric effort to uncover endangered human genomes. Rather, its first goal was to map the genome of the malaria parasite—which kills more people each year than the AIDS virus has killed in the last fifteen—and then to proceed to other parasites whose existence are real matters of life and death to Africans.

For a malaria genome initiative, Cohen estimated he would need some $5 million a year—a drop in the bucket compared to the funding for the Human Genome Project. He began by tossing a substantial sum into the bucket from Genethon, the central French gene-mapping institute, which he headed. Then he challenged the Americans to ante up as well.

At a conference in Dakar, Senegal, in January 1997, a major international collaborative effort in malaria research began to take shape, of which one of the first consequences is further support for a program to map the genome of the malaria virus. One of the strongest voices in support of the initiative has been NIH director Harold Varmus. Since Cohen's plea, the NIH has more than doubled its commitment to malaria research, from $11 million to $25 million.

"We shouldn't forget that we work for 25 percent of humanity," Cohen said at a press conference in 1992. (He meant for the wealthy nations, those people contributing their genomes to the genome project.) "Three-fourths of the world is starving, and we must do everything we can to help them."

Theologist Ronald Cole-Turner would concur. Christian ethics measures moral progress by the treatment given to the weakest and poorest in a community, he observes, and would channel an advance such as genome mapping so that it would primarily serve the needs of the weak, the sick, and the poor. A similar train of thought runs through most major religions.

By this standard, current trends in genetic technology run counter to the deepest moral heritage of developed societies. The first objects of the new genetic research were the rare diseases of children and adults in affluent Western nations, not the malaria that kills millions of destitute African children each year. Even within our own borders, we seem to be moving in the direction of using genetic advances either as "boutique medicine" for the wealthy, as "public health" initiatives designed to eliminate the sick and powerless, or else—at least in the American system, where health insurance is becoming a luxury limited to those who are either healthy, wealthy, or just plain lucky—as a means of discriminating against those who are ill, poor, or just plain unfortunate.

What is the future of gene testing in the United States? Many experts in the field of genetics—the head of research at a major pharmaceutical company, the medical director of a major gene-testing laboratory, a medical geneticist with a major managed care plan, the head of the genome project itself—declare either publicly or privately that the only solution to the conundrums posed by genetic testing here would be the establishment of a single-payer health care system: national health insurance. Only in such a system can the possibility of discrimination be eliminated. But how likely is it to be created in our lifetimes?

An astute observer of the turmoil in our health care system, policy analyst David Blumenthal, M.D., of Harvard University, argues that the only force that will bring a single payer system to fruition is a large nationwide constituency of ordinary people who feel that health care reform, "with all its attendant risks and uncertainties, is preferable to the status quo."

And the only force that can make *that* happen, he continues, is a situation in which the problems of our existing health care system "affect the personal lives of many voters." As more people are forced to learn that they are at genetic risk, a constituency motivated to change the situation may arise. In fact, this seems to be happening already. Several important national politicians, even the president, are now pushing the issue. Perhaps hidden inside the threat of widespread genetic testing is its own solution.

Futurist Clement Bezold, executive director of the Institute for Alternative Futures, boldly spelled out some visions of the future of American health care in his 1996 book *Future Care: Responding to the Demand for Change*. Bezold described four possible scenarios, in each of which genetic progress has a different impact. But one certain consequence of genetic testing is common to all of them: a shift toward forecasting and preventing illness. What happens to individuals as a result of this shift will depend on how it is managed.

In one scenario, things proceed much as they are going today. Providers of health care move ever more into forecasting and managing illness, using powerful tools such as DNA fingerprints that allow people to understand their own risks and promote their own well-being. But those tools are available only to the affluent. Those with adequate financial resources can fix most of their health problems. But widespread poverty persists and expands, while access to health care of any kind for the poor diminishes. The rich stay healthy, the poor cannot.

In the second scenario, federal and state governments eventually take over control of health care and ration its services. Universal access is given to a very limited range of medical care, paid for by a heavy tax that is levied on the expenditures of those rich enough to pay for additional services out of pocket. Again, by and large genetic services are available only to the affluent, except where there is a cost advantage to including these services rather than rationing them away.

The third scenario is brighter. Public policymakers, employers, and

consumer groups ally in an effort to solve the crushing problem of
health care costs and access by taking an active role in determining the
future course of the medical system. They pressure those who provide
care not only to control costs but to learn which treatments are effective and apply them sensibly. (Some moves are being made in this direction already. An entire government entity, the Agency for Health
Care Policy and Research, is devoted to promoting studies of the effectiveness of health care interventions, and in recent years a bevy of independent agencies such as the Foundation for Accountability and the
National Committee for Quality Assurance have emerged with a goal
of setting hard-nosed standards for the quality of medical care, to ensure
that providers supply care that is needed without forcing upon us interventions that are not.)

In this future world, public funding is adjusted to assure basic health
care for everyone. Meanwhile a thriving market emerges for a wide variety of treatments and care providers — including, no doubt, geneticists
and genetic counselors. Because of the diversity of the market, a wide
range of services are available for most consumers, who are thoroughly
informed about their own health. Sophisticated information systems exist to make it easy for them to manage much of their own care, if they
are motivated to make the effort.

Bezold's fourth and final scenario is brightest of all, because it foresees a society that has redefined the meaning of *health*, community
by community. Everyone involved in health care, from the employers
and government who buy its services to providers of all sorts, as well
as the consumers, joins in finding ways to integrate all aspects of quality of life — not just physical health but psychic balance, public safety,
and broad equality of opportunity — in order to improve the health of
entire communities, not just individuals.

In two minor examples, coalitions of hospitals and community
groups join in vital campaigns to control firearms and to encourage bicycle safety among children. Such public-spirited efforts are only sensible, for with health plans so large, they are a way to reduce spending
for emergency care.

This utopian vision, with its focus on community health, has something in common with the motives of the early eugenicists, because it
focuses on the welfare of a population and not on the health of individuals. In fact, many foundations and conferences in the United States
now focus on the same kinds of goals. But Bezold's final scenario sounds
inclusive, not exclusive, supported by the finest of motives and directed

toward improving the environment, not the genome. If only we could assure that the turmoil in our health care system would resolve itself as something like this scenario.

Bezold finds an irony in his studies: When people are surveyed about the scenarios, the one they prefer is the fourth, but the one they predict as most likely to happen is the first.

"The moral and existential gap for health care organizations . . . is that most organizations reinforce the present or the most likely scenario," he writes. ". . . They plan for that future. They make it more likely by not planning to create the future — the local health care system — they prefer."

Were consumers not part of the final scenario, it would be easy to feel distanced from these processes, or even helpless. But there is much we can do beyond merely watching genetic research as it evolves. We can inquire, of ourselves, of our doctors, and probably of other sources too, whether testing for any trait is necessary and what the likely consequences of gaining the information will be. The satisfaction of consumers (that is, patients) has been gaining importance in managed care as health plans seek to attract membership (and avoid censure). We can take courage and demand to know what is being covered or not, and why — and we can respond loudly if we do not like what we hear, or fail to hear.

The more often and the more strongly we voice our intentions about health care, the more likely the system will shape itself to our needs. Many health plans will go to a great distance to avoid lawsuits or negative publicity over coverage policies. Even the federal Health Care Financing Administration, which oversees Medicare, revamped its own policy about responding to complaints about coverage decisions, without waiting for the outcome of its legal appeal of the court decision that had ordered that change of policy. The lawsuit was brought by a Medicare beneficiary aggrieved about a coverage denial.

We can also hold our public policymakers responsible for protecting such basic rights as privacy of medical information and reasonable health care for the indigent. As the medical privacy legislation mandated by the 1996 Kennedy-Kassebaum law is drafted, for instance, our vigilance is needed to ensure that it is effective and is enforced. We could create care for the handicapped that is sufficient to reassure pregnant women that they need not desperately fear giving birth to an "imperfect" baby.

Collectively and individually, we can refuse to abandon efforts to manage the environment—social as well as natural—so that even the underprivileged, and especially their children, have the chance to make the best of what they are born with. Inadequate nutrition, stimulation, parental support, and education wreak far more havoc on the "quality" of human children than do all of the genetic mutations known to medical science.

We can also refuse to accept the assertion that any characteristic—especially one with social consequences, such as intelligence or aggression—is largely hereditary, unless that is proven rigorously. Even then, we can be vigilant in our responses to such information, as careful to encourage potential as we are to place limits and cast blame.

The German geneticist Benno Müller-Hill has spent some time musing about the most likely impact of genome research on the industrialized and information-rich parts of the world, setting aside the hype and the hyperbole. He does not deny that the Human Genome Project "will be truly enlightening about the molecular structure of the human body and brain," and that this knowledge alone is exciting enough to justify the program. But he also foresees the emergence of clubs for the "healthy" that will demand proof of "genetic fitness" for admission, as well as cheap tests that will allow everyone to learn about genetic variations underlying their psychiatric or psychic qualities, outside the doctor's office. Genetic racial injustice, he predicts, will be a fact.

"Progress may be painfully fast or slow," Müller-Hill wrote in the scientific journal *Nature*, "and will be full of contradictions. To master it demands firm values. At the extremes, people will have to choose between the values of the Nazis and those of Moses—that is, racism or an appreciation of equal human rights." We will need to be alert to the imminent potential for gene research to revive old and unwanted forms of discrimination in new guises, and always be prepared to contest them.

It would take many generations to trace a change in our genetic evolution resulting from gene research. But it is quite possible to chronicle how, within barely a single generation, genetic research has prompted a dramatic evolution in our attitudes and our social understanding.

"If we don't pay attention to history, we are likely to repeat it—and we are about to do so again with genetic screening," said geneticist Robert Murray of Howard University at a conference in May 1998. He was reminding an audience of public health officials about the regrettable history of sickle-cell screening in America. The meeting's sponsors included the National Human Genome Research Institute and the

U.S. Centers for Disease Control and Prevention (CDC), the nation's premier public health agency.

Murray had spoken often about sickle-cell screening—in fact, he is almost typecast in the role—but never more importantly than now. The purpose of that meeting was to herald the rebirth of an old and troubled partnership: public health and genetics.

The CDC's major tasks include surveillance and assessment for disease, as well as preventing the spread of transmissible illness. By the time of the meeting a new Office of Genetics and Disease Prevention existed within the agency, and the CDC had a major new grant for prevention in its budget, with an important focus on genetics.

On the face of it, there was good reason to be troubled by the fact that a major government prevention agency, and all those public health officials, were showing a keen interest in the tidal wave of new gene tests surging toward them. Do genetic diseases constitute an epidemic to be eradicated? That would appear to be so, unless you took a close look at the agenda.

Although there were plenty of sessions on ethical questions, nothing on the scheduled program focused on the cases usually held up as triumphs of genetics in public health: Tay-Sachs screening, for instance, or prenatal testing for AFP, or even the recent NIH consensus statement in favor of population screening for cystic fibrosis. Why is that, ethicist Eric Juengst inquired of the audience. "Aren't we interested in primary prevention—that is, preventing the spread of disease from one person to another?" Not anymore, he went on. Not when it comes to genetics. "I think behind this interesting programmatic agenda is a change of philosophy."

The acting director of the CDC's Office of Genetics, Muin Khoury, M.D., had already said as much. Over the previous year, in formulating its strategic plan for genetics, the agency had "made a paradigm shift," Khoury said, "a philosophical paradigm shift in CDC policy, toward what you call phenotypic testing."

In contrast to a genotype or genetic type, a phenotype is the clinical manifestation of the action of a gene. Thus, in medicine it may be a symptom or obvious physical sign that a certain genetic type is present: chest pain in heart attack, for instance, or dementia for Alzheimer's disease—or simply a blood or tissue type. In applying genetics to public health, the CDC had made a momentous decision: not to be involved in efforts to test the unborn for genetic disease, and not to search for disease genes in people who are currently healthy. There's plenty to use genetics for, after all, in people who already show signs of trouble: confirming diagnoses, targeting medications or other therapies, or studying which genetic types foreshadow especially strong reactions to environmental factors such as diet or pollutants, once a disease process has begun.

This policy directive was not a flash of insight from Khoury or a dictum from the top. It had evolved. A CDC task force reached the conclusion after considering the deliberations of numerous other panels mentioned in these pages, including the President's Bioethics Advisory Board, the panel that had advised restructuring ELSI, and the Genetic Testing Task Force, headed by Neil Holtzman.

Henceforth, the CDC would educate the public as to our options and risks in gene testing, and try to protect us whenever a disease reared its head, but it would not organize fishing expeditions simply to find and eradicate deleterious genes among individuals within the general American population. This policy came adorned with numerous underlying value statements, including a recognition of the importance of human diversity and of the need to balance individual interests with those of the population as a whole.

"Prevention carries many meanings," Khoury said. "Prevention is environmental most of the time. The role of the environment is going to be crucial in our prevention strategy." (By "environment" he meant the whole gamut of influences on health, not just pollutants, but also dietary and exercise habits, education, infectious disease history, life events, everything.)

To make his point, Khoury showed a slide defining the difference between genotypic and phenotypic prevention in public health. The former equates with averting undesirable reproduction—the transmission of certain genes from one generation to the next—and is associated with eugenics, he said. Phenotypic prevention equates with preventing disease, disability, and death. But never birth. It is not eugenics, but *euphenics*.

Eric Juengst, who is a professor of ethics and not a public health official, drew the distinction more bluntly: Phenotypic prevention assumes that the person being tested will survive the process, and does not equate the person with the disease or the genetic type with the disease. Genetic prevention, on the other hand, assumes that the patient is nothing more than the disease, that the disease is nothing more than the genetic type, and that all three need to disappear. This is just as true, by the way, for predictive genetic testing of adults by managed care plans or employers as for such testing of fetuses by public health plans—although the CDC has less influence on the former. It was also true of Hitler and Verschuer, of sterilization and the Final Solution.

There's nothing wrong with families making private reproductive decisions about what kinds of inheritance they can or cannot confront, Juengst went on (although he conceded later that society and even medical practice do have an influence on what people feel they can accept). "The error," he said, "comes when we shift to making it public policy."

Besides avoiding the taint of eugenics, the CDC has another good reason to disavow predictive testing. If the public fears genetic testing because of its risks, the agency will never be able to gain the information vital to understanding genetic variations as they emerge: differing responses to pollutants, for instance, or to medications or nutrients, or statistics about the varying importance of genetic subtypes in different ethnic populations, which could be critical to battling infectious epidemics such as AIDS.

Another part of the CDC's strategic plan (as the Genetic Testing Task Force had proposed) is to carry out quality assurance and effectiveness studies of new gene tests. Simple estimates of gene prevalence are critical to this effort, and they're not available yet. That information does not exist for most of the 100,000 genes soon to be identified. "We *should* have it," Khoury said, "and we'd better begin to have it."

There's a message for the rest of us outside that meeting room: Unless we find a way to trust gene testing in some fashion, at some level, we will nullify the work needed to make it safe and effective. At its best, gene testing can prove advantageous in helping us prevent illness once the gene becomes evident. It is in our interest to help assure its quality, as long as the testing is used responsibly.

That the major U.S. government agency responsible for prevention has taken the dramatic step of disavowing widespread mandatory predictive testing is both heartening and fascinating. But it does not protect us completely. Public health agencies, after all, do not govern managed care plans or control the activities of major employers. We will still need to press for better laws.

Nor is it enough to hope that a national health system will someday rescue us from the threat that managed care could bring to genetic testing. In centralized health care systems such as the British National Health Service, after all, geneticists are also asked to justify what they do in terms of cost-effectiveness. Bottom lines are bottom lines, whoever is paying the cost of health care. There are still very tough questions for our policymakers to address as they ponder gene research. How do we, as a society, want to spend our money in order to keep people healthy or even alive?

However, our society has taken an important first step to distance what we are undertaking now from the abuses of the past. Someone at the CDC meeting asked point-blank how the efforts of the new public health genetics will differ from the bad old days of eugenics, and there was an immediate and direct response from John Mulvihill, a geneticist at the nation's only genetics department located within a school of public health, at the University of Pittsburgh.

The legacy of eugenics will always impose itself upon public health, Mulvihill said. The difference, he went on, "is that all of the parties are at the table now, and that we acknowledge the need to articulate as clearly as possible that the focus is not on reducing the incidence of disease, but on being sure that everyone knows the options that are available to them."

There are new responsibilities for us nonexperts, too, as a result of this paradigm shift in public policy. We must be sure that there are effective and informed parties to represent our interests at that table, and that we take full advantage of the opportunity to learn about the options available to us as a result of the new genetics. We must also be alert to public health programs that do not adhere to these lofty standards, because they will surely arise. No society is perfect. Ours? Hardly.

The problem with gene research is the same as its beauty. Its intellectual simplicity, its satisfying resolution of baffling medical puzzles with logical molecular explanations, creates the illusion that it will provide us with easy answers to larger human problems. Although some geneticists may make simplistic statements about the promise of gene research in order to get attention or funding, few among them actually suffer from this illusion.

Researchers in the field well realize aspects of evolution that Charles Darwin could never have imagined: the complex nature of genes, the stutters and interruptions within them, the degree to which they are prey to influences within and outside the body that are inscrutable and sometimes even random, the ease with which they can be vandalized, lost, stolen, or simply misplaced. The rest of us need to understand the rock-bottom truth that most geneticists take for granted — not the molecular esoterica of how genes operate, but the reality that *genetic* only rarely implies "inevitable" or "incurable," and least of all, "fully understood."

Above all, we can look into each other's eyes and see individuals, wondrous and incomprehensible entities, rich with surprise and potential. We are whoever we are not just because of what our genes contain, but because of what has happened to us since our birth and how we use that unique genetic endowment, day after day. The same holds true for the whole population of humanity. Equality is not written into the genes, of course — quite the contrary. It is something we confer upon each other if we wish.

It may turn out, Mr. Darwin, that we are not necessarily to be excused — as individuals, as a vast collection of genomes, as a species — for feeling any particular pride about who we are becoming during the course of human evolution. If we want to feel any pride at all for how we evolve as a species, we shall have to earn it for ourselves. Among ourselves.

ACKNOWLEDGMENTS

MANY PEOPLE HELPED AND ENCOURAGED ME DURING the long and difficult process of completing this book. I am grateful for the interesting and supportive contributions of Richard Benson, professor of moral theology at St. John's Seminary in Camarillo, California, and for the opportunity to read his thesis. I was buoyed by encouragement from many people along the way, especially Erik Parens and other staff members at the Hastings Center. Dorothy Wertz of the Shriver Center was always welcoming and informative.

My heartfelt thanks to Anna, to the Vander Plaats, to Lynne Quittell, and to Jodi Rucquoi for granting me time and allowing me to intrude on their privacy. I also thank Annetta Able for her interest and assistance. Several individuals who took time to read and comment on the manuscript in the early stages have earned a huge debt of gratitude: Leslie Eitzen, Marvin Fast, Bennette Kramer, and Theresa Rijk. A staff member in a health-related government agency who wants to remain anonymous contributed greatly to the quality of the content.

Thanks also to Catriona Fletcher and Laura Newman for assistance with research and preparation of the manuscript, to Donna Cook for vetting the manuscript for scientific accuracy, and to Mary Carol Sullivan of the Midwest Bioethics Center for reading the manuscript and commenting on its accuracy with regard to bioethics matters. Hallie Strohl contributed an important and very heartening suggestion at the last minute. Thanks also to Bernard Harrigan for technical support.

My coworkers and supervisors at Faulkner & Gray, where I worked as I wrote this book, also contributed by giving me the time and emotional space. Special thanks to Spencer Vibbert for his support and to Mike Warner for the leave of absence.

I am grateful to my agents, Cindy Klein and Georges Borchardt, for believing in the concept and seeing me through the years between concept and publication.

Above all, I want to express my regret to Katie and Alex for missing so many moments of their early childhood and for not always being the mother I wanted to be because the "accursed manuscript" got in the way. This book is about the future. I wrote it for you and everyone else who is a child today.

As for my husband Mark, I am not nearly a good enough writer to try to convey in words my gratitude, my admiration, or my love.

NOTES

INTRODUCTION

Page viii: Of some 80,000 human genes . . . : Lee Rowen et al., "Sequencing the Human Genome," *Science* 278 (24 October 1997): 605–7.

Page viii: more than 1,200 gene segments . . . : Clair A. Francomano and Francis Collins, "The Human Genome Project: Implications for Medical Practice," *Today's Internist* (November/December 1997): 11–15.

Page ix: "I have found this to be . . . : Francis Collins, interview, Bethesda, MD, 23 September 1997.

Page xi: A now-famous survey of people . . . : Paul R. Billings et al., "Discrimination as a Consequence of Genetic Testing," *American Journal of Human Genetics* 50 (1992): 476–82.

Page xii: At the time, Kretz's own mother . . . : At a Faulkner & Gray conference on patient-focused health care, Baltimore, MD, June 1996.

CHAPTER 1: Generation of the Upright

Page 3: An evil God would be proud . . . : Jared Diamond, "Curse and Blessing of the Ghetto," *Discover*, March 1991, 60.

Page 4: About 6 million Ashkenazim . . . : Arno Motulsky, *Nature Genetics* 9 (February 1995): 100.

Page 5: Tay-Sachs Disease . . . : Michael Kaback et al., "Tay-Sachs Disease–Carrier Screening, Prenatal Diagnosis, and the Molecular Era," *Journal of the American Medical Association* 270 (17 November 1993): 2307–14.

Page 5: The genetic screening program he founded . . . : Josef Ekstein, presentation at PRIMR conference, Boston, 1 June 1994.

Page 5: By the time he came to Brooklyn . . . : Josef Ekstein, interview, Dor Yeshorim headquarters, Brooklyn, 27 March 1995.

Page 7: The matchmakers' priorities . . . : Jerome Mintz, *Hasidic People: A Place in the New World* (Cambridge: Harvard University Press, 1992).

Page 7: Some rabbis judged that giving . . . : Fred Rosner, "Screening for Tay-Sachs Disease: A Note of Caution," *Journal of Clinical Ethics* 2 (Winter 1991).

Page 8: They call the program Dor Yeshorim . . . : "Dor Yeshorim: Phase II," *Jewish Observer*, September 1993.

Page 8: the genetic counselor and social worker . . . : Frances Berkwits, interview, Kingsbrook Jewish Medical Center, 12 December 1994.

Page 8: At that time it was the only . . . : Michael Herring, "Timely Action Urged in Tay-Sachs Pregnancy," *Medical Tribune*, 16 February 1975.

Page 9: "Basically it was a hospice . . . : Dr. Larry Schneck, interview, Kingsbrook Jewish Medical Center, Brooklyn, NY, December 1994.

Page 11: Does genetic testing indicate . . . : Rabbi Shmuel Lefkowitz, "Dor Yeshorim: A Grass Roots Success Story," *Genesis* (newsletter of the Genetics Network of the New York State Department of Health) 4, no. 2 (n.d.).

Page 11: Two years later the program began mass testing . . . : Ibid.

Page 11: Today Dor Yeshorim's offices in New York . . . : Ekstein presentation at PRIMR conference.

Page 11: "This pamphlet describes a real . . . : Dor Yeshorim Committee for the Prevention of Jewish Genetic Diseases, "Tay-Sachs Disease and Now Cystic Fibrosis Can Be Prevented: Read and Understand This Information for the Sake of Your Family's Health," undated pamphlet.

Page 13: "Why the molecular strands . . . : James Neel, *Physician to the Gene Pool* (New York: John Wiley and Sons, 1994), 271.

Page 14: other misfortunes such as, say, deafness . . . : Ekstein interview, 27 March 1995.

Page 15: the result of an inherited deficiency . . . : "Gaucher Disease: Current Issues in Diagnosis and Treatment," National Institutes of Health Technology Assessment Conference Statement, Bethesda, MD, 27 February–1 March 1995.

Page 16: "While we recognize that Gaucher . . . : Josef Ekstein, speech at NIH Gaucher conference, Bethesda, MD, February 1995.

Page 18: this was a courageous act . . . : Ekstein interview, 27 March 1995.

Page 19: "I do think our society has to . . . : Berkwits, interview, 12 December 1994.

Page 19: "Although this population is unique . . . : Robert J. Desnick, M.D., "Genetic Testing in the Ashkenazi Jewish Population," grant application to the National Institutes of Health, 18 February 1994.

CHAPTER 2: The Stress Test

Page 21: As is ours to Anna W. . . . : All information with reference to Anna W. is drawn from an in-person interview on 26 September 1995 and subsequent telephone conversations.

Page 23: "Mrs. W. is of Polish descent . . . : Letter provided by A. B., dated 29 June 1995.

Page 25: "In medicine you don't usually make . . . : Virginia Corson, press conference, American Society of Human Genetics conference, Washington, DC, 14 October 1994.

Page 26: "the provider may tell the patient . . . : Suzanne Carter, "Genetic Counseling Issues in Maternal Serum Screening Programs," presentation at the American Society of Human Genetics conference, Minneapolis, MN, 25 October 1995.

Page 27: Most clients in genetic counseling . . . : D. C. Wertz and J. C. Fletcher, "Communicating Genetic Risks," *Science, Technology and Human Values* 12 (1987): 60–66.

Page 28: "I was hoping I'd never have . . . : Rayna Rapp, "Chromosomes and Communication: The Discourse of Genetic Counseling," *Medical Anthropology Quarterly* 2 (1988): 143–57.

Page 29: "the mere existence of the new technology . . . : Troy Duster, *Backdoor to Eugenics* (New York: Routledge, 1990), 79.

Page 29: "just a simple blood test . . . : Nancy Press and C. H. Browner, "Risk, Autonomy and Responsibility: Informed Consent for Prenatal Testing," *Hastings Center Report*, May–June 1995, S9.

Page 29: "Society does not truly accept . . . : Abby Lippman, "Screening: Constructing Needs and Reinforcing Inequities," *American Journal of Law and Medicine* 17 (1991): 15–50.

Page 29: "We need to reassess . . . : Robyn Rowland, "Of Women Born, But for How Long: The Relationship of Women to the New Reproductive Technologies," in *Made to Order: The Myth of Reproductive and Genetic Progress*, edited by Patricia Spallone and Deborah Lynn Steinberg (New York: Pergamon Press, 1987).

Page 30: One recent survey of obstetricians . . . : L. Hinds et al., "Obstetricians' Current Use of and Attitudes Toward Maternal Serum Marker Screening," *American Journal of Human Genetics* 57 (suppl.) (1995) abstract 1721. Further information from authors' presentation at American Society of Human Genetics annual conference, Minneapolis, MN, October 1995.

Page 31: "Many women are not given . . . : Golder Wilson, M.D., telephone interview, 22 July 1996.

CHAPTER 3: Choices

Page 34: "I guess I value each day . . . : All details taken from interview with Vander Plaats at their home, 21 January 1995.

Page 35: even people who are tested . . . : Joanna Fanos and John Johnson, "Barriers to Carrier Testing for Adult Cystic Fibrosis Sibs: The Importance of Not Knowing," *American Journal of Medical Genetics* (October 1995).

Page 36: "My view and that of most . . . : Lynne Quittell, M.D., interview, Columbia–Presbyterian Medical Center, New York, 20 January 1995.

Page 36: Today Meghan can expect . . . : "Genetic Testing for Cystic Fibrosis," NIH Consensus Development Conference Statement, 14–16 April 1997.

Page 36: Dr. Ronald Crystal began testing . . . : Symposium at New York Hospital–Cornell Medical Center, New York, 14 November 1995.

Page 38: Some 650 different mutations . . . : T. Bienvenu, "Molecular Basis of Phenotype Heterogeneity in Cystic Fibrosis," *Annales Biologie Clinique* (Paris) 55 (1997): 113–21.

Page 38: Therefore testing will not leave someone . . . : Michael Welsh and Alan Smith, "Cystic Fibrosis," *Scientific American*, December 1995, 52.

Page 39: "how do we understand . . . : Charles Scriver, "Genetic Screening–The Heterozygote Experiment," summary paper for presentation at American Association for Advancement of Science conference, 13 February 1978.

Page 42: a fetus with a "serious defect" . . . : "Abortion: The Rate vs. the Debate," *New York Times*, 26 February 1996, E4.

Page 42: 46 percent of Americans . . . : "1 in 5 Polled Would Outlaw Abortion," *Washington Times,* 23 January 1995.

Page 42: the education brochure prepared by the state . . . : Nancy Press and C. H. Browner, "Risk, Autonomy and Responsibility: Informed Consent for Prenatal Testing," *Hastings Center Report,* May–June 1995, S9.

Page 43: After about 1950 doctors began . . . : Laurence Tribe, *Abortion: The Clash of Absolutes* (New York: W. W. Norton, 1992).

Page 43: people like Michelle and Paul O'Brien . . . : Jeff Lyon and Peter Gorner, *Altered Fates: The Genetic Re-engineering of Human Life* (New York: W. W. Norton, 1994), 498.

Page 44: After that, Hughes recalls . . . : Mark Hughes, conference at Faulkner Reproductive Center, Boston, 4 March 1995.

CHAPTER 4: The Faulkner Conference

Page 46: at a public symposium in Boston . . . : Much of the material in this chapter is taken from the Faulkner Reproductive Center conference, Boston, 4 March 1995.

Page 59: A cloned calf was finally born . . . : "Calf Cloned From Bovine Cell Line," *Science* 277 (15 August 1997): 903.

Page 60: University of Pennsylvania bioethicist . . . : Arthur Caplan, presentation at National Academy of Sciences, 16 January 1997.

Page 61: "Knowing the complete genetic makeup . . . : *Cloning Human Beings: Report and Recommendations of the National Bioethics Advisory Commission,* Bethesda, MD, June 1997, 33.

Page 62: Today the results of amniocentesis . . . : Mark Evans, M.D., "Interphase FISH: A Physician's Viewpoint," *Genetic Viewpoint* (Integrated Genetics) 2 (1995), 1.

Page 62: Newer FISH tests . . . : David Ledbetter, "What Is the Status of FISH in Clinical Cytogenetics?" *Genetic Viewpoint* (Integrated Genetics) 2 (1995), 3.

Page 63: Now it is often used . . . : Brian Ward et al., "Rapid Prenatal Diagnosis of Chromosomal Aneuploidies by Fluorescence In Situ Hybridization: Clinical Experience with 4500 Specimens," *American Journal of Human Genetics* 52 (1993): 854.

Page 63: the hot prospect for the future . . . : Various presentations, American Society of Human Genetics annual conference, Minneapolis, MN, October 1995.

Page 63: a woman whose fetus was misdiagnosed . . . : Peter Benn et al., "A Rapid (But Wrong) Prenatal Diagnosis," *New England Journal of Medicine* 326.

Page 63: FISH was not ready to be . . . : American College of Medical Genetics, "Prenatal Interphase Fluorescence In Situ Hybridization (FISH) Policy Statement," *American Journal of Human Genetics* 53 (1993): 526.

Page 63: "The correct procedure, if you're using . . . : Gorden Dewald, presentation at the American Society of Human Genetics annual conference, Minneapolis, MN, October 1995.

Page 64: Urine-based tests for pregnancy . . . : Wendy Diller, "The Failure and Potential of Home Diagnostics," *In Vivo* 15 (November 1997): 5–10.

Page 64: some researchers have begun experimenting . . . : Harold Nitowsky, "A Look to the Future of Screening for Genetic Disease in Pregnancy," presentation at the

American Society of Human Genetics, annual conference, Minneapolis, MN, 25 October 1995.

Page 64: "the long-awaited non-invasive . . . : Mei-Chi Cheung, James Goldberg, and Yuet Wai Kan, "Prenatal Diagnosis of Sickle Cell Anemia and Thalassemia by Analysis of Fetal Cells in Maternal Blood," *Nature* (14 November 1996), 264.

Page 64: "could usher in a new era . . . : S. Sternberg, "Mother's Blood Shows Baby's Future," *Science News* (2 November 1996), 276.

Page 65: One analyst has estimated . . . : Dorothy Wertz, "DNA Chips: Testing for Thousands of Genetic Conditions on One Sample," *Gene Letter*, August 1997.

Page 66: "I didn't feel the trauma of losing . . . : Esther Fine, "Fetal Test Focuses the Health-Care Debate," *New York Times*, 5 February 1994, 1.

Page 67: In China, where widespread abortions . . . : Nora Frenkiel, "Family Planning: Baby Boy or Girl," *New York Times*, 11 November 1993, C1.

Page 67: sex-screening of fetuses was banned . . . : "New Chinese Law Prohibits Sex-Screening of Fetuses," *New York Times*, 15 November 1994.

Page 68: "The grieving process appears to be . . . : A. Kolker and B. M. Burke, "Grieving the Wanted Child: Ramifications of Abortion after Prenatal Diagnosis of Abnormality," *Health Care Women International* 14 (November–December 1993): 513–26; J. Lloyd and K. M. Laurence, "Sequelae and Support After Termination of Pregnancy for Fetal Malformation," *British Medical Journal* 290 (23 March 1995): 907–909; and P. Donnai, N. Charles, and R. Harris, "Attitudes of Patients After 'Genetic' Termination of Pregnancy," *British Medical Journal* 282 (21 February 1981): 621–22.

Page 69: studies indicate that families whose . . . : Dorothy Wertz, "Families of Children with Mental Retardation and Developmental Disabilities: How Well Are They Doing?" *Gene Letter* I (5 March 1997).

Page 69: "Triple screening is not finally about . . . : Thomas Elkins and Douglas Brown, *Clinical Obstetrics and Gynecology* 36 (September 1993): 532–40.

Page 69: "We didn't understand until recently . . . : James Haddow, "Controversies in Maternal Serum Screening: Utility in Older Women," presentation at the American Society of Human Genetics annual conference, Minneapolis, MN, 25 October 1995.

Page 70: In 1992 some 60 percent . . . : George Cunningham, geneticist at California's Department of Health Services, presentation at "Cost-Benefit/Cost Effectiveness Analyses in Genetics" conference, sponsored by the New England Regional Genetics Group, Boston, Cambridge, MA, 30 March 1996.

Page 70: "In coming to believe that 'individuals' . . . : Troy Duster, *Backdoor to Eugenics* (New York: Routledge, 1990), 34.

Page 71: "Primary prevention . . . : Jane Lin-Fu, presentation at Genetic Testing Task Force meeting, Baltimore, MD, 17 March 1997.

CHAPTER 5: Regarding Borderlines

Page 72: even that observation would generate . . . : Courtney S. Campbell, letter to *Hastings Center Report*, May–June 1995, 5.

Page 73: who could advise the government . . . : Eliot Marshall, "Rules on Embryo Research Due Out," *Science* (19 August 1994), 1024.

Page 73: "Even if competing biases were . . . : Ruth Bulger, Elizabeth Boby, and Harvey Fineberg, eds., *Society's Choices: Social and Ethical Decision Making in Biomedicine*, Institute of Medicine (Washington, DC: National Academy Press, 1995), 187.

Page 73: were implicitly denied permission to study . . . : Howard W. Jones, Jr., "The Status of Regulation of Assisted Reproductive Technology in the United States," *Journal of Assisted Reproduction and Genetics* 10 (1993): 331.

Page 74: In 1992 infertile women underwent . . . : "Infertility and IVF and Other Types of Assisted Reproduction," NIH backgrounder to press briefing, 20 September 1994.

Page 74: responding to reports of abuses at some . . . : Diane Gianelli, "Fertility Scandal Raises Call for Regulation," *American Medical News*, 11 September 1995. Also Steve Jennings, personal communication, in Senator Wyden's office, 24 July 1995.

Page 74: In fact, in order to avoid . . . : Bernard Lo, director of medical ethics at the University of California, San Francisco, quoted in "Commission Proposing Guidelines for Human Embryo Cloning," Associated Press, 4 June 1997.

Page 75: In January 1993, on the twentieth . . . : Bulger, Boby, and Fineberg, *Society's Choices*, 353.

Page 75: The head of the agency that would have . . . : Joseph Palca, "Doing Things with Embryos," *Hastings Center Report*, January–February 1995, 5.

Page 78: "aboriginal subject in bioethics" . . . : Eric Juengst, "Germ-line Gene Therapy: Back to Basics," *Journal of Medicine and Philosophy* 16 (1991): 587–92.

Page 79: "germ-line engineering . . . : Marc Lappe, "Ethical Issues in Manipulating the Human Germ Line," *Journal of Medicine and Philosophy* 16 (1991): 621–39.

Page 79: some enthusiasts have begun to argue . . . : Burke Zimmerman, "Human Germ-Line Therapy: The Case for its Development and Use," *Journal of Medicine and Philosophy* 16 (1991): 593–612.

Page 80: In late 1993 two scientists from George Washington . . . : Gina Kolata, "Scientist Clones Human Embryos, and Creates an Ethical Challenge," *New York Times*, 24 October 1993, 1.

Page 80: The Vatican quickly responded . . . : Gina Kolata, "The Hot Debate About Cloning Human Embryos," *New York Times*, 26 October 1993, 1.

Page 80: A researcher in England had reported . . . : S. M. Willadsen, "Nuclear Transplantation in Sheep Embryos," *Nature* 320 (6 March 1986): 63–65, and references at end.

Page 80: "Guidelines are in place . . . : Howard W. Jones et al., "On Attempts at Cloning in the Human," *Fertility and Sterility* 61 (March 1994): 423–26.

Page 81: revelation about Hall and Stillman . . . : Broadcast transcript, report by Joseph Palca, *All Things Considered*, National Public Radio, 6 December 1994.

Page 83: King was no novice . . . : Robert Cook-Deegan, *The Gene Wars* (New York: W. W. Norton, 1994), 240.

Page 83: "legitimacy of nontherapeutic . . . : Eliot Marshall, "Rules on Embryo Research Due Out," *Science* (19 August 1994), 1024.

Page 86: "The American people will be justifiably . . . : Palca, "Doing Things with Embryos," 5.

Page 90: "I have always felt a nagging . . . : Daniel Callahan, "The Puzzle of Profound Respect," *Hastings Center Report* 25 (1995): 39.

Page 91: It was not clear how long the ban . . . : *Science* 3:271, p. 585.

Page 91: According to a report in *Science* . . . : Eliot Marshall, "Varmus Grilled Over Breach of Embryo Research Ban," *Science* 276 (27 June 1997): 1963.

Page 91: "I believed in good faith . . . : Dr. Mark Hughes, statement following the House Oversight Subcommittee hearing on the NIH enforcement of embryo research ban, 19 June 1997.

Page 93: panel members were defending their work . . . : George Annas et al., "The Politics of Human Embryo Research–Avoiding Ethical Gridlock," *New England Journal of Medicine* 334 (1996): 1329–32. Also see several articles in *Hastings Center Report*, January–February 1995, and replies in succeeding issues.

Page 96: Others felt just as deeply . . . : *Cloning Human Beings: Report and Recommendations of the National Bioethics Advisory Commission*, Bethesda, MD, June 1997.

Page 97: human cloning should be banned . . . : Ibid.

Page 97: "Banning human cloning reflects our humanity . . . : "Remarks by the President at Announcement of Cloning Legislation," 9 June 1997.

Page 97: "Gearhart himself wonders . . . : J. Travis, "Human Embryonic Stem Cells Found," *Science News*, 19 July 1997, 36.

Page 97: Richard Seed, the Chicago physicist . . . : Diane M. Gianelli, "On the Frontier or the Fringe?" *American Medical News*, 26 January 1998, 1.

CHAPTER 6: The New Paradigm

Page 99: an endearing image . . . : Joseph B. Verrengia, "Saliva Test Tracks Down Inherited Disorder," *Rocky Mountain News*, 10 March 1993, 26.

Page 99: One in 1,500 males . . . : Michael Mennuti, M.D., "A 35-year-old Woman Considering Maternal Serum Screening and Amniocentesis," *Journal of the American Medical Association* 275 (8 May 1996): 144.

Page 100: three days later . . . : Correction, *Rocky Mountain News*, 13 March 1993, 4.

Page 102: About a third of girls . . . : American College of Medical Genetics, policy statement, "Fragile X Syndrome: Diagnostic and Carrier Testing," *American Journal of Medical Genetics* 53 (1994): 380–81.

Page 102: informed consent procedures did not . . . : Dorothy Nelkin, presentation to the 1994 Human Genome meeting sponsored by *Science* magazine, Washington, DC, September 1994.

Page 102: "The project will pay for itself . . . : Quoted in Leslie Roberts, "Report Card on the Genome Project," *Science* 253 (26 July 1991): 376.

Page 103: "will be orders of magnitude . . . : David P. Lauria et al., "The Economic Impact of the Fragile X Syndrome on the State of Colorado," 1992 International Fragile X conference, Snowmass, CO, July 1992.

Page 103: The study might have vanished . . . : Jamie Stephenson, "Genetic Discrimination: Causes for Concern," presentation at "Cost-Benefit/Cost-Effectiveness

Analyses in Genetics" conference, sponsored by the New England Regional Genetics Group, Cambridge, MA, 30 March 1996.

Page 104: "It used a worst-case logic . . . : Allen C. Crocker, "Cost Accounting in Developmental Disabilities," presentation at "Cost-Benefit/Cost-Effectiveness Analyses in Genetics" conference, Cambridge, MA, 30 March 1996.

Page 105: A 1996 study comparing adolescents . . . : S. Saigal et al., "Self-Perceived Health Status and Health-Related Quality of Life of Extremely Low Birthweight Infants at Adolescence," *Journal of the American Medical Association* (14 August 1996), 453.

Page 105: self-worth among young people with . . . : G. A. King et al., "Self-valuation and Self-concept of Adolescents with Physical Disabilities," *American Journal of Occupational Therapy* 47 (1993): 132; and P. L. Appleton et al., "The Self-concept of Young People with Spina Bifida: A Population-based Study," *Developmental Medicine and Child Neurology* 36 (1994): 198–215.

Page 105: someone who had been quoted . . . : "Gene Key to Mental Disorder Diagnosis," *Rocky Mountain News*, 23 June 1991, 6.

Page 106: Putting a genetic label . . . : D. Callahan, "Ethics, Law and Genetic Counseling," *Science* 176 (1972): 197–200.

Page 106: six of ten felt parents should . . . : Dorothy Wertz, "Disclosure to Relatives and Testing Children," poster presented at the American Society of Human Genetics annual conference, Montreal, September 1994.

Page 106: a genetics conference in Montreal . . . : American Society of Human Genetics conference, Montreal, September 1994.

Page 107: the next annual conference, in Minneapolis . . . : American Society of Human Genetics conference, Minneapolis, MN, October 1995.

Page 110: The results showed how differently . . . : Kathy A. Fackelmann, "DNA Dilemmas: Readers and 'Experts' Weigh in on Biomedical Ethics," *Science News* 146 (17 December 1994), 408–9.

Page 113: "It's amazing for me to find . . . : I. Arzimanoglou, interview at American Society of Human Genetics annual conference, Montreal, September 1994.

Page 118: from a 1994 article about screening . . . : Darren Shickle and Ruth Chadwick, "The Ethics of Screening: Is 'Screeningitis' an Incurable Disease?" *Journal of Medical Ethics* 20 (1994): 12–18.

Page 120: "There is a tendency of pilot . . . : Neil Holtzman, "What Drives Neonatal Screening Programs?" *New England Journal of Medicine* 325 (1991): 802.

Page 121: "When the CF gene was discovered . . . : Quoted in "The Gene-Testing Boom Is Still Set for Someday," *Business Week*, 21 November 1994, 102.

Page 121: "This represents DNA testing . . . : Quoted in "Panel Backs Widening Net of Genetic Test," *Science News*, 26 April 1997, 253.

Page 125: "If we tell you what your genotype is . . . : Allen Roses, presentation to science writers' conference on neurology, sponsored by American Academy of Neurology, New York City, 5 February 1996.

Page 126: recent studies scanning the entire genomes . . . : Margaret A. Pericak-Vance et al., "Complete Genomic Screen in Late-Onset Familial Alzheimer Disease," *Journal of the American Medical Association* 278 (15 October 1997): 1237; also Roger Rosenberg, M.D., "Molecular Neurogenetics: Settling the Issue," same issue, 1282.

Page 127: By his report she has weathered . . . : Lisa Seachrist, "Testing Genes," *Science News* 148 (1995): 394.

Page 129: "It is one thing already to bring . . . : Robert B. Scott and Robert P.

Gilbert, "Genetic Diversity in Hemoglobins: Disease and Nondisease," *Journal of the American Medical Association* 239 (1978): 2681–684.

Page 131: "the advent of genetic testing . . . : Robert Wachbroit, *Report from the Institute for Philosophy and Public Policy* 16 (Summer/Fall 1996).

Page 131: Myriad set up a confidential . . . : Donna Shattuck-Eidens et al., "BRCA1 Sequence Analysis in Women at High Risk for Susceptibility Mutation," *Journal of the American Medical Association* 278 (15 October 1997): 1242–50.

Page 131: its Center for Bioethics began . . . : *American Medical News*, 12 August 1996, 3.

Page 131: The National Cancer Institute . . . : *Journal of the National Cancer Institute* 88 (1 May 1996): 579.

Page 132: valuable guidance in its position paper . . . : National Society of Genetic Counselors, "Predisposition Genetic Testing for Late-Onset Disorders in Adults," *Journal of the American Medical Association* 278 (15 October 1997): 1217–20.

Page 134: Probably the only thing that is . . . : Ruth Hubbard and R. C. Lewontin, "Pitfalls of Genetic Testing," *New England Journal of Medicine* 224 (1996): 1192.

CHAPTER 7: Missing Links

Page 135: a young graduate student from Ohio . . . : Neel's early experience with human genetics is recounted in James V. Neel, *Physician to the Gene Pool: Genetic Lessons and Other Stories* (New York: John Wiley and Sons, 1994).

Page 136: "People were more confident . . . : Barbara Tuchman, *The Proud Tower* (New York: Macmillan, 1966), xiii.

Page 137: "Davenport deplored the fact . . . : Daniel Kevles, *In the Name of Eugenics* (Berkeley and Los Angeles: University of California Press, 1985), 51.

Page 137: "was to be perceived . . . : Jonathan Marks, "Historiography of Eugenics," *American Journal of Human Genetics* 53 (1993): 650–52.

Page 139: The most visible eugenics efforts . . . : Kevles, *Eugenics*, 62ff. Much of this history is also told in Diane B. Paul, *Controlling Human Heredity* (Atlantic Highlands, NJ: Humanities Press, 1995).

Page 139: transformed birth control from a movement . . . : Paul, *Controlling*, 96.

Page 140: Adults who were "idiots" . . . : Kevles, *Eugenics*, 77ff.

Page 140: the matter of Carrie Buck . . . : Robert Cook-Deegan, *The Gene Wars*, (New York: W. W. Norton, 1994), 249.

Page 144: set about to reform it . . . : Paul, *Controlling*.

Page 145: "unsatisfactory manner . . . : Quoted in Neel, *Physician*, 15.

Page 145: he found only one . . . : James Neel, personal communication.

Page 145: "I see an extraordinary potential . . . : Quoted in "The Gene Hunt," *Time*, 20 March 1986, 63.

Page 146: reporting that biologist Jacques Loeb . . . : Ludger Wess, *Die Träume der Genetik*, 11. My account of Loeb and T. H. Morgan was drawn from Wess, but is available in numerous other sources.

Page 148: "We used to think our fate . . . : Quoted in "Gene Hunt," 67.

CHAPTER 8: Otmar von Verschuer: A Gentleman and a Scholar

Page 152: had committed suicide on the run . . . : Benno Müller-Hill, *Tödliche Wissenschaft* (Reinbek Verlag, 1984), 82.

Page 152: Verschuer had stood at a podium . . . : Monika Daum and Hans-Ulrich Deppe, *Zwangssterilisierung in Frankfurt-am-Main, 1933–1945* (Campus Verlag, 1991), 65.

Page 152: "We stand at the beginning of a new . . . : Otmar von Verschuer, "Aufgaben und Ziele des Institut für Erbbiologie und Rassenhygiene zu Frankfurt am Main," *Erbarzt* 7 (1935).

Page 153: "A good *Volksmaterial* is the greatest . . . : Quoted in Gerda Stucklik, *Goethe in Braunhemd: Universität Frankfurt 1933–1945* (Roederberg Verlag, 1984).

Page 154: including Verschuer's own writings . . . : For instance, "Woran erkennt man die Erblichkeit körperlicher Missbildungen?" *Erbarzt* 21 (May 1938), 61.

Page 154: appeared in a local weekly . . . : Dr. Werner Fischer-Defoy, "Das Gesundheitswesen der Stadt Frankfurt am Main," *Frankfurter Wochenschau*, 7–13 April 1935, 1.

Page 155: The 1933 Law for the Prevention of . . . : "Gesetz zur Verhütung erbkranken Nachwuchses," 14 July 1933 (Reichsgesetzblatt I, 529), reprinted in Daum and Deppe, *Zwangssterilisierung*.

Page 156: Even when Verschuer gave a sterilization . . . : Daum and Deppe, *Zwangssterilisierung*, 75ff.

Page 158: argued for a change in the sterilization . . . . Otmar von Verschuer, "Die Unfruchtbarmachung bei schwerer erblicher geistiger Störung," *Erbarzt* 10 (1938), 125.

Page 158: No records survive to tell us . . . : Klaus Dieter-Thoman, "Rassenhygiene und Anthropologie: Die zwei Karrieren des Prof. Verschuer," *Frankfurter Rundschau*, 20 May 1985, 20.

Page 159: His friends described him as . . . : Ibid.

Page 159: a member of the Bekennende Kirche . . . : Müller-Hill, *Tödliche*, 122, 127.

Page 160: somehow delayed joining . . . : Paul Weindling, "The Survival of Eugenics in 20th-Century Germany," *American Journal of Medical Genetics* 52 (1993): 649.

Page 160: "As a scientist . . . : Notker Hammerstein, *Die Johann Wolfgang Goethe-Universität Frankfurt am Main: Von der Stiftungsuniversität zur Staatlichen Hochschule*, vol. 1, *1914–1950* (Alfred Metzner Verlag, 1989), 316.

Page 160: when he was eight or nine . . . : Müller-Hill, *Tödliche*, 127.

Page 160: "He never said . . . : Ibid., 121.

Page 161: "In the spring of 1924 . . . : Ibid., 106.

Page 161: Several of Verschuer's colleagues . . . : Ibid., 160.

Page 162: a better opportunity . . . : Ibid., 71.

Page 162: One woman who was spared death . . . : Annetta Able, Auschwitz survivor and identical twin, personal communication.

Page 162: Mengele gave the twins . . . : Müller-Hill, *Tödliche*, 113.

Page 163: "It is horrible . . . : Ibid., 130.

Page 163: "We had no doubt . . . : Ibid., 162.

Page 163: "Genetic Endowment as Fate and Responsibility": Otmar von Verschuer, "Erbanlage als Schicksal und Aufgabe," *Prussische Akademie der Wissenschaften: Vorträge und Schriften,* vol. 18, *1944,* 21.

Page 164: "Plasma substrates have been . . . : Müller-Hill, *Tödliche,* 74.

Page 165: Germany's largest institute of human genetics . . . : Heinrich Schade, "Professor O. von Verschuer zum 70. Geburtstag," *Deutsche Medizinische Wochenschrift* 28 (1966), 1281.

Page 165: he was invited as the leader . . . : Ludger Wess, *Träume der Genetik* (Hamburger Stiftung für Sozialgeschichte des 20. Jahrhunderts, 1989), 44.

Page 166: "The author has not to my knowledge . . . : L. C. Dunn, "Cross Currents in the History of Human Genetics," *American Journal of Human Genetics* 14 (1962): 1–13.

Page 166: "Whenever such statements . . . : Letter to the editor, *American Journal of Human Genetics* 14 (1962), 309.

Page 166: a long and glowing eulogy . . . : Heinrich Schade, "Otmar von Verschuer," *Deutsche Medizinische Wochenschrift* 46 (1969), 2407.

Page 166: "The circumstances of human genetics . . . : Otmar von Verschuer, "Bemerkungen zur Genanalyse beim Menschen," *Erbarzt* 7 (September 1939), 59.

CHAPTER 9: What's Wrong?

Page 167: The Nuremberg medical trials: *Trials of War Criminals Before the Nürnberg Military Tribunals* (U.S. Government Printing Office).

Page 168: "No refined questions confront us . . . : Ibid., vol. 1, 70.

Page 170: Nazi scientists in the dock . . . : Arthur Caplan, *When Medicine Went Mad* (Humana Press, 1992), 71.

Page 170: "The dominant tendency . . . : Robert Jay Lifton, *The Nazi Doctors* (New York: Basic Books, 1986), 8.

Page 172: "informed consent" takes on . . . : Troy Duster, *Backdoor to Eugenics* (New York: Routledge, 1990), 86.

Page 173: "It has taken a long time . . . : Caplan, *When Medicine,* 25.

Page 174: The now-infamous Tuskegee "experiment": Many sources used, prominently Duster, *Backdoor,* 83–85.

Page 176: a policy statement that had been issued . . . : "U.S. Guidelines on Human Experimentation–Institutional Guide to the DHEW Policy on Protection of Human Subjects" (U.S. Public Health Service, 1971).

Page 176: those who were exposed to . . . : National Research Council, *Toxicologic Assessment of the Army's Zinc Cadmium Sulfide Dispersion Tests* (Washington, DC: National Academy Press, 1997).

Page 176: "During this century and particularly . . . : Jay Katz, "Do We Need Another Advisory Commission on Human Experimentation?" *Hastings Center Report* 25 (1995), 29–31.

Page 177: a deep distrust of the mainstream . . . : Deborah Shelton, "President Apologizes, Calls Syphilis Study 'Morally Wrong,'" *American Medical News,* 16 May 1997, 1. Also Deborah Shelton, "Legacy of Tuskegee," *American Medical News,* 3 June 1996, 1.

CHAPTER 10: Genes and the Bomb

Page 178: When the war ended in 1945 . . . : All of Neel's recollections in this chapter are taken from his autobiography, *Physician to the Gene Pool*, chaps. 4 and 5.

Page 179: An ordinary medical X ray . . . : Neel, *Physician*, 320ff.

Page 180: It has been estimated that . . . : Daniel E. Koshland, Jr., "Molecule of the Year: The DNA Repair Enzyme," *Science* 266 (23 December 1994): 1925.

Page 180: a newfound class of molecules . . . : Elizabeth Culott and Daniel E. Koshland, Jr., "DNA Repair Works Its Way to the Top," *Science* 266 (23 December 1994): 1926.

Page 181: "In an instant . . . : Paul Boyer, *By the Bomb's Early Light* (New York: Random House, 1985), 133. All post-Hiroshima quotes from the public press in the following paragraphs are taken from this book.

Page 185: "It has been called . . . : *Harbor Transcript*, newsletter of the Cold Spring Harbor Laboratory, Winter 1988.

Page 185: "Man's feeling of self-importance . . . : Robert Cook-Deegan, *The Gene Wars* (New York: W. W. Norton, 1994), 114.

Page 186: MIT historian of science Charles Weiner . . . : Charles Weiner, "Anticipating the Consequences of Genetic Engineering—Past, Present and Future," in *Are Genes Us?* edited by Carl F. Cranor (New Brunswick, NJ: Rutgers University Press, 1994).

CHAPTER 11: The Atlas of Ourselves

Page 188: "The nature of what can . . . : Alvin Toffler, *Future Shock* (New York: Random House, 1970), 203.

Page 189: "physicists and astronomers were not . . . : Roger Lewin, "In the Beginning Was the Genome," *New Scientist*, 21 July 1990, 35.

Page 189: "Genesis: The Sequel": Robert Cook-Deegan, *The Gene Wars* (New York: W. W. Norton, 1994), 79ff.

Page 189: "What it did . . . : Russell Dolittle, presentation at American Society of Human Genetics annual conference, Minneapolis, MN, October 1995.

Page 191: "Suddenly we had these tools . . . : James Watson, testimony before U.S. House of Representatives Appropriations Committee, 28 February 1995.

Page 193: a project to discover the molecular sequence . . . : Renato Dulbecco, "A Turning Point in Cancer Research: Sequencing the Human Genome," *Science* 231 (1986), 1055–56.

Page 193: "But I listened to my friend . . . : James Watson, House Appropriations Committee testimony, 28 February 1995.

Page 196: "mediocre science and terrible . . . : *The Gene Wars*, 171.

Page 197: some so-called junk DNA . . . : Natalie Angier, "Keys Emerge to Mystery of 'Junk' DNA," *New York Times*, 28 June 1995, C1.

Page 197: the prevalence of "pseudogenes" . . . : James Neel, *Physician to the Gene Pool* (New York: John Wiley and Sons, 1994), 255, 266.

Page 201: "the genome project was something . . . : Francis Collins, interview, Bethesda, MD, 23 September 1997.

Page 201: "more than half of the human . . . : Harold Varmus, testimony before U.S. House of Representatives Appropriations Committee, 23 March 1995.

Page 202: "The result will be a flood . . . : From press information provided supplementary to *Nature*, 28 September 1995.

Page 203: a goal of completing the sequence . . . : "Evolution of a Vision," *Human Genome News* (NCHGR newsletter), September–December 1995.

CHAPTER 12: Days of Miracle and Wonder

Page 206: its annual conference . . . : Human Genome Conference, Washington, DC, 2–5 October 1994. The conference heralded the publication of numerous genome-related articles in *Science*, 30 September 1994.

Page 210: The Patent Office had been . . . : S. M. Thomas et al., "Ownership of the Human Genome," *Nature* (4 April 1996), 387–88.

Page 213: had committed to contributing . . . : Press pack with release of the Genome Directory, *Nature* publications, 26 September 1995.

Page 214: the sequence of a bacterium found . . . : Jean-F. Tombs et al., "The Complete Genome Sequence of the Gastric Pathogen *Helicobacter pylori*," *Nature* 388 (7 August 1997): 539–45.

Page 215: "I think what we have . . . : Thomas Caskey, interview, Merck headquarters, 21 May 1996.

Page 215: Some companies were purifying . . . : "GI's Discover Ease Isn't So Easy," *In Vivo* 15 (November 1997): 2–3.

Page 216: the gene doctors and genetic counselors . . . : American Society of Human Genetics, annual conference, Montreal, October 1994.

Page 217: a major report about genetic testing: Ruth Bulger, Elizabeth Boby, and Harvey Fineberg, eds., *Assessing Genetic Risks: Implications for Health and Social Policy*, Institute of Medicine (Washington, DC: National Academy Press, 1994).

Page 222: The gene behind Huntington's . . . : Marcia Barinaga, "An Intriguing New Lead on Huntington's Disease," *Science* 271 (1 March 1996): 1233.

Page 222: HD has a long and troubled . . . : Peter Harper, "Huntington's Disease and the Abuse of Genetics," *American Journal of Human Genetics* 50 (1992): 460–64.

Page 223: He responded by handing her a card . . . : Jane Solomon, American Society of Human Genetics, telephone communication, 28 January 1998.

Page 226: Craig Venter upped the ante . . . : Nicolas Wade, "Scientist's Plan: Map All DNA Within 3 Years," *New York Times*, 10 May 1988.

CHAPTER 13: ELSI, the Gentle Watchdog

Page 227: held its first congress in Frankfurt . . . : "Genome Analysis: From Sequence to Function," first European meeting of the Human Genome Organization, Frankfurt am Main, Germany, 10–12 December 1990.

Page 227: "no other ethically right choice . . . : Richard Benson, "The Human Genome Initiative: A Scientific Prerogative or an Ethical Imperative," *Advances in Molecular Genetics* 4 (1991): 403–14.

Page 228: He had since reordered his thoughts: Richard Benson, interview, 4 October 1994, during Human Genome meeting in Washington, DC. Also: "The Human Genome Projects: The Ethical Implications of the Epistemological Limits of the Molecular Genetic Paradigm," unpublished ms.

Page 228: The Biotechnology Industry Organization . . . : Kathleen Day, "Genetics Research Begets Questions," *Washington Post*, 8 May 1996, A1.

Page 228: The worst thing for science . . . : Lee Hoke, "Researchers and Their Bioethicist Critics Move Toward Better Working Relationship," *Scientist* 9 (2 October 1995): 8–9.

Page 229: "I want to proceed . . . : Robert Cook-Deegan, *The Gene Wars* (New York: W. W. Norton, 1994), 237.

Page 229: "I still don't understand . . . : Eric Juengst, "Self-Critical Federal Science? The Ethics Experiment Within the U.S. Human Genome Project," *Social Philosophy and Policy* (Summer 1996): 63–95.

Page 229: "No one knew where it was going . . . : Elizabeth Thomson, interview, Montreal, 26 October 1995.

Page 230: "Were they supposed to be advising . . . : Francis Collins, interview, Bethesda, MD, 23 September 1997.

Page 230: "She pours on them . . . : Americo Negrette, "La Catira," *Panorama* (Maracaibo, Venezuela, 1990); quoted in Cook-Deegan, *Gene Wars*, 235.

Page 231: By the end of its first five years . . . : Steven Benowitz, "Scientists Struggling with Concerns Raised by Genome Project Progress," *Scientist*, 8 July 1996, 1.

Page 232: many of the one hundred . . . : "States Show Keen Interest in Genetic Policy," *Gene Letter* 1 (March 1997): 5.

Page 233: Medicine, says one ethicist . . . : William Fulford et al., "Introduction: Diverse Ethics," in *Medicine and Moral Reasoning* (New York: Cambridge University Press, 1994).

Page 233: a flowering of advisory bodies . . . : "Business Booms for Guides to Biology's Moral Maze," *Nature* 389 (16 October 1997): 658–62.

Page 233: the results of deliberations between them . . . : Ruth Bulger, Elizabeth Boby, and Harvey Fineberg, eds., *Society's Choices: Social and Ethical Decision Making in Biomedicine*, Institute of Medicine (Washington, DC: National Academy Press, 1995).

Page 236: both organizations continue to insist . . . : Robert Pear, "States Pass Laws to Regulate Uses of Genetic Testing," *New York Times*, 18 October 1997, 1.

Page 237: an "unavoidable political tax" . . . : Quoted in Kathi E. Hanna, "The Ethical, Legal and Social Implications Program of the National Center for Human Genome Research: A Missed Opportunity?" in *Society's Choices*, 432.

Page 237: a sharply critical portrait . . . : Charles Weiner, "Anticipating the Consequences of Genetic Engineering: Past, Present and Future," in *Are Genes Us?* edited by Carl F. Cranor (New Brunswick, NJ: Rutgers University Press, 1994).

Page 238: Trottier says he was told . . . : Ralph Trottier, telephone interview, 9 July 1996.

Page 238: James Watson had stepped down . . . : "Head of Gene Map Threatens to Quit," *New York Times*, 9 April 1992, A26.

Page 238: "Possessing information about women . . . : Francis Collins, interview, Bethesda, MD, 23 September 1997.

Page 239: "I think we have to move . . . : Francis Collins, testimony before U.S. House of Representatives Appropriations Committee, 23 March 1995.

Page 239: "What we find *will* be used . . . : Elizabeth Thomson, interview, Montreal, 26 October 1995.

Page 239: During the 1995 appropriations hearings . . . : Hearings of 104th Congress House of Representatives Appropriations Committee, 23 March 1995.

Page 240: such protections were not completely . . . : Collins interview.

Page 241: a symposium cosponsored with the National . . . : Karen Rothenberg et al., "Genetic Information and the Workplace: Legislative Approaches and Policy Changes," *Science* (21 March 1997), 1755.

Page 241: Collins himself sat up . . . : Collins interview.

Page 241: "One can see it happening . . . : Eric Juengst, personal communication, 11 September 1996.

Page 242: the working group's plan to spend $20,000 . . . : Sally Lehrman, "Genome Ethics Chair Resigns amid Worries over Autonomy," *Nature* (14 March 1996).

Page 242: "There is a hostility to scrutiny . . . : Robert Lee Hotz, "Panels Step Up Efforts to Regulate New Field," *Los Angeles Times,* 27 April 1997.

Page 242: "Serious concerns have been raised . . . : Report of the Joint NIH/DOE Committee to Evaluate the Ethical, Legal, and Social Implications Program of the Human Genome Project, January 1997. Available at http://www.ornl.gov/hgmis/archive/elsirept.htm.

Page 245: In its interim report, issued in January . . . : "Proposed Recommendations of the Task Force on Genetic Testing," *Federal Register* 16 (30 January 1997), 4539.

Page 245: "I am disappointed and alarmed . . . : Comments to the proposed report, Neil Holtzman, private communication.

Page 248: The final report is clearly worded . . . : Task Force on Genetic Testing, "Promoting Safe and Effective Genetic Testing in the United States: Principles and Recommendations," 14 June 1997.

Page 249: At least fifteen genes . . . : "As Discoveries Unfold, A New Urgency to Bring Genetic Literacy to Physicians," *Journal of the American Medical Association* (15 October 1997): 1225–26.

Page 249: a total of some 450 genetic tests . . . : Kathy Hudson, assistant director of the National Human Genome Research Institute, quoted in "States Pass Laws to Regulate Use of Genetic Testing," *New York Times,* 18 October 1997, 1.

Page 250: part of the problem with regulating . . . : Arno Motulsky, telephone interview, 8 April 1996.

Page 250: "You never know the answer . . . : Harold Shapiro, remarks at press conference after inaugural meeting of National Bioethics Advisory Commission, Bethesda, MD, 4 October 1996.

CHAPTER 14: Identity Crisis

Page 251: "We get everything in here . . . : Jodi Rucquoi, interview, Yale Children's Hospital, New Haven, CT, 13 October 1995.

Page 252: A 1995 survey of pediatricians . . . : S. J. Hayflick et al., "Utilization of Genetics Services by Family Physicians," *American Journal of Human Genetics* 57 (October 1995): A57.

Page 252: the proposal that physicians should obtain . . . : C. Kozma et al., "Human Genome Education Model (HuGEM) Project: Ethical, Legal and Social Issues," *American Journal of Human Genetics* 57 (October 1995): A28.

Page 254: the genetic counseling profession . . . : Rayna Rapp, "Chromosomes and Communication: The Discourse of Genetic Counseling," *Medical Anthropology Quarterly* 2 (1988): 143–57.

Page 254: Ethicist Arthur Caplan . . . : Public address at the National Academy of Sciences, Washington, DC, 16 January 1997.

Page 256: "However much the value of neutrality . . . : Daniel Callahan, "Ethics, Law and Genetic Counseling," *Science* 176 (1972): 197–200.

Page 256: "We do not expect doctors . . . : Robert Wachbroit and David Wasserman, "Clarifying the Goals of Nondirective Genetic Counseling," *Report from the Institute for Philosophy and Public Policy* (University of Maryland) 15 (Spring/Summer 1995): 1.

Page 256: "Uncertainty is not related to . . . : Dorothy Wertz and John Fletcher, "Communicating Genetic Risks," *Genetic Technology and Human Values* 12 (1987): 60–66.

Page 257: "A lot of people look at genetics . . . : Golder Wilson, telephone interview, 22 July 1996.

Page 258: A survey funded by the New England . . . : "Reconsidering 'Nondirectiveness' in Genetic Counseling," *Gene Letter* 1 (January 1997) (http://www.geneletter.org/0197).

Page 258: the 44 percent of clients . . . : Wertz and Fletcher, "Communicating Genetic Risks"; Rapp, "Chromosomes and Communication," 154.

Page 259: an example of this dilemma . . . : Troy Duster, *Backdoor to Eugenics* (New York: Routledge, 1990), 142–43.

Page 259: "The counselors I interviewed . . . : Rapp, "Chromosomes and Communication," 146.

Page 260: "What counts as success . . . : Ruth Chadwick, "What Counts as Success in Genetic Counselling?" *Journal of Medical Ethics* (1993): 43–46.

Page 261: "It is immediately apparent . . . : Angus Clarke, "Is Non-directive Genetic Counselling Possible?" *Lancet* 338 (1991): 998.

CHAPTER 15: Genes and Managed Care: The Bottom Line

Page 264: 57 percent of whom . . . : Press release, Project Hope, 5 May 1996.

Page 264: "Geneticists are going to . . . : Peter Rowley, "Evaluating Genetic Services: Analyzing Outcomes and Cost-Effectiveness," presentation at American Society of Human Genetics annual conference, Minneapolis, MN, 25 September 1995.

Page 265: Virtually all the major national . . . : Janet Corrigan et al., "Trends Toward a National Health Care Marketplace," *Inquiry* 34 (Spring 1997): 11–28.

Page 266: "nonmonetary costs and benefits . . . : New England Regional Genetics Group (NERGG), Ethical and Social Concerns Committee, "Draft Statement on Cost-Effectiveness and Cost-Benefit Analysis," background papers for the conference "Cost-Benefit/Cost-Effectiveness Analyses in Genetics," Cambridge, MA, 30 March 1996.

Page 266: A recent study compared two . . . : Peter Ubel et al., "Cost-Effectiveness Analysis in a Setting of Budget Constraints: Is It Equitable?" *New England Journal of Medicine,*" 334 (2 May 1996): 1174–77.

Page 267: In the real world . . . : Theodore Ganiats, "Justifying Prenatal Screening and Genetic Amniocentesis Programs by Cost-Effectiveness Analyses: A Reevaluation," *Medical Decision Making* 16 (1996): 45.

Page 268: "Eventually I think that's . . . : Francis Collins, interview, Bethesda, MD, 23 September 1997.

Page 269: "The viability of a voluntary . . . : White Paper on Genetic Testing, Genetic Testing Working Group of the Life Insurance Committee, National Association of Insurance Commissioners, 4 June 1996.

Page 269: "The decision has got to be made . . . : John Mann, presentation at conference on cost-effectiveness analysis in genetics, Cambridge, MA, 30 March 1996.

Page 269: "inherent conflict of interest . . . : Marcia Angell and Jerome Kassirer, "Quality and the Medical Marketplace–Following Elephants," *New England Journal of Medicine* 335 (1996): 883–85.

Page 270: "almost total failure to address . . . : Geraldine Dallek et al., "Consumer Protections in State HMO Laws," *Center for Health Care Rights* 1 (November 1995), 157.

Page 270: state legislatures began to adopt . . . : Tracy E. Miller, "Managed Care Regulation in the Laboratory of the States," *Journal of the American Medical Association* 278 (1 October 1997): 1102–09.

Page 271: about 30 percent of Americans . . . : Thomas O. Pyle and Gerry Brunk, "The Reformation of the Health Care System," *Internist* (January 1995), 13.

Page 271: the proportion of the nonelderly population . . . : Employee Benefits Research Institute, "Trends in Health Insurance Coverage," *Issue Brief* no. 185 (May 1997).

Page 272: "Even if employers do not use . . . : Karen Rothenberg et al., "Genetic Information and the Workplace: Legislative Approaches and Policy Changes," *Science* (21 March 1997), 1755.

Page 273: "We can't buy everything . . . : Michael Garland, "Role of Economics in Setting Health Practices and Priorities: The Oregon Plan," presentation at conference on cost effectiveness analysis in genetics, Cambridge, MA, 30 March, 1996.

Page 273: "on a budgetary tightrope": Thomas Bodenheimer, "The Oregon Health Plan–Lessons for the Nation (Part II)," *New England Journal of Medicine* (September 1997), 720–23.

Page 273: The protections provided by . . . : Robert Pear, "States Pass Laws to Regulate Uses of Genetic Testing," *New York Times,* 18 October 1997, 1.

Page 274: it seems unlikely that any broad-based new protections . . . : "Hill Staff Forecast for '98: Cloudy Prospects for Managed Care Law," *Medicine and Health,* 28 January 1998, 1.

Page 275: "At the heart of our approach . . . : "Optimized Healthcare Outcomes: Our Focus Is Your Future" (Integrated Disease Management, 1994).

Page 275: "This is all about cost containment . . . : Sheila Shuster, at exhibition booth for Genetrix, American Society of Human Genetics annual conference, Montreal, September 1994.

Page 276: "efficacy proven in outcomes": Genetrix brochure "The Genetic Health Network: The Key to Patient Outcome" (Scottsdale, AZ, 1994).

Page 276: "will initiate a major change . . . : SmithKline Beecham Genetic Testing Backgrounder (n.d.), 22.

Page 277: "We've never had a specialty . . . : Jean Amos, interview, American Society of Human Genetics conference, Minneapolis, MN, October 1995.

Page 277: "Although the current market . . . : "Vysis Inc. Molecular Disease Management: Company Background," 24 October 1995.

Page 277: "Theoretically there is no limit . . . : Integrated Genetics press release, "Integrated Genetics Announces Technological Breakthrough: New Test Can Simultaneously Detect More than One Hundred Mutations in Hundreds of Patient Samples," 26 October 1995.

Page 278: By 1997 more than one hundred . . . : Philip Reilly, "States Show Keen Interest in Genetic Privacy," *Gene Letter* 1 (March 1997) (http://www.geneletter. org/0397).

Page 278: "this is the beginning . . . : Quoted in Jocelyn Kaise, "Privacy Rules Set No New Research Curbs," *Science* 277 (19 September 1997): 1751.

Page 278: The Kennedy-Kassebaum Health Insurance . . . : Karen Rothenberg et al., "Genetic Information and the Workplace: Legislative Approaches and Policy Changes," *Science* (21 March 1997), 1757.

Page 279: "the latest in a long line . . . : Quoted in *American Health Line*, 8 August 1996.

Page 279: the pharmaceutical giant Glaxo-Wellcome . . . : "Informatics: Integrating Healthcare Networks," *Datamonitor* (April 1996), 146.

Page 279: "Preventable illness accounts for . . . : Quoted in "The State of Health Care in America 1995," supplement to *Business and Health*, 17.

Page 280: some thirty states have now enacted . . . : Karen Rothenberg, "Genetic Information and Health Insurance: State Legislative Approaches," *Journal of Law, Medicine and Ethics* 23 (1995): 312–19.

Page 280: nine states enacted new legislation . . . : Barbara Fuller, J. D., personal communication.

Page 280: A law passed in New Jersey . . . : Philip Reilly, "New Jersey Privacy Bill Offers Broader Protection Than Most," *ASHG Newsletter* (July 1996).

Page 280: The Health Insurance Portability . . . : "Health Reforms Enacted," *Milliman & Robertson Perspectives* (update), September 1996; "New Employer Requirements for Health Plans," *Hewitt Special Report to Clients*, Hewitt Associates LLC, 22 April 1997.

Page 281: "If you think about the future . . . : Philip Boyle, interview, 31 January 1995.

Page 281: set much higher rates for new policies . . . : Robert Pear, "Health Insurers Skirting New Law, Officials Report," *New York Times*, 4 October 1997, 1.

Page 281: Moreover, the provisions of this law . . . : Editorial in the *Baltimore Sun*, 2 August 1997, quoted in "How's It Playin? Kassebaum/Kennedy Reviews Are In," *American Health Line* 88 (6 August 1996): 5.

Page 281: only 37 percent of health care organizations . . . : Bruce Bunschoten, "Striking a Balance Between Access and Security," *Health Data Management* (May 1996), 69–71.

Page 282: "Our system lacks strong institutions . . . : Marc Rodwin, "Consumer Protection and Managed Care: The Need for Organized Consumers," *Health Affairs* 15 (Fall 1996): 110–23.

Page 282: "What you're seeing over and over . . . : Vincent Riccardi, interview, 28 March 1996.

Page 283: "The characteristically unique quality . . . : Maimon Cohen, "The Impact of the Current Legislative Climate on Genetic Services" (p. 141) and F. Desposito et al., "Clinical Genetic Services and Their Relevance to Public Health" (p. 64), in Sallie Freeman, Cynthia Hinton, and Louis Elsas, eds., *Genetic Services: Developing Guidelines for the Public's Health*, proceedings of a conference sponsored by the U.S. Department of Health and Human Services Maternal and Child Health Bureau and the Council of Regional Networks for Genetic Services, 16–17 February 1996.

Page 284: "pay very close attention . . . : Jewell Ward et al., "Impact of Medicaid Managed Care on Implementation of Genetic Services Guidelines: The Tennessee Experience," in Freeman, Hinton, and Elsas, *Genetic Services*, 70.

Page 284: "When motives are mixed . . . : Diane Paul, *Controlling Human Heredity* (Atlantic Highlands, NJ: Humanities Press, 1995), 134.

Page 285: "It's more productive, in my view, . . . : Diane Paul, at conference on cost-effectiveness analysis in genetics, Cambridge, MA, 30 March 1996.

CHAPTER 16: Pandora's Box

Page 287: "The costs of illness . . . : Daniel Koshland, editorial, *Science* 246 (13 October 1989), 189.

Page 288: a startling report about genes . . . : Dean L. Hamer et al., "A Linkage Between DNA Markers on the X Chromosome and Male Sexual Orientation," *Science* 261 (16 July 1993): 321–27.

Page 288: an autopsy study published two years earlier . . . : Simon LeVay, "A Difference in Hypothalamic Structure Between Heterosexual and Homosexual Men," *Science* 253 (30 August 1991): 1034–37.

Page 288: a joint report of their research . . . : Simon LeVay and Dean Hamer, "Evidence for a Biological Influence in Male Homosexuality," *Scientific American* (May 1994).

Page 288: an autobiography depicting his trials . . . : Dean Hamer and Peter Copeland, *The Science of Desire* (New York: Simon and Schuster, 1994).

Page 288: trying to confirm Hamer's results . . . : Eliot Marshall, "NIH's 'Gay Gene' Study Questioned," *Science* 268 (30 June 1995): 1841.

Page 289: a 231 percent increase in articles . . . : Troy Duster, *Backdoor to Eugenics* (New York: Routledge, 1990), 93.

Page 289: "seemed one of the most promising . . . : David Wasserman, telephone interview, 20 July 1995.

Page 289: goaded by outraged objections . . . : Philip Hilts, "U.S. Puts a Halt to Talks Tying Genes to Crime," *New York Times*, 5 September 1992, 1. The topic is also covered extensively in Pat Shipman, *The Evolution of Racism* (New York: Simon and Schuster, 1994).

Page 290: "On a radio talk show . . . : David Wasserman, "Science and Social Harm: Genetic Research into Crime and Violence," *Report from the Institute for Philosophy and Public Policy* 15 (Winter 1995): 14–19.

Page 291: One of the most controversial . . . : H. G. Brunner et al., "Abnormal Behavior Associated with a Point Mutation in the Structural Gene for Monoamine Oxidase A," *Science* 262 (22 October 1993): 578–80. Also reported at American Society of Human Genetics conference, New Orleans, LA, 5–9 October 1993.

Page 292: "I'm not sure what they've found . . . : Robert T. M. Phillips, telephone interview, 15 October 1993.

Page 293: researchers in France stumbled on . . . : "Aggressive Behavior and Altered Amounts of Brain Serotonin and Norepinephrine in Mice Lacking MAOA," *Science,* 23 June 1995.

Page 296: Heritability is a fraction . . . : Daniel J. Kevles, *In the Name of Eugenics* (Berkeley and Los Angeles: University of California Press, 1985), 280.

Page 296: height is the most heritable . . . : Stephen Jay Gould, *The Mismeasure of Man* (New York: W. W. Norton, 1981), 156.

CHAPTER 17: Traces

Page 305: photograph, reproduced . . . : Luigi Cavalli-Sforza, "Genes, People and Languages," *Scientific American* 265 (1991): 104–10.

Page 306: "Many of them are very brave . . . : Luigi Cavalli-Sforza and Francesco Cavalli-Sforza, *The Great Human Diasporas: A History of Diversity and Evolution* (Reading, MA: Addison-Wesley, 1995). Except for the material gained during interviews, most of the quotes and biographical information about Cavalli-Sforza come from this book.

Page 306: as a child, when his father . . . : Luigi Cavalli-Sforza, telephone interview, 8 January 1993.

Page 307: "a vanishing opportunity" . . . : L. L. Cavalli-Sforza et al., "Call for a Worldwide Survey of Human Genetic Diversity: A Vanishing Opportunity for the Human Genome Project," *Genomics* 11 (1991): 490–91.

Page 308: a British television documentary . . . : *The Gene Hunters*, Luke Holland/ZEF productions, 1994.

Page 308: an unrelated biomedical experiment . . . : Gary Taubes, "Scientists Attacked for 'Patenting' Pacific Tribe," *Science* (17 November 1995): 1112.

Page 308: "stealing genes": Ibid.

Page 308: "a distinct political society" . . . : Timothy Egan, "New Prosperity Brings New Conflict to Indian Country," *New York Times*, 8 March 1998, 1.

Page 308: "As a student from Berkeley . . . : Mary Claire King, "Human Genome Diversity," presentation at Human Genome Conference, Washington, DC, 3 October 1994.

Page 313: This entire literature has been . . . : Stephen Jay Gould, *The Mismeasure of Man* (New York: W. W. Norton, 1981).

Page 314: blood types as markers for various . . . : William H. Schneider, "Blood,

Crime and Genetics: The Search for Genetic Markers of Criminal and Other Deviant Human Behavior," presentation at University of Maryland conference on genetics and criminal behavior, University of Maryland, 23 September, 1995.

Page 314: analyzing variations in the inheritance . . . : A. M. Bowcock et al., "Study of 47 DNA Markers in Five Populations from Four Continents," *Gene Geography* 1 (1987): 47–64.

Page 315: "isolated human populations are . . . : Cavalli-Sforza et al., "Call for a Worldwide Survey."

Page 315: a series of workshops . . . : Leslie Roberts, "How to Sample the World's Genetic Diversity," *Science* 257 (28 August 1992): 1204–05; and "Anthropologists Climb (Gingerly) on Board," *Science* 258 (20 November 1992): 1300–1301. See also Patricia Kahn, "Genetic Diversity Project Tries Again," *Science* 266 (4 November 1994): 720–22.

Page 316: detailed maps of human migrations . . . : L. Cavalli-Sforza, P. Menozzi, and A. Piazza, "Demic Expansions and Evolution," *Science* 259 (1993): 639–46.

Page 317: "21st century technology . . . : Quoted in Roger Lewin, "Genes from a Disappearing World," *New Scientist* (29 May 1993), 25–29.

Page 318: a talk that began . . . : Jonathan Marks, personal communication.

Page 318: "needs to reformulate itself . . . : Jonathan Marks, "The Human Genome Diversity Project: Good for If Not Good as Anthropology?" *Anthropology Newsletter,* April 1995, 72.

Page 319: "One of the exciting aspects . . . : Luigi Cavalli-Sforza, "The Human Genome Diversity Project," address to UNESCO, Paris, 12 September 1994.

Page 321: "an aspect of our diversity . . . : Georgia Dunston, interview, National Institutes of Health, 21 September 1995.

Page 324: searching for pairs of siblings . . . : "Science Scope," *Science* (11 April 1997), 187.

Page 325: Officials in other areas of the NIH . . . : Douglas Steinberg, "NIH Jumps Into Genetic Variation Research," *The Scientist,* 19 Jan. 1998, p.1.

Page 325: As a result of these concerns . . . : "A Resource for Discovering Human DNA Polymorphisms," NHGRI Request for Proposals HG-98-001.

CHAPTER 18: On Human Evolution

Page 328: the eminent Australian immunologist: McFarlane Burnet, *Endurance of Life: The Implications of Genetics for Human Life* (Cambridge: Cambridge University Press, 1978), 205.

Page 328: "Randomness, like determinism, shapes . . . : Sara Maitland, *A Big Enough God* (New York: Henry Holt, 1995), 58–59.

Page 329: Writing on the subject in 1967 . . . : Joshua Lederberg, "Genetic Intervention Is a Way of Improving Our Species," *New York Times,* 4 November 1967, A13.

Page 329: "with the new genetic markers . . . : Thomas Caskey, interview, Merck headquarters, 21 May 1996.

Page 330: "learning how the disease develops . . . : Henri Begleiter, interview, 24 July 1995.

Page 331: "we are quite ignorant . . . : Kurt Hirschhorn, presentation at American Society of Human Genetics conference, Minneapolis, MN, 28 October 1995.

Page 332: diabetes may have survived . . . : James Neel, "Diabetes Mellitus: A 'Thrifty' Genotype Rendered Detrimental by 'Progress'?" *American Journal of Human Genetics* 14 (1962): 353–62.

Page 333: "enormous genetic heterogeneity . . . : Susan Wolf, "Beyond 'Genetic Discrimination': Toward the Broader Harm of Geneticism," *Journal of Law, Medicine and Ethics* 23 (1995): 345–53.

Page 334: "reproductive cells, one or both . . . : See H. J. Muller, *Man's Future Birthright: Essays on Science and Humanity* (Albany: State University of New York Press, 1973).

Page 334: One single mother who bore a son . . . : Mark Stuart Gill, "The Genius Babies," *Ladies Home Journal*, March 1995: 79.

Page 335: The earth's population is 5.7 billion . . . : James Neel, presentation at American Society of Human Genetics conference, Minneapolis, MN, 28 October 1995.

Page 336: "we must be able to operate . . . : Alvin Toffler, *Future Shock* (New York: Random House, 1970), 13–14.

Page 337: He predicts that if the means existed . . . : Luigi Cavalli-Sforza and Francesco Cavalli-Sforza, *The Great Human Diasporas* (Reading, MA: Addison-Wesley, 1995), chap. 8.

Page 338: There aren't even any genetically "pure" families . . . : Pat Shipman, *The Evolution of Racism* (New York: Simon and Schuster, 1994), 95.

Page 339: Cavalli-Sforza's gene map . . . : L. L. Cavalli-Sforza et al., "Reconstruction of Human Evolution: Bringing Together Genetic, Archaeological and Linguistic Data," *Proceedings of the National Academy of Sciences* 85, (August 1988): 6002–6006.

Page 340: "There's something fundamental about . . . : Georgia Dunston, interview, 21 September 1995.

Page 341: An emerging theory in population . . . : David Sloan Wilson, "Human Groups as Units of Selection," *Science* 276 (20 June 1997): 1816–17.

Page 342: the NIH has more than doubled . . . : Nigel Williams, "Consensus on African Research Projects," *Science* 278 (21 November 1997): 1393.

Page 342: Christian ethics measures moral progress . . . : Ronald Cole-Turner, *The New Genesis: Theology and the Genetic Revolution* (Westminster/John Knox Press, 1993).

Page 343: Clement Bezold, executive director . . . : Excerpted in *Medicine and Health Perspectives*, 15 January 1996, 1–4.

Page 345: The lawsuit was brought by a Medicare . . . : Mark Fuerst, "HCFA Loosens Up on Coverage Decisions," *1998 Medicare Managed Care Sourcebook* (Faulkner & Gray, 1997).

Page 346: "Progress may be painfully fast . . . : Benno Müller-Hill, "The Shadow of Genetic Injustice," *Nature* 362 (1993): 491–92.

Page 346: He was reminding an audience of public health officials . . . : First Annual Conference on Genetics and Public Health: Translating Advances in Human Genetics into Disease Prevention and Health Promotion, Decatur, 13–15 May 1998.

FOR FURTHER READING

Andrews, Lori, et al., eds. *Assessing Genetic Risks: Implications for Health and Social Policy.* Institute of Medicine. Washington, DC: National Academy Press, 1994.

Bulger, Ruth, Elizabeth Boby, and Harvey Fineberg, eds. *Society's Choices: Social and Ethical Decision Making in Biomedicine.* Institute of Medicine. Washington, DC: National Academy Press, 1995.

Cavalli-Sforza, Luigi Luca, and Francesco Cavalli-Sforza. *The Great Human Diasporas: A History of Diversity and Evolution.* Reading, MA: Addison-Wesley, 1995.

Cook-Deegan, Robert. *The Gene Wars: Science, Politics, and the Human Genome.* New York: W. W. Norton, 1994.

Cranor, Carl F., ed. *Are Genes Us? The Social Consequences of the New Genetics.* New Brunswick, NJ: Rutgers University Press, 1994.

Drlica, Karl. *Double-Edged Sword: The Promises and Risks of the Genetic Revolution.* Reading, MA: Addison-Wesley, 1994.

Duster, Troy. *Backdoor to Eugenics.* New York: Routledge, 1990.

Gould, Stephen Jay. *The Mismeasure of Man.* New York: W. W. Norton, 1981.

Holtzman, Neil. *Proceed with Caution: Predicting Genetic Risks in the Recombinant DNA Era.* Baltimore: Johns Hopkins University Press, 1989.

Holtzman, Neil, and Michael Watson, eds. *Promoting Safe and Effective Genetic Testing in the United States.* Final Report of the Task Force on Genetic Testing. National Human Genome Research Institute, September 1997.

Hubbard, Ruth, and Elijah Wald. *Exploding the Gene Myth: How Genetic Information Is Produced and Manipulated by Scientists, Physicians, Employers, Insurance Companies, Educators, and Law Enforcers.* Boston: Beacon Press, 1993.

Kevles, Daniel J. *In the Name of Eugenics: Genetics and the Uses of Human Heredity.* Berkeley and Los Angeles: University of California Press, 1985.

Kitcher, Philip. *The Lives to Come: The Genetic Revolution and Human Possibilities.* New York: Simon and Schuster, 1996.

Lifton, Robert Jay. *The Nazi Doctors: Medical Killing and the Psychology of Genocide.* New York: Basic Books, 1986.

Neel, James V. *Physician to the Gene Pool: Genetic Lessons and Other Stories.* New York: John Wiley and Sons, 1994.

Paul, Diane B. *Controlling Human Heredity, 1865 to the Present.* Atlantic Highlands, NJ: Humanities Press, 1995.

Shipman, Pat. *The Evolution of Racism: Human Differences and the Use and Abuse of Science.* New York: Simon and Schuster, 1994.

Waldholz, Michael. *Curing Cancer: The Story of the Men and Women Unlocking the Secrets of Our Deadliest Illness.* New York: Simon and Schuster, 1997.

White, Michael, and John Gribbin. *Darwin: A Life in Science.* New York: Dutton, 1995.

Wilkie, Tom. *Perilous Knowledge: The Human Genome Project and Its Implications.* Berkeley and Los Angeles: University of California Press, 1993.

RESOURCES

(Internet addresses valid as of February 1998)

Alliance of Genetic Support Groups
35 Wisconsin Circle, Suite 440
Chevy Chase, Maryland 20815
800-336-4363
http://medhlp.netusa.net/www/agsg.htm

American Society of Human Genetics
9650 Rockville Pike
Bethesda, Maryland 20814-3998
301-571-1825
http://www.faseb.org/genetics/ashg

Cystic Fibrosis Foundation
6931 Arlington Road
Bethesda, Maryland 20814
301-951-4422
800-FIGHT-CF
http://www.cff.org

FRAXA Research Foundation, Inc.
(Nonprofit foundation dedicated to research into Fragile X syndrome)
P.O. Box 935
West Newbury, Massachusetts 01985
978-462-1866
http://www.FRAXA.org

Hereditary Disease Foundation
1427 7th Street, #2
Santa Monica, California 90401
310-458-4183
http://www.hdfoundation.org

Huntington's Disease Society of America
140 West 22nd Street, 6th floor
New York, New York 10011-2420
212-242-1968
800-345-HDSA
http://neuro-www2.mgh.harvard.edu/hdsa/society.nclk

March of Dimes
(provides a very broad range of resources about hereditary diseases and birth defects)
1275 Mamaroneck Avenue
White Plains, New York 10605
914-428-7100
http://www.modimes.org

National Down Syndrome Society
666 Broadway, 8th floor
New York, New York 10012-2317
212-460-9330
800-221-4602
http://www.ndss.org

National Organization for Rare Disorders
P.O. Box 8923
New Fairfield, Connecticut 06812-8923
203-746-6518
800-999-6673
http://www.pcnet.com/~orphan

National Society of Genetic Counselors
233 Canterbury Drive
Wallingford, Pennsylvania 19086-6617
610-872-7608
http://members.aol.com/nsgcweb/nsgchome.htm

INTERESTING INTERNET SITES

CDC Office of Genetics and Disease Prevention
Very rich site with news, literature, and links about genetics
http://www.cdc.gov/genetics

Ethics & Genetics: A Global Conversation
Chat-group Web site run by the University of Pennsylvania's Center for Bioethics
http://www.med.upenn.edu/~bioethic/genetics.html

ELSI Task Force on Genetic Testing: Final Report
http://www.nhgri.nih.gov/ELSI/TFGT_final

The Gene Letter
Online newsletter about genetics, ethics, and policy issues sponsored by the Shriver
Center in Waltham, Massachusetts
http://www.geneletter.org

Gene Saver
(Private company offers to extract and archive your DNA)
http://www.genesaver.com

Genetics & Ethics
Web site coordinated by a student at the University of British Columbia's Centre for
    Applied Ethics
http://www.ethics.ubc.ca/brynw/

Human Genome Diversity Project
http://www-leland.stanford.edu/group/morrinst/HGDP.html

hum-molgen
Newsgroup and chat group about human molecular genetics. Contains a site about
    ethics and genetics of special interest because many molecular scientists contribute.
http://linkage.rockefeller.edu/hum-molgen

U.S. Human Genome Project—Department of Energy Branch
http://www.ornl.gov/hgmis

U.S. Human Genome Project—National Institutes of Health Branch
http://www.nhgri.nih.gov

ABOUT THE AUTHOR

LOIS WINGERSON is editor in chief of *HMS Beagle* (www.hmsbeagle. com), an Internet magazine for biomedical scientists, published by Elsevier Science, and the author of *Mapping Our Genes* (1990). She has written for *The Economist, Science Digest, Discover,* and other prestigious lay and professional scientific publications. She lives in Brooklyn, New York.

INDEX